The
Problem Knee

Malcolm Macnicol

MBChB, BSc (Hons), MCh, FRCS, FRCSEd (Orth), FRCP, Dip Sports Med

Previously Consultant Orthopaedic Surgeon and Senior Orthopaedic Lecturer, Royal Hospital for Sick Children, Royal Infirmary and Murrayfield Hospital, Edinburgh, UK

and Franky Steenbrugge

MD, PhD, MChOrth, FRCSEd

Professor in Orthopaedics, Department of Orthopaedic Surgery and Traumatology, Ghent University Hospital, University of Ghent, Belgium; Co-founder of the Belgium Knee Society

The
Problem Knee

Diagnosis and management in the younger patient

3rd Edition

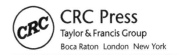

CRC Press
Taylor & Francis Group
Boca Raton London New York

CRC Press is an imprint of the
Taylor & Francis Group, an **informa** business

CRC Press
Taylor & Francis Group
6000 Broken Sound Parkway NW, Suite 300
Boca Raton, FL 33487-2742

First issued in paperback 2018

ISBN-13: 978-1-4441-2011-0 (hbk)
ISBN-13: 978-1-138-37246-7 (pbk)

British Library Cataloguing in Publication Data
A catalogue record for this book is available from the British Library

Library of Congress Cataloging-in-Publication Data
A catalog record for this book is available from the Library of Congress

Commissioning Editor:	Francesca Naish
Project Editor:	Joanna Silman
Production Controller:	Joanna Walker
Cover Design:	Julie Joubinaux
Indexer:	Laurence Errington

Typeset in 10.5/12 pt Goudy Old Style Regular by Datapage

What do you think about this book? Or any other Hodder Arnold title?
Please visit our website: www.hodderarnold.com

Visit the Taylor & Francis Web site at
http://www.taylorandfrancis.com

and the CRC Press Web site at
http://www.crcpress.com

Contents

Preface

The knee is a complex and crucial joint, vulnerable in the daily round as well as during sports and in transport or industrial accidents. While the causes of acute or chronic knee symptoms are not always apparent, it is to be hoped that, at very least, an informed questioning and examination of the patient or injured athlete will ensure that needless morbidity is avoided. Whether the sometimes inextricable mix of reactive synovitis, soft tissue and osteochondral damage can be teased apart may eventually depend on the experience and investigative skills of the surgeon; but assuredly a lack of cooperation and free communication with colleagues in other disciplines will retard both the speed and success of treatment.

This monograph emphasizes the basic principles in managing a 'problem knee' in the younger patient. The interrelationship between skeletal and soft tissues injuries is acknowledged, but in the interests of a simplified and rational approach, separate chapters deal with the different components of the joint, albeit with some repetition. Details about most surgical approaches have been kept to a minimum because these can be learnt effectively only in the operating theatre. Scanning the knee with magnetic resonance imaging, ultrasound or computed tomography has augmented the clinical value of history taking, careful and standardized physical examination, and conventional radiography. However, the unconditional and excessive use of investigations of this sort cannot be condoned. Clinical assessment is still the bedrock of management.

Operative intervention for patellar pain, with or without maltracking, is less frequently advised than in the past. The subtleties of patellar instability make surgical procedures prone to patient disappointment. Cruciate ligament reconstruction, on the other hand, is now a relatively safe and satisfactory procedure, particularly for the acute anterior cruciate rupture. The benefits of this intervention are now convincing, not least the protection of other structures in the knee that has been stabilized. Meniscal repair and (osteo)chondral grafting are appropriate in selected cases, and after all forms of surgery a more rapid rehabilitation is espoused.

The text now incorporates recent advances in surgical management and newer concepts in conservative treatment. As before, systemic conditions are described as they relate to the knee in younger patients but degenerative disease is excluded. An overview of fracture care is presented without elaboration.

The first edition of *The Problem Knee* appealed especially to physiotherapists, family doctors and casualty officers. The second edition broadened its appeal to surgical trainees and those in orthopaedic practice. With the welcome assistance of Professor Franky Steenbrugge, who has extensively revised Chapters 5 and 6, it is hoped that this third edition will prove of further value. Chapter 4 on paediatric conditions has also been modernized.

Acknowledgements

The authors thank Ian Beggs, Michael Devlin, Alison Green, Robb Kidd and Morag Lunn for their contributions to the third edition.

We dedicate the book to our wives and children.

The mechanism and presentation of injuries to the knee

Introduction

The knee joint is designed for rapid and complex movements, often when encumbered by the weight of the body. These two requirements, speed and strength, place stresses upon the knee structures, which may in turn produce symptoms. Another characteristic is the exposed position of the knee, which makes it vulnerable in many occupations and sports. The combination of this vulnerability to trauma and its underlying sophistication must be kept in mind not simply when identifying the mechanism of injury but also when planning a return to normal activities and to the repetitive demands of sport.

There are four principal groups who may present with symptoms:

- Those who are relatively unfit and in whom a mild congenital weakness may make the knee slightly unstable and subsequently troublesome
- Athletic individuals who subject their knees to repeated stresses and significant loading, with subsequent fatigue not only of the soft tissues but of the skeleton and surfaces of the joint
- Otherwise normal individuals whose knees are subjected to a sudden, high-velocity collision or fall, which exceeds the strength of the components of the knee, for example, those involved in motorcycle accidents
- Those in whom injuries seem inextricably and frustratingly linked with a personality disorder or neurosis.

The knee joint is supported by its capsule, the ligaments and surrounding muscles, with assistance from the menisci and the patellofemoral joint. The configuration of the femoral and tibial articular surfaces is principally concerned with weightbearing, since the relatively unconstrained hinging and gliding that occurs between them is designed for speed of movement. That temperamental sesamoid – the patella – improves the efficiency of the quadriceps muscle group and hence the strength of extension and anti-gravity control. The biological trade-off between mobility and stability is largely governed by the proprioceptive loop formed by the sensors in the ligaments and their companion muscles (Figure 1.1). A break in this protective arc affects function and long-term recovery. The balance between stability and free movement is easily upset.

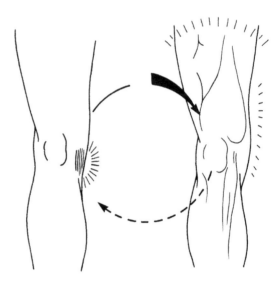

Figure 1.1 A protective reflex arc links the ligaments and muscles of the knee; when a ligament, such as the medial collateral, is stretched, impulses are referred by the afferent nerves to the spinal cord. Efferent nerves then transmit the signal to the muscles, which contract appropriately, thus enhancing the stability of the knee. Proprioception is also afforded by other structures in the knee (see Table 5.1, p. 96).

History

Obtaining a clear history of the events leading up to an injury of the knee may be difficult but is of importance. A careful questioning about the onset of the problem leads the clinician to examine and investigate the knee more accurately. Contributory spinal, hip and other pathologies are more likely to be exposed. It also allows an assessment of the personality and reaction of the patient to the mishap. Unfortunately, the memory of acute events is often blurred by the speed of the accident or by the time that has elapsed following a more chronic complaint. On rare occasions the patient may conceal the nature of an injury or its circumstances if litigation or intentional concealment colour the event.

Since the knee can be stressed in any direction, the mechanism of injury may include valgus or varus angulation, excessive flexion or extension, and extremes of internal or external rotation, often in combination. Forced anterior or posterior movement of the tibia in relation to the femur, and axially directed stresses may damage both bone and soft tissue. Malfunction of the patellofemoral mechanism may confuse matters further and may persist after the original injury has resolved.

Anatomy

Understanding the surface anatomy of the knee is essential if the extent of the structural damage or pathological process is to be assessed accurately. Certain landmarks of surface anatomy are relatively prominent and thus palpable: the condyles and joint lines, patellar outline, tibial tuberosity and Gerdy's tubercle, and the fibular head (Figure 1.2). The extent of the suprapatellar pouch, dimensions of the patellar tendon, trailing edge of the iliotibial band, collateral ligament attachments and popliteal structures are identifiable. Further details about the anatomy of the patellofemoral mechanism, the ligaments and the menisci are given in Chapters 4–7.

The cutaneous nerves are important to appreciate and are relatively constant (Figure 1.3). Surgical incisions and percutaneous procedures may endanger these nerves, most commonly the infrapatellar branch of the saphenous and the sural. Troublesome numbness and

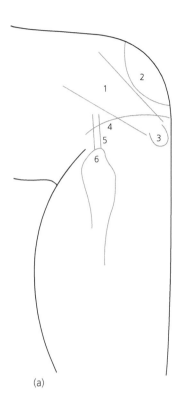
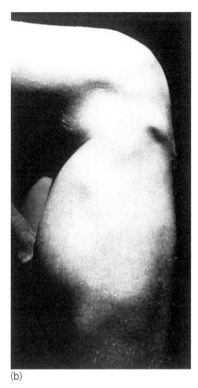

Figure 1.2a,b Surface anatomy of the lateral side of the knee: 1, iliotibial band; 2, patella; 3, Gerdy's tubercle, where part of the band inserts into the tibia; 4, lateral joint line (defining the peripheral rim of the lateral meniscus); 5, lateral (fibular) collateral ligament; 6, fibular head.

(a) (b)

dysaesthesia in the affected nerve distribution may cause significant complaints from those affected.

Medial side of the knee

Figures 1.4 and 1.5 show the structures that overlie the medial side of the knee. These may be injured in sequential fashion by a valgus force applied to the leg, including the medial collateral ligament, the medial capsule and its important posteromedial corner, the medial meniscus and the anterior cruciate ligament. Greater disruption produces subluxation and dislocation of the joint, with tearing of more distant structures such as the medial patellar retinaculum, the posterior cruciate ligament and capsule, and possibly the lateral compartment components.

Rotational stresses combined with valgus force produce different patterns of disruption. Some structures will tear completely whereas others will remain 'in continuity' but weakened. Fractures of the joint surfaces or avulsion of ligament attachments to the skeleton are seen in the child (Chapter 4) because the strength of cancellous bone is less than that of connective tissue.

Lateral side of the knee

A similar cascade of injuries may occur when a varus force is applied to the knee. The damaged structures include the fibular (lateral) collateral ligament, the lateral capsule and arcuate complex posteriorly, the lateral meniscus, the cruciate ligaments, the iliotibial band, the biceps tendon and peroneal nerve and the popliteus tendon (Figures 1.6, 1.7, p. 6). Compressive lesions in the medial compartment may coexist, including bone bruising and osteochondral fractures, and medial meniscus lesions. Anatomical structures in the thigh and calf (Figures 1.7–1.9, pp. 6–7) may also be injured.

Figure 1.3 The distribution of the cutaneous nerves of the lower limb with relevance to the knee: (a) anterior knee; and (b) posterior knee.

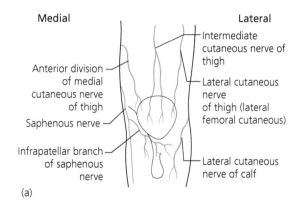

(a)

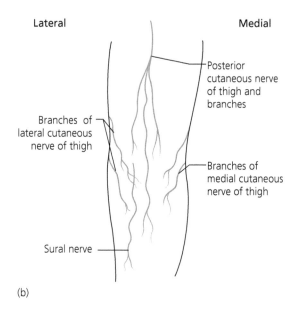

(b)

Clinical presentation

When taking a history, specific questions should be asked about:

- pain
- loss of normal movement
- locking
- swelling
- abnormal mobility (instability).
- personality
- age-related symptoms

■ Pain

Pain is not often well localized (Figure 1.10, p. 8), although associated tenderness tends to be. However, secondary but mild injuries to other structures may even make the relevance of the apparently focal tenderness uncertain, such as patellar subluxation producing pain

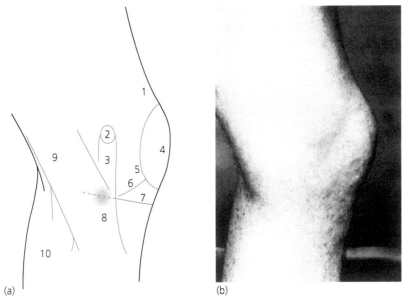

(a) (b)

Figure 1.4a,b Surface anatomy of the medial side of the knee: 1, suprapatellar pouch; 2, adductor tubercle; 3, medial (tibial) collateral ligament; 4, patella; 5, parapatellar synovium; 6, anterior edge of the medial femoral condyle; 7, medial joint line (defining the peripheral rim of the medial meniscus); 8, 'no man's land' where the medial ligament and medial meniscus overlap; 9, the 'pes anserinus' (sartorius, gracilis and semitendinosus tendons); 10, semimembranosus and medial head of the gastrocnemius muscles.

Figure 1.5 Soft tissue anatomy of the medial side of the knee.

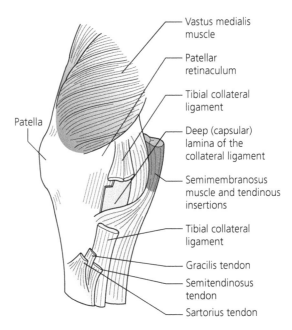

Vastus medialis muscle

Patellar retinaculum

Tibial collateral ligament

Deep (capsular) lamina of the collateral ligament

Semimembranosus muscle and tendinous insertions

Tibial collateral ligament

Gracilis tendon

Semitendinosus tendon

Sartorius tendon

Patella

and tenderness over the medial side of the knee, suggesting medial ligamentous or meniscal damage; or tears in one meniscus referring symptoms, and even signs, to the contralateral compartment of the knee. Despite these difficulties, it is important to describe pain as precisely as possible, noting site, periodicity, precipitating factors and any referral of the symptom.

Figure 1.6 Soft tissue anatomy of
the lateral side of the knee.

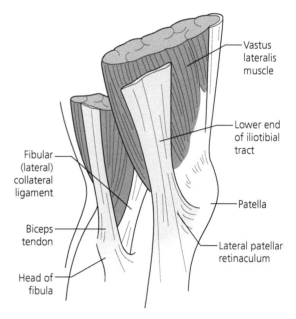

Vastus
lateralis
muscle

Lower end
of iliotibial
tract

Fibular
(lateral)
collateral
ligament

Patella

Biceps
tendon

Lateral patellar
retinaculum

Head of
fibula

Figure 1.7 Soft tissue anatomy of
the posterior surface of the knee.

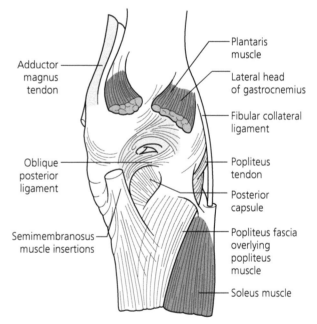

Plantaris
muscle

Adductor
magnus
tendon

Lateral head
of gastrocnemius

Fibular collateral
ligament

Oblique
posterior
ligament

Popliteus
tendon

Posterior
capsule

Semimembranosus
muscle insertions

Popliteus fascia
overlying
popliteus
muscle

Soleus muscle

■ Loss of normal movement

Loss of normal movement is usually described by the patient as a feeling of stiffness, or as a
'block' to the full range of knee extension or flexion. Both these forms of restriction may be
painful, accompanied by a limp or alteration in gait pattern. Rotation of the tibia below the
femur is also reduced.

Stiffness indicates that the periphery and possibly also the articular cartilage surfaces
are abnormal. This increased resistance to movement throughout the range of flexion is
characteristic of an inflammatory condition, with or without the presence of an effusion.
A more unyielding form of stiffness develops in time, particularly if muscle and soft tissue

contractures occur, or if the osteoarthritic process alters the articular surfaces markedly and reduces the compliance of soft tissues.

■ Locking

True locking may be intermittent or persistent. A relatively painless block to extension, or flexion deformity, and the loss of flexion resulting from chronic arthritis should be distinguished from the springy and often exquisitely painful block produced by a torn meniscus or loose body. Locking may also be produced by an impinging anterior cruciate ligament stump or synovial impingement, especially if affected by an inflammatory process or neoplasm.

The circumstances that cause the knee to feel restricted or locked should be identified. A synovitis will cause the knee to stiffen after a night's sleep or after prolonged sitting. Locking tends to be noticed during activity more than at rest, although it may be accompanied by a sense of restriction when the knee has been kept in flexion, during crouching or sitting. Certain unguarded movements, particularly twisting on the flexed knee, are not only potent causes of meniscal tears but also produce further episodes of locking and increased displacement of the tear (Figure 1.11).

Trillat (1962) described the progression of a vertical tear which may either proceed through the central portion of the meniscus, forming a 'bucket handle', or may rupture through the posterior horn, producing a flap. The bucket handle may tear across centrally, resulting in various sizes of anterior and posterior flaps, or may rupture through the anterior horn. Locking may then become intermittent or cease, although the patient may feel something intermittently moving within the knee or protruding at the joint line. Dandy (1990) also described his experience with different meniscal tears, and offered an alternative classification, although the nature of the lesions is basically the same.

The presence of a pathological meniscus usually causes some loss of passive movement, even in the chronic stages. However, peripheral tears in the vascular zone may heal with time, if stable, and smaller flaps and tags may be thinned out to the extent that they cease to trouble the patient. The horizontal cleavage lesion, and certain oblique degenerative tears, may also become asymptomatic (Noble and Hamblen 1975; Noble and Erat 1980). It can be surprising to encounter the occasional case of a displaced bucket handle tear in a

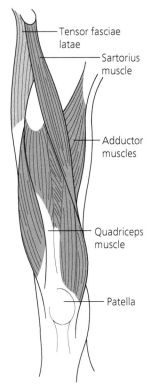

Figure 1.8 The anterior thigh muscles.

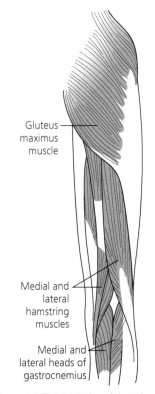

Figure 1.9 The posterior thigh and superficial calf muscles.

7

patient with minimal symptoms. Certain types of work will of course highlight any restriction and thus an athlete or a manual worker will be unable to tolerate the functional deficiencies that may be accepted by someone in sedentary employment.

■ Swelling

Rapid swelling of the knee after injury is usually noted accurately by the patient, whereas more gradual swelling may be misinterpreted with regard to both the site and extent of the swelling. An acute and tense swelling almost always means that bleeding has distended the joint, and this haemarthrosis is a sign that a vascular structure has been torn. Synovial and ligament tears will produce a haemarthrosis, as will intra-articular fractures. A peripheral tear through the vascular outer zone of the meniscus will be an occasional cause in the younger patient. In severe knee disruptions blood leaks out through the synovial and capsular tear. An ecchymosis develops, resulting in widespread bruising that may track down the leg. These characteristics are described more fully in Chapters 2 and 3.

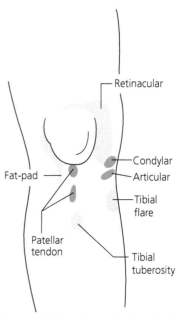

Figure 1.10 Typical sites of referred pain and local tenderness over the anterior aspect of the knee.

Gradual swelling from meniscal injury or a sprain will fill the synovial cavity over a 24-hour period. The associated enlargement of the suprapatellar pouch (Figure 1.12, see also Figures 2.6, p. 17, and 2.7, p. 18) may be a source of confusion. Discrete swellings (Figure 1.13) develop insidiously but vary in size less than an effusion.

Classically, a mild effusion occurs after a twisting injury of the knee. In patients with inflammatory disease or a bleeding condition such as haemophilia minor trauma may produce

Figure 1.11 (a) The approximate incidence of traumatic tears at various sites in both menisci; (b) the three diagrams to the left show the typical progression of a posterior, vertical meniscal tear to a 'bucket handle' lesion and eventually to a pedunculated tag; the three diagrams to the right show an inner rim tag, a peripheral split causing slight meniscal displacement and a 'parrot beak' radial tear.

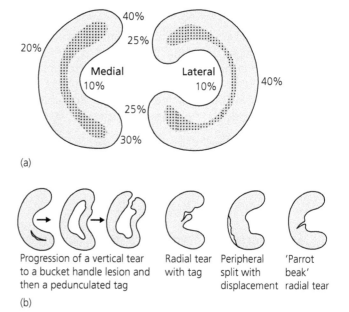

a disproportionately large swelling. Normally the swelling disappears with rest and reoccurs with further activity or stress. Detection of this fluid is an important part of knee examination (Chapter 2), allowing a gradation from mild, to moderate (lax), to major (tense). The physiotherapist or doctor can use the presence or absence of an effusion after exercise as the monitor of the progress of a patient, the promotion of an effusion indicating that the speed of rehabilitation is too fast for that stage of healing. If a synovitis with its associated effusion becomes established it may respond to a non-steroidal anti-inflammatory agent (Chapter 9). Magnetic resonance (MR) scanning or arthroscopic review of the pathological lesion may eventually be indicated to assess the stage of healing after injury or earlier surgery.

If a patient states that the knee regularly becomes swollen, but no convincing effusion or discrete swelling can be detected on the day of examination, it is often instructive to request that the patient returns on a day when the swelling is apparent, perhaps provoked by exertion. Defining the site, nature and periodicity of the swelling is an important aspect of careful clinical examination.

◼ Instability

Direct or indirect trauma may make the knee joint incompetent when bearing the weight of the body. Buckling or instability is the symptom, pathological laxity the sign. Angulatory and rotational stress cannot be resisted. Instability of this sort can be very troublesome as the knee gives way in an unexpected and often dangerous way. Anterolateral instability, when the convex lateral tibial condyle and lateral meniscus sublux under the lateral femoral condyle, causes a feeling of two knuckles rubbing against each other and a painful buckling results (Chapter 5).

Ligament tears in various combinations account for most instances of gross instability but the knee may also give way under load if the patella subluxes/ dislocates laterally or if the axis of motion is impeded by an obstructive meniscus or a loose body. Additional causes of buckling include chronic quadriceps weakness or a reflex inhibition of thigh muscle contraction owing to an obstructive and painful lesion in the joint. This functional instability may occur when a person is climbing ladders or negotiating rough ground, when the quadriceps mechanism is under greater load. Chronic angular deformity, whether congenital or acquired, may also lead to instability, often compounded by ligament laxity or muscle weakness.

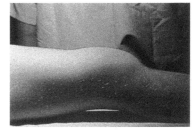

Figure 1.12 Generalized swelling of the knee in juvenile chronic arthritis.

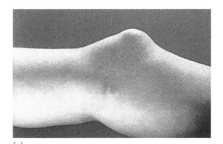

(a)

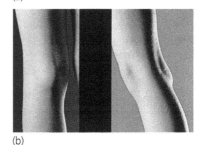

(b)

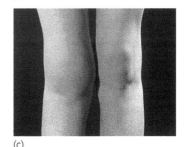

(c)

Figure 1.13 (a) The discrete swelling of prepatellar bursitis ('housemaid's knee'); (b) the popliteal cyst in childhood usually disappears; (c) a left quadriceps ganglion.

Personality

The perception of the cardinal symptoms – pain, loss of movement and instability – will be influenced by the demands placed on the joint by individuals as well as their personality and expectations of physical fitness. Highly tuned athletes tolerate poorly a relatively minor impairment that a less active person may accept perfectly readily. A clicking sensation in the joint and patellofemoral crepitus are common features but may provoke considerable anxiety in the introspective individual. One patient may shrug off a symptom or adapt to it, whereas for another the persistence of a minor disability may preoccupy the mind. During adolescence, pains in the knee may prove very troublesome for not only the patient but also the parents, and eventually the doctor and physiotherapist. There may come a time when the patient is asked 'to live with the pain' if diagnostic efforts have drawn a blank.

Such counsel is often hard to give and even harder to accept. But if all investigations have proved unconvincing for pathology, and the possibility of referred pain ruled out, advice that the patient will have to endure the symptoms is often accepted if there has been a frank explanation of the position (Sandow and Goodfellow 1985). In childhood the 'growing pains' experienced may lessen with stretching exercises and with time (Chapter 4). During adolescence some hope should also be entertained that the condition may resolve at the end of skeletal growth or in early adult life. A change in lifestyle and sporting interests may prove beneficial.

Age-related symptoms

The age of the patient is an important factor and will indicate the likely causes of the symptoms (Table 1.1). In children, problems usually relate to patellar malalignment syndromes, congenital abnormalities (such as a discoid lateral meniscus), stress or avulsion fracture, and

Table 1.1 Common causes of knee symptoms related to the age and sex of the patient

Age (years)	Sex	
	Female	Male
5–10	Discoid lateral meniscus	Discoid lateral meniscus
	Synovitis or arthropathy	Synovitis, arthropathy, haemophilia
	Fractures	Fractures
	Patellar instability	Soft tissue tumours
	Soft tissue tumours	Patellar instability
10–20	Patellar instability	Osteochondritis dissecans
	Patellar pain (?stress)	Meniscal tears
	Ligament rupture	Osteochondroses
	Osteochondritis dissecans	Patellar instability
	Fracture	Fracture
	Arthropathy	Ligament rupture
		Arthropathy
20–30	Patellar instability	Meniscal tear
	Cystic lateral meniscus	Ligament rupture
	Arthropathy	Fracture
	Ligament rupture	Arthropathy
	Meniscal tear	Cystic lateral meniscus
30+	The problems detailed above, often superimposed on increasing degenerative changes	

arthropathies, including juvenile chronic arthritis. Meniscal tears are relatively rare so other causes of apparent knee locking should be considered, including osteochondritis dissecans.

After puberty, girls are prone to patellar pain; this may be related to compression stresses or instability of the knee cap secondary to torsional abnormality of the legs, to ligament laxity or to a growth spurt. The source of symptoms may be so puzzling and inextricably linked with emotional factors that intervention by the surgeon may do more harm than good (Figure 1.14).

With juvenile athletes, patellar tracking, an apophysitis, a discoid meniscus or osteochondritis dissecans may be responsible. Ligament injuries are unusual but stress fractures are not. Bone bruising often shows up on the MR scan. The possibility of significant alternative pathology, such as infection or neoplasia should be considered. Meniscal tears are more frequent in later adolescence and a traumatic synovitis or traction apophysitis can prove troublesome. Lastly, in the 'mature' athlete, between the ages of 20 and 70 years these days, ligament sprains and ruptures, synovial fringe and fat pad lesions and degenerative changes must be added to the list of possible diagnoses.

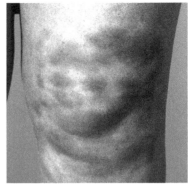

Figure 1.14 Factitious bruising produced by the patient striking the knee in the region of the anterior 'window' of a canvas knee splint.

The ensuing chapters will outline the approach to a knee injury or repetitive stress lesion. Many associated conditions have to be considered as they will influence susceptibility and recovery. Both the patient and the therapist must accept that some injuries and acquired dysfunction will not be completely cured. Early, and appropriate, treatment should nevertheless speed recovery and minimize the risk of long-standing morbidity.

References

Dandy DJ (1990) Arthroscopic anatomy of symptomatic meniscal lesions. *J Bone Joint Surg Br* **72**, 628–31.

Noble J and Erat K (1980) In defence of the meniscus: a prospective study of 200 meniscectomy patients. *J Bone Joint Surg Br* **62**, 7–11.

Noble J and Hamblen DL (1975) The pathology of the degenerate meniscus lesion. *J Bone Joint Surg Br* **57**, 180–6.

Sandow MJ and Goodfellow JW (1985) The natural history of anterior knee pain in adolescents. *J Bone Joint Surg Br* **67**, 36–9.

Trillat A (1962) Lésions traumatique du ménisque interne du genu. Classement anatomique et diagnostic clinique. *Rev Clin Orthop* **48**, 551–63.

2

Methods of clinical examination

Introduction

Careful examination of the knee is essential before enlisting additional tests or arranging arthroscopic and other forms of surgery. The history very often suggests the diagnosis. If the physical features are elicited precisely, the diagnosis may be clinched and the patient will have greater confidence in the therapist. Attention to the details of examination may also save the patient an unnecessary number of investigations and should allow the examiner an authoritative approach to the problem.

The routine

It is always helpful to follow a routine as it will make errors of omission less likely and also helps in the layout of the subsequent clinical notes and letter. At the beginning, determine if the dynamic tests of walking, squatting, 'duck-waddling' and extension of the knee against gravity should be carried out before or after examination of the patient on the couch. A limp may be caused by symptoms in the knee or weakness, and may also indicate that an abnormality affects the hip or the rest of the leg. It is important to assess the locomotor system more generally to rule out obvious neurological disease and to consider medical conditions that may influence knee function. This applies to the arthropathies, haematological conditions and to congenital or inherited diseases. Particular attention should be paid to abnormalities of the lumbar spine, hip joint, leg musculature, ankle and foot, and to possible leg-length discrepancy.

The patient should be undressed sufficiently to allow a comprehensive review of the spine, hip and lower limb. Valgus, varus and torsional deformities should be noted and compared with the contralateral leg. Hip stiffness and losses or increases of rotation may affect knee function adversely. Pain may radiate to the medial side of the knee by referral along the anterior branch of the obturator nerve, as seen in slipped capital femoral epiphysis (SCFE). Radiographs of the knee are therefore sometimes found in the case notes of a patient with obvious shortening and external rotation of the leg resulting from SCFE. The patellofemoral joint may become symptomatic secondary to a number of abnormalities, as discussed in Chapter 7.

Inspection

Looking at the knee from both the front and the back is a logical first inspection. The appearance of the skin, the presence of scars and their width, the position of any swellings

(Figure 2.1) and the bulk of both thighs should be noted. Bruising or an ecchymosis indicates the site and severity of injury, a boggy, ill-defined swelling suggesting major ligament and capsular disruption. Other, more discrete, swellings include the lateral (or sometimes medial) meniscal cyst, prepatellar or infrapatellar bursae, ganglia, a popliteal cyst or semimembranosus bursa, swellings in relation to the pes anserinus (sartorius, gracilis and semitendinosus muscle insertions) and saphena varix. Acute injuries may be accompanied by blistering, contusions and haematoma, and abrasions or lacerations.

The chronically injured or inflamed knee will show a classical reversal of contour, in that the thigh muscles waste, while the synovial and capsular envelope enlarges owing to fluid or synovial hypertrophy.

Patella alta (see Figure 4.4, p. 61) may predispose the patient to both patellar pain and lateral subluxation so the positioning and tracking of the patella should be carefully observed during

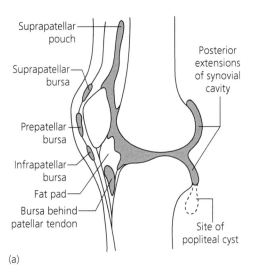

Figure 2.1 Cystic swellings around the knee: (a) from the side (cross-section), (b) from the front.

Suprapatellar pouch
Suprapatellar bursa
Prepatellar bursa
Infrapatellar bursa
Fat pad
Bursa behind patellar tendon
Posterior extensions of synovial cavity
Site of popliteal cyst

(a)

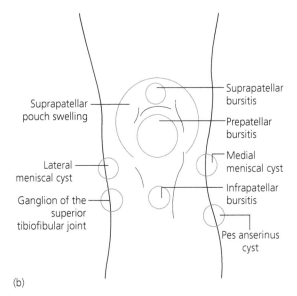

Suprapatellar pouch swelling
Lateral meniscal cyst
Ganglion of the superior tibiofibular joint
Suprapatellar bursitis
Prepatellar bursitis
Medial meniscal cyst
Infrapatellar bursitis
Pes anserinus cyst

(b)

13

the course of the clinical examination (Figure 2.2). Linked with any patellar problem is the functioning of the quadriceps muscles, most accurately measured by:

- Comparison (from the foot of the couch) with the opposite thigh and palpation of the tone of the quadriceps muscles, particularly vastus medialis, when the patient forcibly extends the knee
- Assessment of thigh circumference, using a tape measure at two defined levels above the tibial tuberosity or the upper edge of the patella (Figure 2.3).

Measurement of the calf girths in both legs is also recommended and may indicate whether the affected leg is being favoured or is primarily weaker.

During the assessment of the knee it is possible to form certain opinions about not merely the physique of the patient but also something of the personality. The response of the patient to questioning and examination often gives vital clues about the manner in which each individual is likely to react to injury, pain and life in general. Small grimaces of discomfort are more helpful in deciding where tenderness is located than loud and sometimes unconvincing exclamations from the patient. This is open to misinterpretation, of course, but the interplay between the personality of the patient and the examiner has a greater influence on the diagnosis, and the eventual outcome, than is generally admitted.

Figure 2.2 (a) The left patella lies above the femoral sulcus but is centrally positioned; and (b) on contracting the quadriceps (or flexing the knee) the patella shifts laterally.

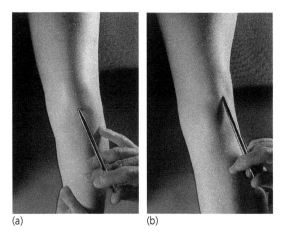

(a) (b)

Figure 2.3 Measurement of the thigh circumference with a tape. The technique is only slightly more accurate than assessing the girth of the thigh by eye.

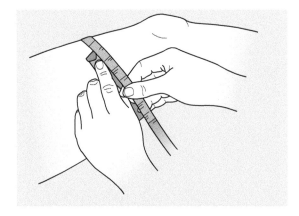

At this stage the presence of generalized ligament laxity and of skin conditions such as psoriasis and eczema should be noted as these may not only be important aetiologically but may also exert an adverse effect on recovery from synovitis. The stigmata of juvenile chronic arthritis and haemophilia are usually clear and documented in the past history of the younger patient (Chapter 9). Yet an injury or spontaneous symptom may be the first manifestation of a systemic condition so that arthropathies, including those secondary to venereal disease, should be remembered in the assessment.

Finally, it is important to stress that both the normal and symptomatic legs should be properly reviewed. The contralateral leg is the baseline from which to work and the problem knee must be compared with its fellow throughout the examination. Alignment and other subtle characteristics will be more obvious through careful comparison.

Palpation

Feeling the temperature and texture of the skin and the tone of muscle groups offers clues to the diagnosis. Roughened skin overlying the patella may have resulted from kneeling a great deal occupationally, with dire effects upon the retropatellar surface. Hypersensitivity may be due to a cutaneous neuroma. Inflammatory conditions produce increased warmth and thickening of the soft tissues. Normal synovium, when picked up between finger and thumb, is barely discernible. However, when engorged and oedematous, a distinct sensation of two slightly rubbery layers moving against each other can be felt. Effusions of varying degree may be encountered. The swollen knee may be principally the result of synovial hypertrophy, a haemarthrosis or effusion, or a combination of both.

▮ Swellings

Swellings may be localized or generalized. The common sites for discrete swelling are over the lateral joint line, in relation to the patella, in the popliteal fossa and arising from muscles such as the semimembranosus and pes anserinus. Some swellings are more obvious when the knee is straight, such as effusions and popliteal cysts (which often co-exist), while others are made obvious by flexing the knee (Figure 2.4).

Before assessing the volume of an effusion it is of value to determine the likely contents of any smaller swelling. Hard lumps which do not transilluminate light are usually bony excrescences and may be overlain by a bursa. Chondral loose bodies may be palpated around the joint margins although in synovial chondromatosis the fragments are very small. An osteochondral loose body of any size may be palpable intermittently, and often by the patient, within the confines of the capsule. In contrast, osteochondromas are present at the metaphysis, a few finger-breadths away from the joint line.

Ganglia and cysts related to tendons may feel firm or even hard when tense, but have a habit of varying in size, a fact often commented on by the patient. Cystic swellings are considered classically to transilluminate, yet many such cysts are deeply placed and loculated, so that convincing transillumination is impossible. Lipomas and other soft tissue lumps may also transmit light in a non-specific manner and hence ultrasound scanning proves to be a very useful discriminant when clinical examination identifies these superficial swellings.

Some swellings may also empty when compressed because a valve-effect is present. This accounts for the periodicity of discomfort in, for example, the popliteal cyst, which is connected to the cavity of the joint (Figure 2.1a).

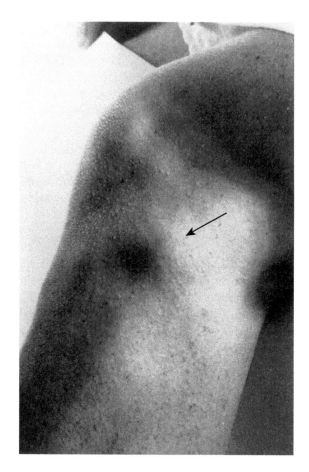

Figure 2.4 A lateral meniscal cyst made obvious by flexing the knee. A tear of the meniscus is often associated.

■ Extended knee

When the knee is extended, skin sensation, the presence of an effusion and the retropatellar surface can be assessed.

Sensation

Cutaneous nerve distribution is shown in Figure 2.5. A common problem arises when the infrapatellar branch of the saphenous nerve is severed during a medial arthrotomy or longitudinal anterior incision. This cutaneous branch may also be injured by impaction against the anteromedial aspect of the knee, such as when the knee strikes the dashboard of a car in a collision. Following severance or crushing of the nerve and its branches loss of sensation and neuropathic pain may prove troublesome.

Paraesthesiae may develop with partial recovery, and heightened sensation (dysaesthesia or hyperpathia), can impede recovery. Neuroma formation may be detected by a positive Tinel's sign over the affected nerve, amenable to treatment by steroid injection or exploration, neuroma excision and burying of the proximal nerve stump.

Effusion

- *Major effusion*: gradation of the volume of an effusion is of value, a major effusion visibly distending the suprapatellar pouch and causing enlargement of the capsule anterior to the condyles when the knee is straight (see Figure 1.12, p. 9). It is unnecessary to attempt to produce a 'patellar tap' against the femur as this sign may be wrongly interpreted.

- *Moderate effusion*: this is present when the volume of fluid is sufficient to fill the hollow medial to the patella and may be made clearer if any medial fluid is swept up to the suprapatellar pouch with the palm of the hand (Figure 2.6). The subsequent, downward fluid shift can be seen when the examining hand is released.
- *Minor effusion*: the trace of fluid present does not fill the medial hollow visibly unless, after sweeping upwards with the hand the examiner then empties the suprapatellar pouch. This shift of fluid is best achieved by compressing the lateral gutter, followed by the suprapatellar pouch, using the back of the hand in a sweeping motion (Figure 2.7). The hand should not be taken too far medially as it may obscure the medial hollow. With experience the examiner develops an individual technique. When the fluid is hard to detect it may help to flex the knee several times, thereby pumping fluid forwards from the posterior recesses of the joint. Remember also to assess the opposite knee for fluid.

◼ Patellofemoral joint

The final assessment with the knee extended concerns the patellofemoral joint. When the patient relaxes completely, the quadriceps muscles will no long tether the patella within the femoral sulcus or trochlea. The knee cap can be moved from side to side (less so in the arthritic knee) and this permits the examining fingers to palpate up to half of its posterior surface, partly medially and partly laterally. Tenderness may be remarked upon by the patient and apprehension is produced both by this manoeuvre and by deviating the patella laterally, forcing it against the lateral sulcus.

Patellar apprehension

The patellar apprehension may be so strongly positive that the patient withdraws the leg rapidly as the examiner approaches the knee with the hand, thus preventing any contact. The interpretation of such a florid response is difficult. It may mean that the patella is the source of symptoms. Alternatively, the patient may be responding in an inappropriate way emotionally. The surgeon should then be wary about eventually recommending a surgical solution.

Patellar grind and restraint tests

If the patient permits the patella to be palpated, discomfort can be assessed by compressing or grinding the posterior patellar surface against the sulcus, comparing the response to the opposite knee. A more vigorous test of retropatellar pain is afforded

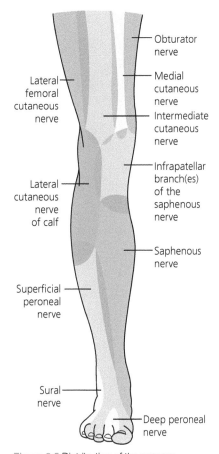

Figure 2.5 Distribution of the sensory cutaneous nerves supplying the leg.

Obturator nerve

Medial cutaneous nerve

Intermediate cutaneous nerve

Infrapatellar branch(es) of the saphenous nerve

Saphenous nerve

Lateral femoral cutaneous nerve

Lateral cutaneous nerve of calf

Superficial peroneal nerve

Sural nerve

Deep peroneal nerve

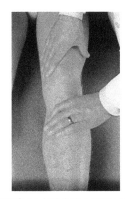

Figure 2.6 Synovial fluid is swept up into the suprapatellar pouch by the flat of the hand; the return of fluid into the medial patellar hollow will be seen in a moderate effusion, if the patient is not obese.

17

by the 'patellar restraint test'. The patella, with the knee still extended, is trapped in the femoral groove with the thumb or hand of the examiner. While the superior patellar pole is being pushed distally the patient is asked to straighten the knee forcibly, as in straight-leg raising (Figure 2.8). Since the patella is not free to move upwards in the femoral groove, a resultant force is generated backwards, thus compressing the patella against the femur. The test is sometime referred to as the 'Osmond Clark test'.

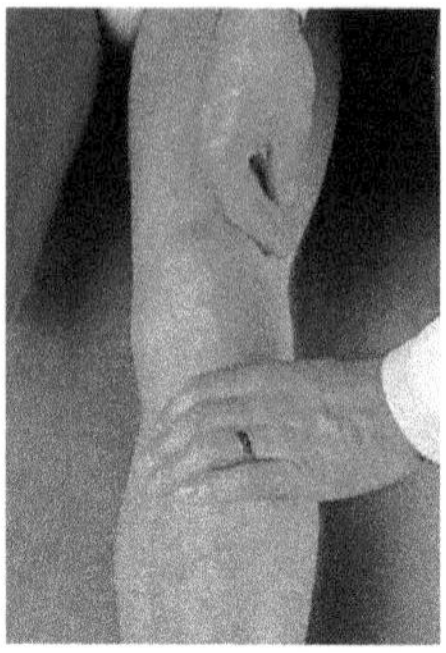

Acute pain is felt if patellar malfunction or pathology is present but the opposite side should always be tested as the sign is often positive bilaterally. This indicates that mild abnormality is present on the apparently asymptomatic side also.

Figure 2.7 When the effusion is minor, the lateral gutter and patellar pouch must be emptied by using the back of the right hand, again sweeping upwards.

Movement (tracking and crepitus)

The hand should now be placed, palm downward, upon the knee cap and the joint flexed and extended actively by the patient. Crepitus may be both felt and heard, but is so regularly evident in asymptomatic knees that this feature is of limited diagnostic value on its own. Indeed, patients with marked patellofemoral crepitus are often found to have normal articular surfaces at arthroscopy although the sign may arise from subtle degrees of synovial engorgement.

An assessment of patellar tracking should be made at this stage, initially by passively moving the knee from extension to flexion and back again. Deviation of the patella laterally may occur in extension particularly if patella alta is present, preventing full 'capture' of the patella as it exits the sulcus proximally. Rarely, the patella shifts medially in full extension, a deviation that may be iatrogenic after excessive medial patellar realignment (Chapter 7). If the quadriceps mechanism is tight or there are lateral tethers, the patella may shift laterally in flexion rather than in extension. A more dynamic test of patellar tracking is afforded if the patient extends the knee under load.

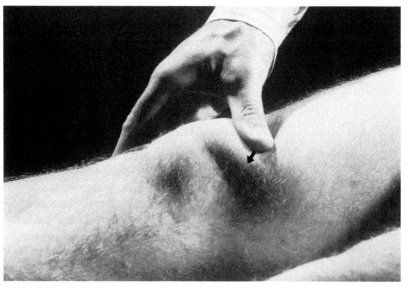

Figure 2.8 The patellar restraint test.

The easiest method is to sit the patient on the couch with both legs flexed over the side. Extension against gravity is then attempted and patellar tilting and tracking carefully reviewed.

■ Flexed knee

The knee is now flexed to a right angle. This throws into relief the joint lines, the contours of the femoral and tibial condyles and the surface marking of the ligament attachments. The underlying anatomy is largely palpable and important for accurate assessment (Chapter 1).

Joint lines

These lie at 90° to the shin and are level with the lower pole of the patella. If the leg is plump it is difficult to feel the small indentations of the joint edges but using surface landmarks and firm palpation should allow reasonable precision. Since this line represents the peripheral margin of each meniscus and their anchoring meniscotibial ligaments it is essential to be certain of its position.

Ligaments

There is a 'no man's land' medially where the medial (tibial) collateral ligament crosses the joint line and hence the meniscal margin. Tenderness here or posterolaterally over the fibular collateral ligament may arise from the relevant ligament, from the meniscus, or from both structures. A tear of the ligament is more likely if tenderness can be traced along the line of the ligament. Medially the adductor tubercle and the medial tibial flare define the attachments of the medial ligament (Figure 1.4, p. 5). Laterally the ligament runs distally from the lateral femoral condyle to the fibular head (Figure 1.2, p. 3). Injury to the iliotibial tract is rarely a solitary lesion. Capsular tenderness may be widespread or localized. The articular margins of the patella, femur and tibia should be palpated thoroughly for the possibility of symptomatic synovial 'fringe lesions' caused by synovitis and entrapment. The fat pad may occasionally be tender or thickenings of synovial 'shelves' or 'plicae' may be present (Figure 2.9).

The largest of these plicae runs over the medial femoral condyle from the upper pole of the patella to the fat pad. When inflamed or thickened by fibrosis this structure may cause local tenderness or clicking. It can be felt as a tender band when the knee flexes and extends. The medial discomfort it produces may be mistaken for a medial meniscal tear. Within the suprapatellar pouch are the medial and lateral suprapatellar plicae, which represent the residual portions of a diaphragm across the synovial cavity that separated the pouch from the rest of the knee in embryonic life. The ligamentum mucosum, or alar ligament, is also a synovial fold or prolongation normally found in the knee, supporting part of the fat pad. These structures can only be deemed pathological when they become sufficiently thickened to cause a catching sensation, or pain as they rub against the condyle, which may be roughened by this abrasion.

Bone

Palpation of the femoral and tibial condyles sometimes elicits acute tenderness, the differential diagnosis including

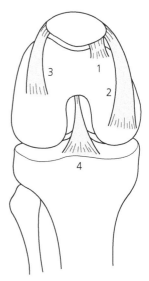

Figure 2.9 Sites of the synovial folds or plicae: 1, medial suprapatellar plica; 2, medial synovial shelf; 3, lateral synovial shelf; 4, ligamentum mucosum (alar ligament). Other synovial fibrous bands may form as a result of direct trauma.

19

osteomyelitis, osteochondritis dissecans or neoplasia (Chapter 9), bone bruising and fracture (Chapter 8). Tenderness which spreads into the femoral and tibial shafts should alert the examiner to the possibility of a more extensive lesion, although after injury the patient may find it difficult to localize tenderness precisely. In some apprehensive individuals tenderness may be commented on anywhere one palpates, and obviously this hypersensitivity must be recognized and placed in perspective.

Movement

The final stage in examining a knee while the patient is on the couch is to assess movement and laxity. Motion may be pathologically increased or decreased in each or several of these ranges:

- Extension to flexion (an arc of approximately 150°)
- Rotation (normally no more than 20°)
- Coronal tilting into valgus and varus (a few degrees each way)
- Sagittal glide (rarely more than 2–3 mm).

The opposite knee should always be used as a comparator, if normal.

◼ Extension

The degree of extension or hyperextension is accurately measured with the patient lying prone. This also reminds the examiner to inspect the posterior aspect of the knee as a routine. The patient is asked to hang the legs straight out, with the front of the knees at the edge of the examination couch (Figure 2.10). It is essential that the edge of the couch is firm and that the legs are placed symmetrically so that the comparison is accurate. Slight elevation of the heel on the affected side indicates loss of full extension, and the eye is far better equipped to assess a distance of this sort than in attempting to detect a minor alteration in knee angle. Small but significant losses of extension, in many instances from a locking knee, will be missed if the legs are examined only in the supine position or on a soft bed.

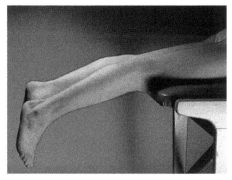

Figure 2.10 The prone-lying test on a firm surface identifies minor restrictions of extension (as in the locked knee) and hyperextension (after ligament rupture).

Increased extension, or hyperextension, is encountered in the patient with hypermobility. If the hyperextension is confined to the affected knee it suggests acute or chronic laxity of the cruciate ligaments and other soft tissue restraints.

◼ Flexion

The range of flexion is measured with the patient supine or prone, using the heel-to-buttock distance on each side, measured in finger-breadths rather than attempting to estimate an angle (Figure 2.11). Viewed from the side these distances are measured for the two knees, and both knees can be flexed together for precision. Variable losses of flexion during this testing suggests that the patient may be anxious or fabricating the restriction.

■ Collateral ligament laxity

Knee in slight flexion

Coronal laxity implicates the collateral ligament and capsule initially. If the laxity is major, other structures, including the cruciate ligaments, may be injured. Valgus and varus stress should at first be applied with the knee in 20° of flexion (Figure 2.12). This relaxes the posterior capsule and means that stability is principally reliant upon the medial and lateral structures. Ruptures of the lateral restraints – the lateral collateral ligament, the fascia lata, the biceps femoris and popliteus muscles, and the arcuate complex – result in moderate varus laxity; this increases perceptibly when the cruciate ligaments are stretched or torn.

It is difficult to grade laxity precisely as the knee tends to rotate and flex during these assessments but the following grading is usually accepted:

> Grade I (minor) – the joint tilts by up to 5 mm more than the contralateral side, with a slight suction sign (a 'jog' of movement).
> Grade II (moderate) – abnormal movement of between 5 and 10 mm is possible, with an obvious suction sign (laxity with an 'end point') (Figure 2.13).
> Grade III (severe) – more than 10 mm of opening up is possible, with no feeling of a resistant 'end point' since tissue tension is absent (laxity with no 'end point').

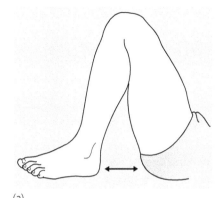

(a)

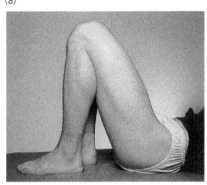

(b)

Figure 2.11 (a) Minor losses of knee flexion are best measured by the heel-to-buttock distance, comparing each leg in turn. Greater restriction of flexion should be measured with a goniometer. (b) The heel-to-buttock distance is the best measure of minor losses of knee flexion, commonly seen in posterior compartment pathology.

Examination under anaesthesia will give a clearer picture at the time of operative reconstruction, augmented by the preoperative magnetic resonance scan.

Knee in extension

When the knee is extended, the medial side will only hinge open if there is a torn cruciate ligament. More than just the circumferential structures have given way. Commonly it is the anterior cruciate ligament that has ruptured, and if the posterior cruciate ligament is progressively torn the valgus laxity will increase, with subluxation of the knee joint. Although the brunt of an injury may be borne by one structure, causing macroscopic tearing, other tissues are invariably stretched and partially ruptured. Thus, tears of the medial ligament are often accompanied by synovial stretching, rents in the posteromedial capsule, damage to the attachment of the medial meniscus and interstitial tearing of the anterior cruciate ligament.

Since ligaments are not simply passive restrainers of abnormal movement but also contain nerve fibres concerned with proprioception and pain, complex tears may render the knee relatively painless when it is examined. In these cases the synovial envelope is usually incompetent and the haemarthrosis leaks out subcutaneously producing a boggy swelling with a spreading ecchymosis but no evidence of a tense knee enlargement. The knee feels unstable when examined and weightbearing is impossible. The long-term deficit reflects the proprioceptive loss in addition to any chronic laxity. These aspects will be discussed more fully in Chapter 5.

■ Cruciate ligament laxity

Laxity in the sagittal plane was classically taught as a differentiation between the anterior and posterior drawer tests with the knee flexed to 90°. The anterior contour of the knee should first be viewed from the lateral side (Figure 2.14). If there is tibial 'drop-back', a concavity is seen below the patella as the upper tibia sags back posteriorly. This indicates that the posterior cruciate ligament has been partially or completely torn. The mechanism of injury may be a direct blow to the upper shin from a collision, forced hyperextension or complex disruption involving the medial and posterior structures. The drop-back may be wrongly interpreted as a positive anterior drawer sign so the contour of the normal knee should always be compared.

The drawer test

After assessing the lateral tibiofemoral relationship, the hamstrings should be palpated to ensure they are relaxed. The proximal tibia is moved firmly, anteriorly and posteriorly, by grasping it with both hands just below the joint lines (Figures 2.15, 2.16). The foot of the leg being examined should be secured by the examiner, who either sits on the side of it or applies the elbows against the dorsum of the foot. Increased movement of more than a few millimetres anteriorly or posteriorly, compared with the other knee, indicates that abnormal laxity is present. A positive anterior drawer sign rarely results from a solitary anterior cruciate tear and usually there has to be associated laxity of the posteromedial corner of the joint. A more specific test of anterior cruciate deficiency is the 'Lachman' test, which can be combined with dynamic assessment of tibiofemoral subluxation under load (the 'pivot shift' test – which may not be positive in the acute situation).

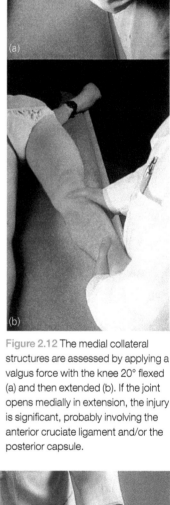

(a)

(b)

Figure 2.12 The medial collateral structures are assessed by applying a valgus force with the knee 20° flexed (a) and then extended (b). If the joint opens medially in extension, the injury is significant, probably involving the anterior cruciate ligament and/or the posterior capsule.

Figure 2.13 A medial joint line suction sign indicates a grade II tear with a definite firm end point.

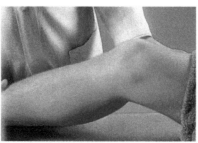

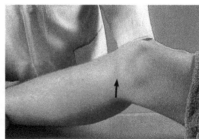

Figure 2.14 The anterior drawer test fixes the foot and assesses the knee in 90° of flexion after checking that the hamstrings are relaxed.

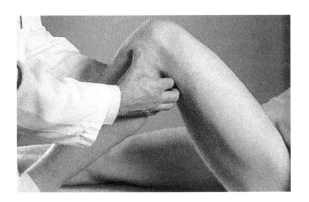

Figure 2.15 (a) Stretching of the posterior cruciate ligament allows the tibia to sublux posteriorly ('drop-back'). (b) When anterior laxity is present the hamstrings will involuntarily contract.

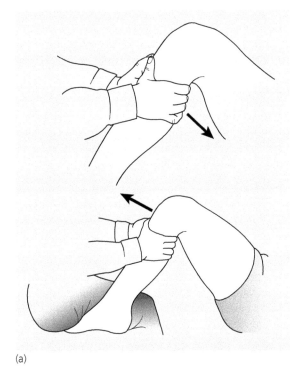

(a)

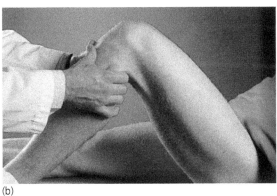

(b)

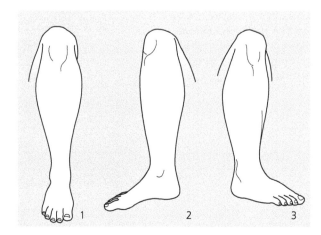

Figure 2.16 Anterior drawer tests with modifications to show rotatory laxity. 1, tibia in a neutral position; 2, tibia in external rotation (assessing anteromedial laxity); 3, tibia in internal rotation (assessing anterolateral laxity).

Ritchey–Lachman test

This test allows the examiner to assess anterior laxity accurately, comparing it with the contralateral knee. In 20-30° of flexion the restraint afforded by the posterior meniscal contour and the collateral structures is reduced to a minimum, unlike the 90° drawer test. Torg *et al.* (1976) popularized the test, which was recognized as early as 1875 by Georges Noulis (Passler 1993) and reported by Ritchey (1960) as a useful means of confirming anterior cruciate ligament disruption.

Anterior stress is applied manually (Figure 2.17) or with a standardized 89 N force. Normally there should be no more than 3 mm variation between the knees. A distance less than this is difficult to judge on standard, clinical examination. Four grades of increasing laxity are recognized (Gurtler *et al.* 1987):

Grade I (3-6 mm) – palpable subluxation with a soft end point
Grade II (6-9 mm) – visible subluxation with a soft end point
Grade III (9-16 mm) – passive subluxation when the proximal tibia is supported
Grade IV (16-29 mm) – active subluxation produced by quadriceps and gastrocnemius muscle contraction.

The test is usually performed with the patient supine. The examiner uses both hands, but this may prove difficult if the leg is large and muscular or if the examiner has small hands. Modification have therefore been proposed, including the supported test (Figure 2.18) (Strobel and Stedtfeld 1990) and by testing the patient when lying on the uninjured side. This may also

Figure 2.17 The standard Ritchey–Lachman test.

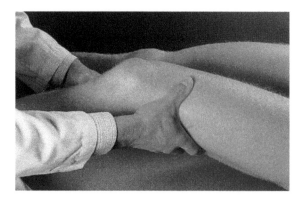

allow the patient to show active (grade IV) subluxation more readily. If the laxity is gross, the crossed knee test is positive (Figure 2.19) (Macnicol 1995) and has the advantage that both knees can be compared under similar load, namely the weight of the leg, and the patient is willing to relax fully in a familiar, sitting posture.

The prone-lying Lachman test (Feagin 1988) and the Hackenbruch modification (Hackenbruch and Muller 1987) rely on the thigh being stabilized while the tibia is being manipulated with one or both hands, respectively. The test can be carried out at the time of the prone-lying assessment of joint extension.

Finochietto (1935) recognized the snapping sensation caused by a torn or hypermobile posterior meniscal horn as an additional characteristic of the pathological anterior tibial glide. This sensation can sometimes be reinforced by rotation of the tibia internally or externally, either with the patient prone or supine. The joint lines should be palpated concurrently.

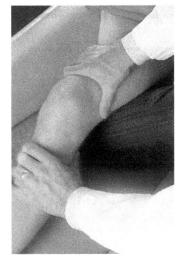

Figure 2.18 If the thigh is supported under the examiner's knee, anteroposterior and collateral laxity can be assessed accurately as the patient relaxes.

The pivot shift (jerk) test

This test is pathognomonic of symptomatic anterolateral laxity as the sense of lateral tibial condylar subluxation is unnerving and ultimately disabling. The knee buckles or collapses with the sensation of the knuckles of one fist moving forcibly over the knuckles of the opposite fist. In children with hypermobility it may be present without symptoms but during adolescence this degree of laxity is usually lost.

The resultant instability was recognized by Amedee Bonnet in 1845 (Passler 1993) and later by Hey-Groves (1919). Lemaire (1967) demonstrated the subluxation, but it only became extensively recognized in the English literature after the paper by Galway et al. (1972). A number of variations have been described but may prove bewildering.

Figure 2.19 The 'crossed knee test' allows the hamstrings to relax naturally, demonstrating anterior laxity.

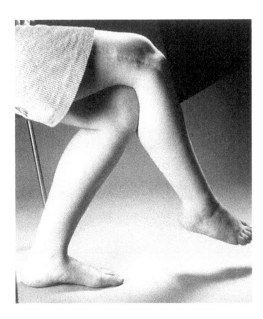

Slocum test (Slocum *et al.* 1976)

1 The patient lies on the normal side with that hip and knee flexed
2 The knee to be examined is extended fully with the medial side of the foot resting on the couch
3 A valgus force is applied to the knee with the tibia internally rotated
4 As the knee is flexed actively to 30°, the anterior subluxation of the lateral tibial condyle is reduced (Figure 2.20).

McIntosh test (Galway *et al.* 1972)

1 The patient lies supine
2 The knee to be examined is extended by supporting the leg with a hand under the heel
3 The lateral tibial condyle subluxes anteriorly and this is made more obvious by applying a valgus force to the knee with the other hand
4 Passive flexion of the knee will reduce the subluxation.

Losee test (Losee 1983)

1 The patient lies supine
2 With the knee flexed 50–60° a valgus force is applied
3 The knee is slowly extended and pressure is applied behind the head of the fibula
4 A clunk occurs as the lateral tibial condyle subluxes forward during the last few degrees towards extension.

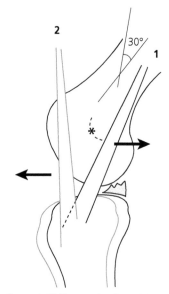

Figure 2.20 The mechanism of the anterior pivot (jerk) test relies upon the forward subluxation of the lateral tibial plateau under the convexity of the femoral condyle. (The asterix represents the centre of rotation of the knee.)

Noyes test (Noyes and Grood 1988) ('flexion-rotation drawer test')

1 The patient lies supine
2 The examiner supports the extended leg at the calf, allowing the femur to rotate externally and drop posteriorly if laxity is present
3 The anterior subluxation of the lateral tibial plateau relative to the femur is corrected by gently flexing the knee while pushing the upper shin posteriorly
4 A clunk may be felt.

These tests produce a clunk or 'pivot shift' as the lateral tibial condyle alters its arc of movement in relation to the femur (Figure 2.20). The essential components of all of these tests are:

- A relaxed patient (hamstring spasm may prevent the subluxation)
- Sufficient laxity to allow the lateral tibial condyle to alter its relationship to the femur during the last 30° of knee flexion
- An additional valgus force to make the subluxation more obvious. The application of an axial force to the foot, directed upwards, mimics weightbearing and will accentuate the abnormal subluxation (Figure 2.21). The convex surface of the lateral tibial condyle (which varies from patient to patient) promotes the nature of the subluxation or jerk (Figure 2.22).

It is important to become familiar with one form of the test and to practise it regularly. The flexion-rotation drawer test may allow a clear assessment of the jerk in the acutely injured knee; the essential feature is that protective hamstring spasm or tone should be minimized. In

Figure 2.21 The pivot shift or jerk test is positive when the iliotibial band comes to lie behind the pivot of the femur while the knee is flexed from 0° to 30°, thus producing a palpable (and usually visible) reduction of the anteriorly subluxed lateral tibial condyle. This forward and backward motion eventually damages the secondary restraints.

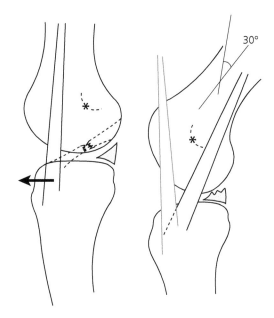

Figure 2.22 (a) Axial loading of the leg is achieved by pushing upwards on the foot, or by applying pressure through the knee to the stabilized hip.

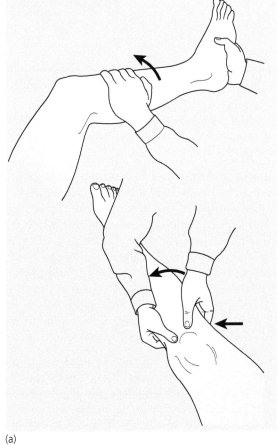

(a)

Figure 2.22 (Continued) (b) The pivot shift may be demonstrated from the flexed position to extension. (c) With the knee in extension, the subluxed lateral tibial condyle will be reduced by a return to the flexed position.

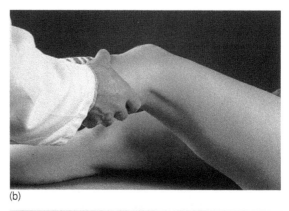

(b)

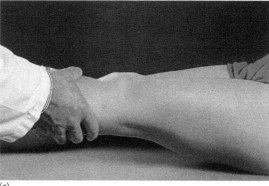

(c)

order to emphasize the subluxation, valgus stress and axial loading are required, together with internal rotation of the tibia. Rupture of the iliotibial tract, obstruction from a meniscal tear or degenerative changes may prevent the pivot shift. This sometimes occurs in children with a discoid lateral meniscus, as the prominence of that structure affects the mechanics of the lateral compartment.

In assessing the pivot shift test, conventional grading describes a negative shift (grade 0), a pivot slide (grade I), where the tibial subluxation is checked before it extends beyond the zenith of the lateral tibial condyle, and a complete shift or jerk (grade II). The grade III pivot is gross, with 'hang-up' during reduction and significant discomfort. Jakob et al. (1987) graded the test in relation to the position of the tibia and suggest that this helps to demonstrate disruption of the posteromedial and posterolateral structures (grade III). Their grade I pivot shift is palpable rather than visible tibial subluxation, present only when the tibia is internally rotated. Grade II subluxation is evident with the tibia in internal or neutral rotation, but absent with external rotation. The grade III test is markedly positive even with the tibia externally rotated and indicates a significant degree of laxity of the secondary restraints. A reverse pivot shift (Jakob et al. 1981) is also demonstrable when complex laxity is present.

Control of the pivot shift, whether by improved hamstring tone or by anterior cruciate ligament reconstruction, correlates closely with successful elimination of instability. Increased medial laxity and complex instability patterns make it increasingly difficult to prevent the pivot shift phenomenon although the patient may learn to avoid the episodes of subluxation. Proprioceptive education (Barrett 1991) and a 'quadriceps avoidance' gait pattern (Berchuck et al. 1991) may be sufficient to deal with lesser degrees of anterolateral laxity. The provoking sporting activity should be avoided and a trial of conservative management allowed. However, surgical reconstruction (Chapter 5) is advisable if episodes of giving way occur in the professional athlete, in those who rely on a dependable knee during work and when everyday activities are enough to promote the instability.

Genu recurvatum external rotation test

This test assesses the integrity of the posterolateral structures. It augments the reverse pivot shift as a sign of major and often permanent rotatory laxity, including damage to the posterior cruciate ligament. The reverse pivot can be demonstrated with the patient lying on the uninjured side. The lateral tibial condyle is directed backwards and the resistance assessed. The genu recurvatum external rotation test (Figure 2.23) confirms the posterolateral laxity but this time with the patient lying supine. If the injured leg is lifted in extension by the hallux or heel the knee may hyperextend and the tibia will externally rotate perceptibly.

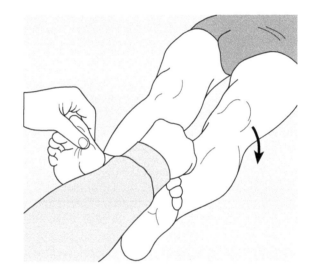

Figure 2.23 The genu recurvatum external rotation test. The leg is suspended in extension as shown and the test is positive if the knee hyperextends with increased external rotation.

◼ Tests of meniscal integrity

A torn meniscus produces tenderness at a localized portion of the joint line. The other cardinal signs are an effusion and loss of movement. A locked knee will demonstrate not just a loss of extension but also reduced flexion and rotation. The loss of extension is rarely more than 10–20° so that a greater restriction suggests an obstructive loose body or voluntary resistance.

Joint line fullness, or a discrete swelling, also suggests meniscal pathology. A lateral meniscal cyst is far more likely than a medial meniscal cyst although a pedunculated tag may lodge in the medial gutter above or below the meniscotibial ligament, producing a variable, firm swelling. The snapping knee produced by a discoid lateral meniscus is discussed in Chapter 4.

Stress can be applied to the meniscus by Bragard's sign, in which medial meniscal tenderness is accentuated by externally rotating and extending the tibia, at the same time as compressing the anterior horn with a finger. Valgus or varus stress may also elicit meniscal tenderness on the side of compression (Bohler's sign) although the test is ambiguous. When combined with altering flexion of the knee (the 'D' test) a more convincing meniscal assessment is possible.

Finochietto's 'jump sign' (Finochietto 1935) is positive in the lax knee when anteroposterior drawer movement (glide) causes a snap or jerk.

McMurray test

Described by McMurray in 1928, this test has a time-honoured place in the examination of the knee. The examiner should palpate the joint line with the fingers of one hand (Figure 2.24) while at the same time the tibia is rotated beneath the femur. The heel of the foot can be grasped conveniently to ensure internal and external rotation while the knee is extended progressively. Internal rotation and a varus stress examine the medial meniscus although an angulatory force can be applied only when the knee incompletely flexed. External rotation and valgus compress the lateral meniscus.

A positive test is present when a clunk is felt, produced by a posterior third tear as the joint is fully flexed. When truly positive the patient becomes apprehensive as the abnormal meniscal movement threatens to lock up the knee. A negative test does not rule out meniscal pathology since the manoeuvre depends on meniscal instability, the state of relaxation of the patient and the experience of the examiner. Magnetic resonance scanning has made the value of this test much less important.

Thessaly test

This is undertaken with the patient standing. The normal knee is assessed first by weightbearing on that side alone with the knee flexed 5° and then 20°. The patient is asked to rotate the knee internally and externally, three times each, lightly balancing with the hands placed on a piece of furniture. On the side with a meniscal lesion, apprehension and pain may be elicited. The test may also reproduce a sense of clicking or instability.

The Apley test (Apley and Solomon 1994), whereby an attempt is made to distinguish between a ligamentous injury (by distracting the joint) and a meniscal tear (by axial compression and rotation of the joint), is open to misinterpretation and is therefore not recommended. The 'bounce(out) test' (Figure 2.25) assesses the feel of the knee as it is dropped into full extension with the patient supine and the foot supported. Loss of the normal screw-home action of the femur on the tibia may be detected as a painful 'bounce' of the joint out of its fully extended

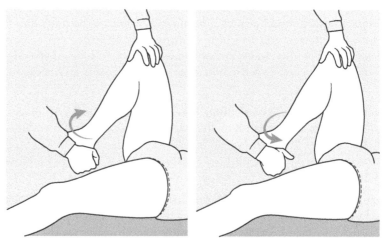

Figure 2.24 The McMurray test for an obstructing posterior meniscal tear. The joint line should be palpated for a clunk, while the tibia is rotated with the knee in different degrees of flexion.

Figure 2.25 The bounce test assesses whether the knee extends fully by means of its 'screw home' action. Anterior meniscal tears, loose bodies and chondral lesions impede the sense of the knee dropping out straight as the right hand releases its support (a and b).

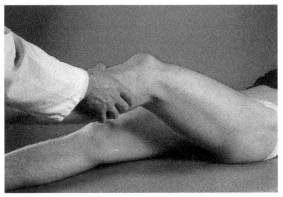

(a)

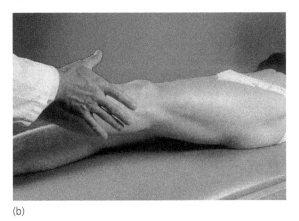

(b)

position. Passive loss of flexion, measured by the heel-to-buttock distance (Figure 2.11b, p. 21), and extension measured by the prone-lying test (Figure 2.10, p. 20), are important discriminators between the presence or absence of obstructive pathology although tense effusions, synovitis, arthritis, loose bodies and protective muscle spasm may result in similar losses of movement.

■ Squatting and weightbearing tests

A full squat is impossible when a displacing meniscal tear is present (Figure 2.26). The distance between the heel and the buttock during squatting should be compared to the normal side. This loss of flexion during loadbearing is almost pathognomonic of a posterior meniscal tear if it persists for more than 6–8 weeks, when most ligament sprains are settling.

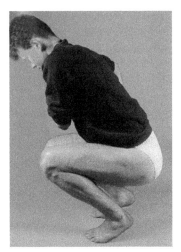

Figure 2.26 Squatting and 'duck-waddling' prove impossible in the presence of a displacing meniscal tear.

A 'duck waddle' requires the fully flexed knee on one side to cope with the full body weight and is generally impossible when a meniscal lesion is present. The test can also be performed with the knee flexed less fully. The patient is asked to rotate the

31

loaded knee internally and externally as detailed above in the Thessaly test, p. 30. Apprehension, pain, local tenderness and the presence of a clunk are noted.

Conclusion

Examination of the knee should include inspection, careful palpation of all anatomical landmarks, and a detailed review of the passive and active ranges of the knee compared with the opposite side. Meniscal and other obstructive lesions produce losses of movement, whereas ligament tears, particularly after the acute phase, result in pathologically increased ranges of movement. Laxity in all planes should be determined, including rotation, although subtle variations from normal are hard to quantify. It is best to become familiar with a few of the tests described in the orthopaedic literature as this should ensure an accurate portrayal of the injuries and lead on to a more thorough use of appropriate investigations. This in turn will lead to improvements in the surgical intervention and subsequent rehabilitation.

References

Apley AG and Solomon L (1994) *A System of Orthopaedics and Fractures*, 7th edn. Oxford: Butterworth-Heinemann.

Barrett DS (1991) Proprioception and function after anterior cruciate reconstruction. *J Bone Joint Surg Br* **73**, 833–7.

Berchuck M, Andriachi TP and Bach BR (1991) Gait adaptations by patients who have a deficient anterior cruciate ligament. *J Bone Joint Surg Am* **73**, 871–7.

Feagin JA (1988) Principles of diagnosis and treatment. In: Feagin JA (ed.) *The Crucial Ligaments. Diagnosis and Treatment of Ligamentous Injuries About the Knee*. New York: Churchill Livingstone, pp. 3–14.

Finochietto R (1935) Semilunar cartilages of the knee. The 'Jump Sign'. *J Bone Joint Surg Am* **17**, 916–18.

Galway R, Beaupre A and McIntosh DL (1972) Pivot-shift – a clinical sign of symptomatic anterior cruciate insufficiency. *J Bone Joint Surg Br* **54**, 763–4.

Gurtler RA, Stine R and Torg JS (1987) Lachman test evaluated – quantification of a clinical observation. *Clin Orthop* **216**, 141–50.

Hackenbruch W and Muller W (1987) Untersuchung des Kniegelenkes. *Orthopäde* **16**, 100–12.

Hey-Groves E (1919) The crucial ligaments of the knee joint; their function, rupture and the operative treatment of the same. *Br J Surg* **7**, 505–15.

Jakob RP, Hassler H and Stäubli HU (1981) Observations on rotatory instability of the lateral compartment of the knee: experimental studies on the functional anatomy and the pathomechanism of the true and reversed pivot shift sign. *Acta Orthop Scand* **52**(Suppl. 191), 1–32.

Jakob RP, Stäubli HU and Deland JT (1987) Grading the pivot shift. *J Bone Joint Surg Br* **69**, 294–9.

Lemaire M (1967) Ruptures anciennes du ligament croisé antérior du genou. *J Chir (Paris)* **93**, 311–20.

Losee RE (1983) Concepts of the pivot-shift. *Clin Orthop* **172**, 45–51.

Macnicol MF (1995) *The Problem Knee*, 2nd edn. Oxford: Butterworth-Heinemann Ltd, p. 26.

McMurray TP (1928) The diagnosis of internal derangements of the knee. In: *Robert Jones Birthday Volume*. Oxford: Oxford Medical Publications, pp. 301–5.

Noyes FR and Grood ES (1988) Diagnosis of knee ligament injuries: clinical concepts. In: Feagin JA (ed.) *The Crucial Ligaments. Diagnosis and Treatment of Ligamentous Injuries About the Knee*. New York: Churchill Livingstone, pp. 261–85.

Passler HH (1993) The history of the cruciate ligaments: some forgotten (or unknown) facts from Europe. *Knee Surg Sports Traumatol Arthroscopy* **1**, 13–16.

Ritchey SJ (1960) Ligamentous disruption of the knee. A review with analysis of 28 cases. *US Armed Forces Med J* **11**, 167–76.

Slocum DB, James Sl, Larson RL and Singer KM (1976) Clinical test for anterolateral instability of the knee. *Clin Orthop* **118**, 63–9.

Strobel M and Stedtfeld HW (1990) *Diagnostic Evaluation of the Knee*. Berlin: Springer-Verlag, p. 121.

Torg JS, Conrad W and Kalen V (1976) Clinical diagnosis of anterior cruciate ligament instability in the athlete. *Am J Sports Med* **4**, 84–91.

3

Investigations

Blood tests

The investigation of a patient with a painful knee, particularly if swelling and stiffness are present, should attempt to exclude systemic disease. When an inflammatory arthritis is suspected, the full blood count, erythrocyte sedimentation rate, C-reactive protein, rheumatoid and antinuclear factors, and titres against various antigens should be obtained. Metabolic abnormalities may also produce an arthropathy and therefore electrolytes, blood glucose and uric acid levels should be measured. If a blood dyscrasia is suspected, tests for clotting, including factors VIII and IX, and for sickle cell anaemia, should be conducted. Occasionally, venereal arthropathy may produce symptoms so that serological tests to exclude gonococcal, syphilitic and other venereal infections should be carried out. The medical implications of these conditions are discussed further in Chapter 9. A multidisciplinary approach is advised and relevant family history or other contributory factors carefully obtained.

Synovial fluid analysis

Synovial fluid can be analysed after aspirating a few millimetres from the knee. The pH of fluid, together with its contents of lactate, fat or blood, are important in the differential diagnosis (Table 3.1). The presence of crystals should be sought if a uric acid (gouty) or pyrophosphate (crystal) arthropathy is suspected.

The white cell count in the synovial fluid is of some differential diagnostic value in that osteoarthritis produces a monocytic picture, with $<2 \times 10^9$ cells per litre and relatively normal complement levels. Rheumatoid arthritis results in a predominance of polymorphonuclear white cells, with a count of $4\text{-}50 \times 10^9$ cells per litre, and low levels of complement. In septic arthritis the polymorphonuclear cell count is very much higher, usually exceeding 60×10^9 cells per litre. An inflammatory condition also lowers the

Table 3.1 Synovial fluid analysis as an aid to diagnosis

Blood	Fracture, ligament rupture, synovial tear (haemophilia, haemangioma)
Fat	Osteochondral fracture, fat pad lesion
Debris	Articular cartilage damage including chondromalacia, meniscal tear
Cells	Monocyte predominance in osteoarthritis
	Polymorphonuclear cell predominance in inflammatory synovitis including rheumatoid arthritis and septic arthritis
Crystals	Gout (urate) – feathery crystals
	Pseudogout (monophosphate) – rectangular crystals
Lactate, acidity and lysosomal enzymes	Increased in inflammatory conditions
Complement	Increased in Reiter's syndrome and gout
	Increased in osteoarthritis
	Decreased in rheumatoid arthritis

viscosity of the synovial fluid and increases the total protein content, such that there is a tendency to form a spontaneous clot.

Synovial fluid should be subjected to microscopy, using both the standard Gram stain and Ziehl–Nielsen staining for acid-alcohol fast bacilli. When infection is suspected, the microscopic appearances may be of great value in early diagnosis, with later confirmation of the bacterial cause of the infection by means of culture. Both pyogenic and tuberculous organisms should be suspected, with the use of appropriate culture media. The specimen must be transported to the microbiology laboratory urgently, preventing drying out and allowing analysis of the fresh specimen. Blood cultures may also be obtained if systemic upset is marked, although they are less likely to be positive than synovial fluid or a soft tissue biopsy.

Biopsy

The arthroscope has made 'closed' synovial and articular cartilage biopsy relatively simple (see Chapter 9). Bone biopsy is only possible by means of an operation under general anaesthesia, and with a tourniquet in place. Bone should be obtained both from the lesion and from the contiguous border of the normal bone after appropriate preoperative investigations including both magnetic resonance imaging (MRI) and computed tomography (CT). The skin incision should be placed in such a way that a wider surgical excision or possible amputation can be planned, incorporating the initial wound. Esmarch compression of the limb should be avoided as the crushing effect may liberate malignant cells from the lesion and a tourniquet should be used sparingly.

Radiography

Radiographs of the knee complement the history and clinical examination, and are an essential part of many assessments, despite Smillie's (1980) contention: 'It should be

Figure 3.1 Radiographic lesions apparent on an anteroposterior radiograph.

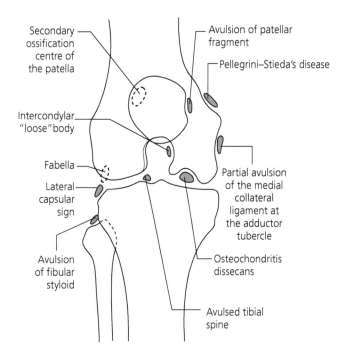

Secondary ossification centre of the patella

Avulsion of patellar fragment

Pellegrini–Stieda's disease

Intercondylar "loose" body

Fabella

Lateral capsular sign

Partial avulsion of the medial collateral ligament at the adductor tubercle

Avulsion of fibular styloid

Osteochondritis dissecans

Avulsed tibial spine

stated, and repeated, that there is no human joint less related, in terms of function, to radiographic findings than the knee joint'. After any significant injury which produces persisting symptoms, radiographs are advisable, and should precede investigations such as arthroscopy. MR scanning, if readily available, is reducing the role of X-rays, but in the acute situation radiographs are still of value. A standard anteroposterior view (Figure 3.1) is often augmented by a standing film of the leg, showing femorotibial alignment during weightbearing.

A lateral film is usually taken with the knee in 30° of flexion (Figure 3.2; see also Figure 7.4, p. 150), although a view of the knee fully extended may be indicated when the position of the patella is being assessed in relation to the femoral condyles or if the severity of a flexion contracture merits definition. A true lateral also allows an estimate of the depth of the sulcus and a possible 'crossing sign' if the sulcus is deficient proximally.

Subtle radiographic signs, such as a lipohaemarthrosis can be demonstrated using a horizontal beam when the patient is lying supine or standing, the fat layer separating from the more dense blood (Figure 3.3a). The Segond fracture, caused by lateral capsular tibial avulsion during rupture of the anterior cruciate ligament, is another example of an unusual but tell-tale radiographic lesion (Figure 3.3b).

The radiographic features of an effusion include:

- An anterior shift or tilting of the patella
- Widening of the suprapatellar pouch
- Anterior bulging of the patellar ligament
- Distension of the posterior capsule.

However, the volume of fluid required to produce these signs is usually quite gross and clinical assessment remains the best method of defining the volume of fluid within the knee.

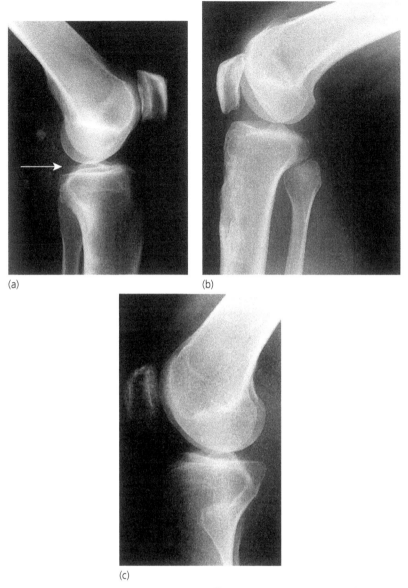

(a)

(b)

(c)

Figure 3.2 A popliteal cyst is outlined by radio-opaque calcified bodies (arrow) (a), patella baja (b) and a plasmacytoma of the patella (c).

▨ Skyline view

The axial, tangential or 'skyline' patellar view shows the retropatellar space and the relationship between the patella and the femoral condyles at one particular level (Table 3.2). Too much can be made of the patellar characteristics and the congruency of the patellofemoral joint since these are known to vary according to the amount of knee flexion and the presence or absence of quadriceps contraction. A variety of patellar outlines have been described (Figure 3.4, p. 40) but these are a poor indicator of true patellar shape and the dynamics of the patellofemoral joint. The same criticism can be levelled against single views of patellar position within the femoral condylar notch or sulcus, although much has been made of

Figure 3.3 (a) A haemarthrosis is evident from the fluid level that has formed in the suprapatellar pouch.

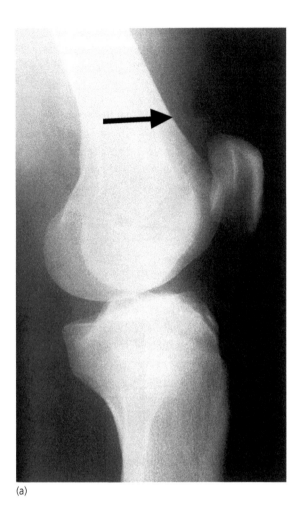

(a)

the congruency and tilting of the patella within the sulcus (Figure 3.5, p. 40). Recent CT studies have confirmed that the radiographic appearance of the patella is inaccurately demonstrated by means of the skyline view, although this radiographic projection is useful in cases where an osteochondral fracture is suspected. One view of the patellofemoral joint may not in itself be sufficient and skyline views with the knee in varying degrees of flexion improve accuracy.

Tunnel, oblique and stress views

The intercondylar or 'tunnel' view of the knee shows whether a radio-opaque loose body is present in that region of the joint, and may give further information about the size and position of an osteochondritis dissecans involving the femoral condyle. The inferior pole of the patella may sometimes be shown clearly on the intercondylar view, as may an osteochondral fracture.

Oblique views of the knee are useful in revealing less obvious fractures, and anteroposterior and lateral 'stress' radiographs (see Figure 8.11, p. 178), preferably obtained when the patient is anaesthetized, are of value in recording epiphyseal displacement and ligament laxity or rupture. The use of an image intensifier and a video recorder for the stress views will afford a dynamic assessment of the ligament injury which can then be stored.

Figure 3.3 (Continued) (b) The Segond fracture (lateral capsular avulsion; arrow) seen after anterior cruciate ligament injury.

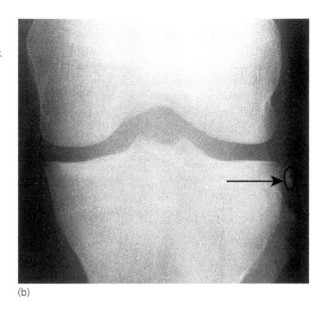

(b)

Table 3.2 Tangential ('skyline') radiographic views of the patellofemoral joint

Knee fully flexed ('sunrise view')	Shows 'odd facet' of patella articulating with medial femoral condylar groove
Knee flexed 45° (Hughston [1968] view) (tube angle of 30°)	Shows patellofemoral articulation and intercondylar notch, but some distortion occurs due to the angulation
Knee flexed to 30° (Merchant *et al.* [1974] view) (radiographic plate on shin)	Useful demonstration of the intercondylar notch and congruence angle
Knee flexed 30° (Laurin *et al.* [1979] view) (radiographic plate on anterior thigh)	Easier to obtain than the Merchant view, and as useful but the dose of radiation is higher

Normal congruence angle (Merchant view) = 8.2°.
Normal intercondylar groove angle (Merchant view) = 139°±6.3°.
Lateral patellar subluxation more likely when the intercondylar angle approaches 150° or more.

■ Schuss view

'Schuss radiographs' are posteroanterior weightbearing views of the knee taken in 30° of flexion (Figure 3.6). Several studies have shown them to be more sensitive detectors of osteoarthritic changes in the knee than standard, extension anteroposterior views. The Schuss radiograph is a valuable tool in the assessment of knee osteoarthritis and may alter clinical management. By reducing non-therapeutic arthroscopies it may significantly restrict the total number of interventions performed in this patient group (Ritchie *et al.* 2004).

■ Tomography

Tomograms of the knee can help to define lesions within the depth of the femoral condyles or proximal tibia, and reduce the artefacts caused by the superimposition of structures seen in the normal radiograph. Figure 9.13 (p. 203) indicates the value of tomography in the case of a young man who presented with a painful knee. Routine investigations, including conventional radiography and arthroscopy, were normal. However, a tomogram revealed the pathological lesion, in this example a chondroblastoma.

◼ Xeroradiography

Xeroradiography converts radiographic images to a blue-white detail based on the photoconductor selenium, and gives a high-definition image of any soft-tissue changes in lesions such as neoplasm and infection. Soft tissue shadows may be shown by abnormal swellings on the radiograph, and are best identified by comparison with the opposite knee. The uses of this technique are limited, however, and it is rarely used nowadays.

Magnetic resonance imaging

Magnetic and electromagnetic fields interact with tissues according to their different densities, producing measureable signals (Table 3.3; Figures 3.7, 3.8). Magnetic resonance imaging does not define cortical changes as readily as CT scanning and oedema produces an abnormal signal which may be confusing. But axial, coronal and sagittal displays are highly accurate and help to detect intraosseous and extraosseous pathology (Berquist 1989).

The visualization of the anatomical relationships of soft tissue masses and the delineation of vascular structures are so good that angiography is little indicated. Lipogenic tumours produce

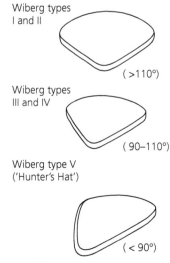

Wiberg types
I and II
(>110°)

Wiberg types
III and IV
(90–110°)

Wiberg type V
('Hunter's Hat')
(< 90°)

Figure 3.4 Three basic patellar shapes are recognizable, but are of dubious relevance to clinical conditions.

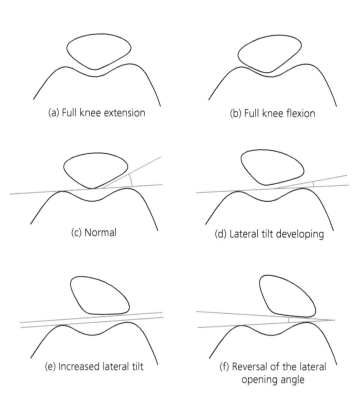

Figure 3.5 Different facets of the patella articulate with the femoral condyles during knee flexion (a,b). Increasing lateral patellar tilt may be associated with lateral subluxation (c–f) and is measured by the lateral opening angle on a skyline view with the knee in 30–40° of flexion.

(a) Full knee extension

(b) Full knee flexion

(c) Normal

(d) Lateral tilt developing

(e) Increased lateral tilt

(f) Reversal of the lateral opening angle

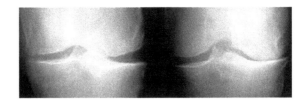

Figure 3.6 The Schuss anteroposterior radiographic projection is taken with the knee slightly flexed.

higher intensity signals than muscle on T_1- and T_2-weighted images, whereas other tumours have low signals on T_1-weighted images and high signals on T_2-weighted images. Malignancy produces a more heterogeneous mass and may be surrounded by the high signal of oedema on the T_2-weighted scan. Magnetic resonance imaging is superior to CT scanning in the evaluation of most soft-tissue tumours and lesions about the knee (Slattery and Major 2010) (see also Chapter 9).

Meniscal tears (Figure 3.9) and cruciate ruptures (Figure 3.10), the discoid lateral meniscus (Figure 3.11) and other meniscal pathology (Figure 3.12, p. 44) are detected with an accuracy of between 75 and 95 per cent (Fischer *et al.* 1991), although a negative MR scan does not rule out intra-articular (Raunest *et al.* 1991) or periarticular pathology. Arthroscopy may miss grade II (incomplete) meniscal tears (Table 3.3), although many of these may heal. Quinn and Brown (1991) considered that the error rate between the two investigations also reflected the experience of the surgeon and the difficulties inherent in visualizing the posterior horn of the menisci. Inner third tears are often minor and asymptomatic so that the surgeon may discount them as insignificant. It should also be appreciated that grades I and II lesions may not progress appreciably with time (Dillon *et al.* 1991) and that stable lesions are common and consistent with satisfactory knee function. More alarmingly, progression in the signal intensity is seen as a result of a season playing American football (Reinig *et al.* 1991) although some lesions may subsequently heal.

Previous meniscectomy, meniscal repair and degenerative change affect the MR scan, making its clinical relevance less defined. Bone marrow oedema and articular cartilage lesions inevitably develop in conjunction with anterior cruciate

Table 3.3 Magnetic resonance scan high-intensity signal (meniscal)

Grade I	Central and globular
Grade II	Primarily linear, not extending to surface
Grade III	Linear and extending to surface

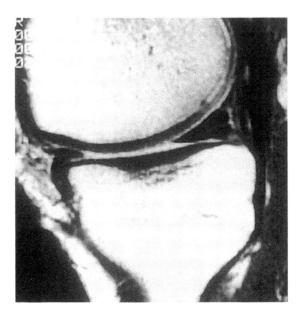

Figure 3.7 Magnetic resonance image of a normal meniscus.

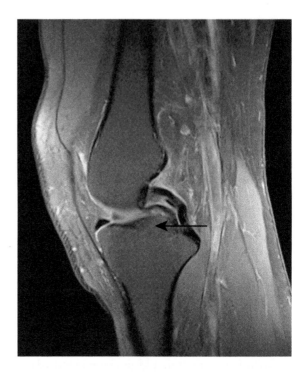

Figure 3.8 'Double posterior cruciate ligament' sign on magnetic resonance scanning, produced by a displaced medial meniscal fragment lying alongside an intact posterior cruciate ligament.

Figure 3.9 A medial meniscal tear on magnetic resonance scanning.

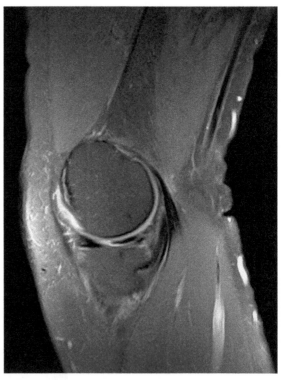

disruption or other injuries (Speer *et al.* 1991). Changes are also detectable in chondromalacia patellae (Hodler and Resnick 1992), although Spiers *et al.* (1993) considered that the MR scan afforded a low sensitivity of only 18 per cent for articular cartilage lesions. This sensitivity is improving with the new generation of MR scanners.

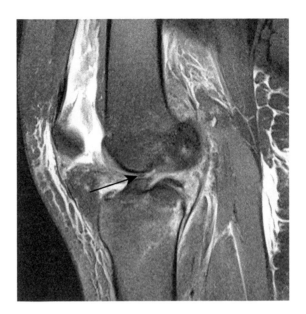

Figure 3.10 A tear of the anterior cruciate ligament on magnetic resonance scanning.

Figure 3.11 Magnetic resonance scan of a discoid lateral meniscus.

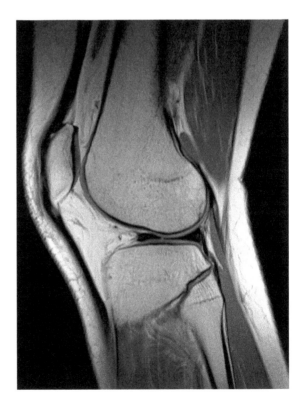

The cruciate ligaments are structures of low signal intensity although the anterior, in contrast to the posterior, is not invariably seen on sagittal scans. A torn anterior cruciate ligament presents with an undulating or irregular anterior margin, high signal intensity within its substance on T_2-weighted images, or a gap. Oedematous intercondylar soft tissue is seen with acute tears (Vahey *et al.* 1991) and the knee laxity may cause anterior bowing of the posterior cruciate ligament. Chronic tears show up with disruption of the contour, atrophy or absence, 43

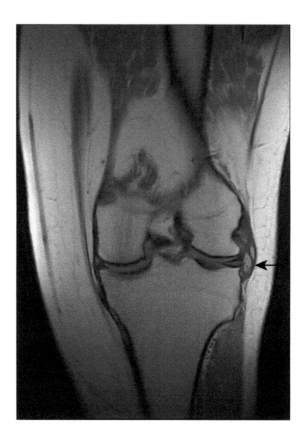

Figure 3.12 Magnetic resonance scan of a peripheral meniscal cyst.

although scar tissue may bridge across or the anterior cruciate remnant may adhere to the posterior cruciate ligament. After reconstruction, increased signals (T_1- and T_2-weighted) may still be consistent with an intact neoligament, although gross focal changes and a wavy outline suggest laxity or rupture. Impingement produces a high-intensity signal in the distal one-third of the graft.

Scanning does pick up continuing pathology within the substance of a sutured meniscus, which is hardly surprising since Negendank *et al.* (1990) and Recht *et al.* (2001) have also reported meniscal degeneration in the, as yet, asymptomatic, contralateral knee of patients with meniscal symptoms. The sensitivity of MR scanning, therefore, makes it an ideal preoperative test, only curtailed by cost or when this facility is unavailable. It augments radiographs and other imaging techniques when the pathological process merits further definition (Figures 3.13, 3.14) but its indiscriminate use cannot be condoned. When the knee is acutely locked or in other urgent situations, MR scanning may not be applicable although this has to be weighed against diagnostic error and possible medicolegal implications.

Bone marrow oedema is revealed not only in a number of conditions (Fowkes and Andoni 2010), most commonly in degenerative disease (McQueen 2007) including chondromalacia patellae (Yulish *et al.* 1987), but also following direct trauma to the articular surfaces (Figure 3.15), in the inflammatory arthropathies, and in association with neoplasias or metastatic tumour deposits. Oedema is often revealed in avascular necrosis from a number of causes and in the painful transient bone marrow oedema syndrome, the pathogenesis of which is unknown. It may be a normal finding in childhood (Pal *et al.* 1999). Whereas water and fluid-containing tissues appear bright on T_2-weighted images and dark on T_1-weighted images,

Figure 3.13 Magnetic resonance scans of a single loose body (a) and multiple posterior loose bodies (b).

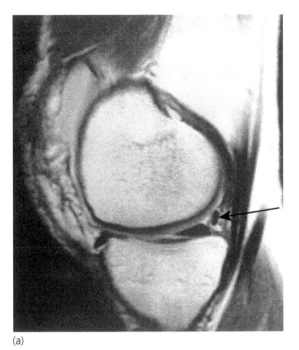

(a)

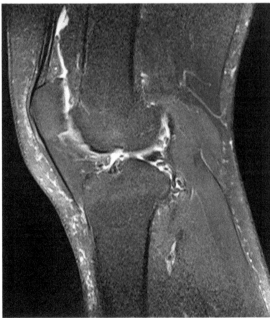

(b)

bone marrow oedema produces a grey image on the T_1-weighted scan and a white image on the T_2-weighted scan.

Ultrasound

Although ultrasound is diagnostically useful in outlining structures within the abdomen and pelvis, and the unstable hip joint in the neonate, its use in the knee is limited. Soft tissue tumours and effusions or cysts can be detected, and the investigation is both cheap

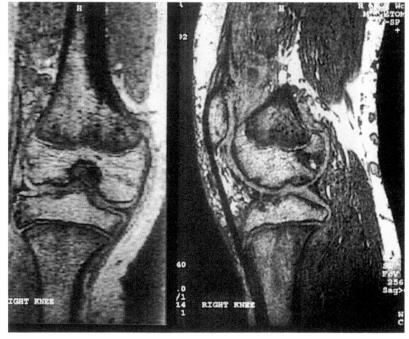

Figure 3.14 Magnetic resonance scan showing articular irregularity and the formation of bone cysts resulting from multiple haemarthroses from an arteriovenous malformation.

Figure 3.15 A subchondral fracture with associated bone bruising/oedema on magnetic resonance scanning.

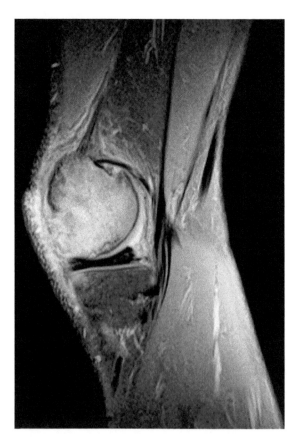

and non-invasive (Finlay and Friedman 2006). Congenital dislocation of the knee, the iliotibial band friction syndrome and patellar tendonitis can also be defined. As a relatively quick assessment of an undiagnosed swelling in the clinic, such as the popliteal cyst, it is of considerable value, reassuring the parent and child (Kuroki *et al.* 2008).

Arthrography

Arthrograms are produced by injecting a positive-contrast medium into the joint, giving particularly good definition. With the increasing availability and sophistication of MR scanning, arthrography is of largely historical interest. Repeated tangential views of the medial and lateral menisci will reveal tears or abnormality within their structure (Figure 3.16), and the cruciate ligaments, articular surfaces of the knee and the size of any popliteal cyst can be defined (Stoker 1980). Synovial folds are demonstrable and one of them, the ligamentum mucosum, should be differentiated from the anterior cruciate ligament. Absence or rupture of the cruciate ligament can be defined, but with less precision than by MR scans.

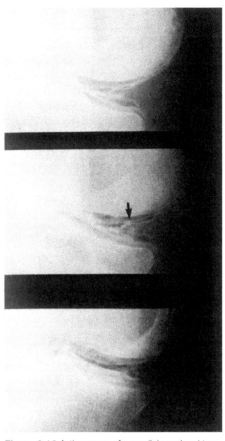

Figure 3.16 Arthrogram of a medial meniscal tear.

Tears of the meniscus allow the contrast medium into the abnormal space, and if double contrast is used a filling defect is revealed. Vertical, longitudinal tears are readily seen, particularly if there is separation of the meniscal segments, but a transverse tear may be missed owing to the projection of the X-ray beam. Nevertheless arthrography affords a diagnostic rate of over 80 per cent with such tears (Nicholas *et al.* 1970; Ireland *et al.* 1980).

Horizontal cleavage lesions of the meniscus usually show up clearly and are only difficult to interpret when there is a superimposition of other structures, such as in the posterolateral aspect of the knee where the popliteus tendon causes an artefact. The presence of degenerative changes throughout the knee may also make interpretation difficult, as may the combination of both vertical and horizontal tears within the meniscus. Lastly, a discoid meniscus, which is quite commonly the site of a tear, can be diagnosed by its bulk and rectangular outline (Figure 3.17).

Osteochondritis dissecans, with a separating fragment, and other irregularities of the articular cartilage, can be visualized by arthrography. However, the accuracy of diagnosis in cases of chondromalacia and early arthritis is less than 70 per cent. Abnormal structures within the knee, such as meniscal remnants, synovial tumours and loose bodies, can be identified, whereas they are often invisible on the standard radiograph as they are radiolucent. But the availability of MR scanning, which is non-invasive, has made arthrography obsolete apart from a few hospitals where MR scanning is lacking.

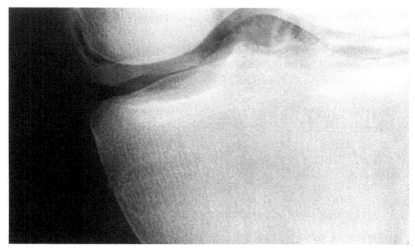

Figure 3.17 Arthrogram of a discoid lateral meniscus.

Arthroscopy

Arthroscopic surgery of the knee is an integral part of orthopaedic practice (Boxes 3.1, 3.2; Table 3.4), although it did not become established as a useful diagnostic aid until the early 1960s. Whereas clinical diagnosis of soft tissue lesions in the knee offers an accuracy rate of approximately 65 per cent, arthroscopy improves this figure to 80 or 90 per cent and has the following advantages:

- More precise assessment of all three compartments of the knee
- Reduced morbidity following meniscal, ligamentous and patellofemoral surgery
- Facility for monitoring conditions affecting the knee (now largely superseded by MR scans).

A patient admitted with a locked knee should be assessed by means of the arthroscope if MR scanning is unavailable since a meniscal tear accounts for locking in less than half of the cases encountered (Gillquist *et al.* 1977). For instance, a block to extension may be produced by ruptures of the anterior cruciate ligament or an anterior synovitis of the knee. In a proportion of cases no obvious abnormality is seen. Arthroscopic examination is particularly important in children where the clinical diagnosis is often erroneous and MR scans may be harder to interpret.

The arthroscope affords a clear portrayal of the following conditions (McGinty and Matza 1978; Dandy 1981):

- Meniscal lesions, particularly vertical tears with displacement
- Anterior and posterior cruciate ligament ruptures

> **Box 3.1** Use of arthroscopy
>
> - Meniscectomy
> - Anterior cruciate reconstruction
> - Arthrolysis
> - Meniscal repair
> - Lateral patellar release
> - Synovectomy
> - Removal of loose body
> - Resection of plica
> - Lavage/drainage
> - Articular cartilage excision/abrasion
> - Synovial biopsy
> - Tibial fracture reduction
> - Osteochondritis drilling/fixation
> - Excision of synovial lesion
> - Removal of implant

48

- Synovial lesions (synovitis, synovial shelf impingement and synovial adhesions) (Patel 1978)
- Articular cartilage changes and osteochondral fractures
- Loose bodies
- Fat pad lesions and miscellaneous conditions such as haemangiomata and cysts.

Certain loose bodies are hard to identify as they may be hidden in the recesses of the knee posteromedially, posterolaterally near the popliteus tendon, and in the periphery of the synovial cavity. Box 3.3 lists the sites in the knee where a good view may be difficult to obtain. These regions may require the use of the 70° telescope and an alteration in technique before a diagnostic view can be obtained. Tears of the retrosynovial posterior cruciate ligament are difficult to identify, even with the 70° arthroscope, and partial tears of the anterior cruciate ligament may be missed if the synovial covering of the ligament appears intact. Probing or pulling on these structures with a blunt hook is of value in this context. Horizontal cleavage and peripheral tears of the menisci are not readily seen, and the numerous causes of patellar pain are rarely apparent, partly because many of them are extra-articular and also because the mechanics of the patellofemoral joint cannot readily be assessed in the totally relaxed, anaesthetized patient. While the arthroscope usually gives a convincing picture of abnormalities which are obstructing knee movement, the diagnosis of chronic, painful conditions, unassociated with abnormal mechanical function, is difficult if not impossible.

The various portals of entry for the arthroscope are shown in Figure 3.18a. Each surgeon will adopt procedures of his own choice and there are advantages to each approach. Certainly, no single site of insertion is superior and the surgeon should be prepared to utilize multiple portals.

A blunt hook is invaluable for probing structures under examination and allows undisplaced tears in the meniscus to be identified accurately, together with the stability of the meniscus. Cutting instruments and the various types

Table 3.4 Complications of arthroscopy*

Complication	Per cent
Haemarthrosis, haematoma	60.1
Infection	12.1
Thromboembolism	6.9
Anaesthetic problems	6.4
Instrument breakage	2.9
Reflex sympathetic dystrophy	2.3
Ligament tear	1.2
Fracture	0.6
Nerve injury	0.6
Other	6.9
	100.0

*Other complications include synovial fistula, compartment syndrome, portal wound tenderness and introduced drape fibres or talc; articular scuffing occurs regularly but is hard to quantify and often poorly recorded.

From Small (1988), with permission.

Box 3.3 Potential arthroscopic 'blind spots'

- Posterior recess including the posterior cruciate ligament
- Posterior capsule
- Posteromedial corner between the medial collateral ligament and the posterior horn of the medial meniscus
- Beneath both menisci
- Popliteus recess
- Periphery of the patella and parts of the suprapatellar pouch

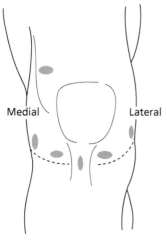

Medial   Lateral

(a)

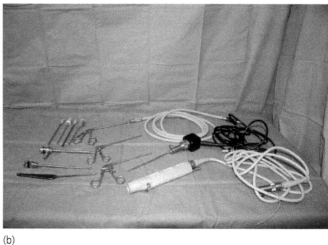

(b)

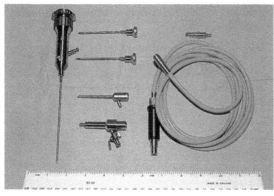

(c)

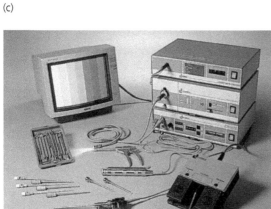

(d)

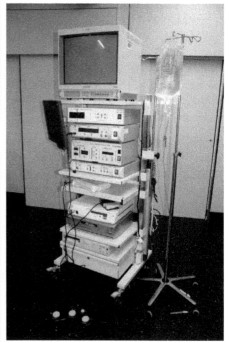

(e)

Figure 3.18 (a) Portals of entry for the arthroscope. The anterolateral approach is usually preferred at the outset of the procedure, combined with a supplementary medial portal. Posterolateral, posteromedial and suprapatellar portals are helpful, but the transpatellar tendon portal may produce postoperative morbidity. (b) and (c) Instruments used when performing arthroscopy. (d) and (e) Television monitor with camera light source, shaver motor and printing device.

of shaver are necessary if arthroscopic surgery is to be carried out, combined with the use of grasping forceps with ratchet handles, rongeurs and biopsy forceps (Figure 3.18b). The television monitor linked to a colour camera (Figure 3.18c) is essential for modern arthroscopic techniques and is a useful aid when instructing theatre staff or informing the patient. The latter may be achieved if the patient is awake during the procedure, or reviews the photographs or video recording postoperatively.

A leg holder and fluid pump to distend the joint capsule aid in access to difficult areas. Since arthroscopy is often undertaken without a surgical assistant, these advances are well established, as is the use of increasingly sophisticated power shavers and cutting instruments. Laser surgery, however, is flawed by complications and is not recommended.

Radioisotope imaging

This technique is sensitive, but relatively non-specific (Box 3.4) (Lisbona and Rosenthal 1977). It tends to overestimate the size of lesions in the region of the knee but does give dynamic information relating to the blood flow characteristics of a pathological process (Figure 3.19).

A variety of radioisotopes are concentrated in bone, and currently technetium-99m labelled compounds, such as methylene diphosphonate,

> **Box 3.4** Radioisotope imaging
>
> - Sensitivity – ability of a test to detect pathology
> - Specificity – ability of a test to detect normality
> - Accuracy – ability of a test to detect the true appearances

are predominantly used for this purpose. After an intravenous injection, distribution of the isotope is identified on radiographic or Polaroid film using a gamma camera to detect the radiation emitted. Bone can be scanned at various periods after injection of the isotope, a triple phase scan constituting: (1) images available after a half-minute, representing blood flow; (2) a blood pool phase, indicating vascularity; and (3) a static phase obtained 2 hours after the bolus injection, defining the sequestration of the absorbed isotope.

Figure 3.19 Isotope bone scan showing pathological uptake at the knee.

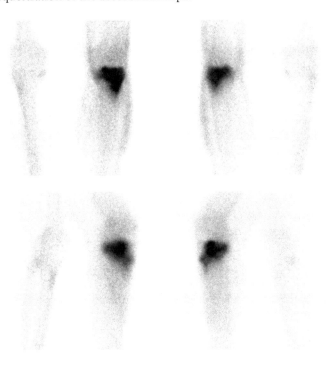

A septic arthritis will produce increased uptake on both sides of a joint, whereas lesions within the bone will be concentrated on the affected side of the knee. Soft tissue lesions tend to produce both increased flow and vascularity phases, with little bone absorption, whereas a synovitis increases isotope emission in all three phases.

When there is a chronic infection present, the triple phase scan may be negative if technetium is used, and in these instances a gallium 67-citrate scan may be diagnostic. The gallium scan gives a more precise picture of local intraosseous involvement than technetium scintigraphy, but with the advent of CT and MRI, this technique is rarely used. Indium-labelled white cells may afford a slightly more specific definition of an infective process than the triple phase technetium scan, but there is a minor increase in the dose of radiation. Bone tumours can be delineated by both the triple phase scan (Simon and Kirchner 1980) and by monoclonal scans.

In conclusion, the following conditions cause increased uptake of radioisotope:

- Infection, including osteomyelitis
- Osteoarthritis where the features are detected earlier than with a radiograph
- Arthropathies, including rheumatoid arthritis and traumatic arthritis
- Tumours
- Fractures.

Although bone scanning is sensitive to early pathological changes in bone it is a non-specific test and the diagnosis may still rest with radiographic, MRI and CT scanning, and histological features.

Computed tomography

This sophisticated method, based on X-rays, converts by computerization a succession of transverse radiographic sections of the knee to a three-dimensional view of the joint from 'within the tissues'. The technique is useful in assessing deeply placed swellings, such as tumours, as there is little or no superimposition of other tissues on the image under examination. A more accurate rendering of the patellofemoral joint can be obtained, and has shown how poorly the skyline radiographs define congruency of the patellofemoral joint and the various patellar shapes (Boven *et al.* 1982).

Cruciate ligament tears can also be identified, and a combination of double-contrast arthrography with CT scanning adds greatly to the precision with which structures in the knee joint can be outlined. Soft tissue, osseous and calcified masses can be seen, as may the three-dimensional patterns of fractures (Figure 3.20) prior to decisions about internal fixation. CT scanning shows mineralization well, so that it offers superior images than MRI in the detection of fracture, cortical destruction, intraosseous spread and soft tissue calcification or ossification. The punctate calcification in chondromatous tumours and the reactive bone shell around an aneurysmal cyst are particularly clearly identified. CT scanning does not differentiate reliably between benign and malignant soft tissue tumours, but their size and location can be defined and a benign lipoma (homogeneous fat density) qualitatively distinguished from a liposarcoma (heterogeneous fat density).

Venography and arteriography

The injection of radioisotope contrast materials into the veins and arteries of the leg is diagnostic in a number of conditions. Deep venous thrombosis can be reviewed accurately, and can be differentiated from a ruptured popliteal cyst, both conditions producing calf pain and swelling.

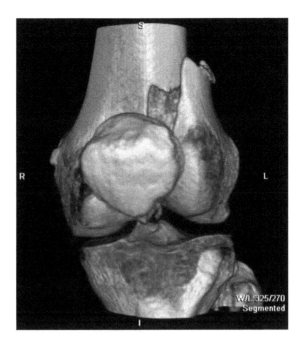

Figure 3.20 Three-dimensional computed tomography scan of distal femoral fracture.

Arteriography is an essential investigation in the severely injured limb with compromised vascularity. The site of arterial injury, whether a laceration, thrombosis or embolism, can be identified with precision, and appropriate surgical treatment instituted. This facility is also valuable in the treatment of certain tumours with extensive arteriolar and capillary networks. Thus the arteriogram will outline the size and spread of the neoplastic mass, allowing appropriate surgery to be planned. If a tumour such as an aneurysmal bone cyst or haemangioma merits embolization, arteriography will define the feeder vessels and the pattern of venous drainage. The vascular characteristics of arteriovenous malformations, aneurysms and fistulae can also be defined (see also Chapter 9).

Radionuclide scintigraphy

Single photon emission computed tomography (SPECT) is a useful means of ruling out lesions in the knee which might give rise to anterior knee pain (Murray *et al.* 1990). Arthroscopic intervention becomes unnecessary and sympathetic blockage may be considered in those with increased uptake on the scan, despite a lack of the features normally associated with complex regional pain syndrome (reflex sympathetic osteodystrophy) (Butler-Manuel *et al.* 1992). True chondromalacia patellae can be detected accurately by combining T_1-weighted (proton-density) images with T_2-weighted images (McCauley *et al.* 1992) but correlates poorly with anterior knee pain.

Thermography

Thermographic assessment of the anterior knee pain syndromes provides colourful but non-specific appearances (see Figure 9.5, p. 194). The investigation is helpful in monitoring the response of an arthropathic knee to medical or surgical treatment. During the early, vasodilatory phase of chronic regional pain syndrome, temperature changes of 2 °C or more are recorded and may help in the earlier diagnosis and management of this troublesome condition. However, the investigation is principally recording from surface blood vessels and its role in knee conditions is therefore somewhat limited and rarely improves upon careful clinical examination and more conventional investigations.

Cybex dynamometry

Muscle power in the hamstrings and quadriceps can be measured by means of the Cybex dynamometer or KinCom apparatus. The effort produced by the patient is calculated in terms of work output and thus the recovery from injury and the power in various muscle groups can be monitored regularly (see Chapter 10).

Optical coherence tomography

Optical coherence tomography is a novel imaging technology that can generate microscopic resolution, cross-sectional images of articular cartilage in near real-time. It can be used clinically to identify early hyaline cartilage alterations. Such quantitative and non-destructive methods for the clinical diagnosis and staging of articular cartilage degeneration are important in the evaluation of potentially disease-modifying treatments for osteoarthritis (Chu *et al.* 2010).

Exercise tests

Simple walking tests are of value in assessing basic gait patterns and loss of walking speed. Measurements of stride length and cadence can be obtained easily, and the patient may be filmed during walking. The hip joint is better assessed than the knee, although bench step-ups and stair-climbing help to quantify knee disability. More sophisticated gait analysis laboratories define the characteristics of each walking pattern. These results can be combined with the use of force-plate studies of the weightbearing foot, offering a more dynamic but at times very complex picture of the mechanics of walking or running.

References

Berquist TH (1989) Magnetic resonance imaging of musculoskeletal neoplasms. *Clin Orthop* **244**, 101–18.

Boven F, Bellamans MA, Geurts J, *et al.* (1982) The value of computed tomography scanning in chondromalacia patellae. *Skeletal Radiol* **8**, 183–5.

Butler-Manuel PA, Justins D and Heatley FW (1992) Sympathetically mediated anterior knee pain: scintigraphy and anaesthetic blockade in 19 patients. *Acta Orthop Scand* **63**, 90–3.

Chu CR, Williams A, Tolliver D, *et al.* (2010) Clinical optical coherence tomography of early articular cartilage degeneration in patients with degenerative meniscal tears. *Arthritis Rheum* **62**, 1412–20.

Dandy DJ (1981) *Arthroscopic Surgery of the Knee.* Edinburgh: Churchill Livingstone.

Dillon EH, Pope CF, Joki P, *et al.* (1991) Follow-up of Grade II meniscal abnormalities in the stable knee. *Radiology* **181**, 849–52.

Finlay K and Friedman L (2006) Ultrasonography of the lower extremity. *Orthop Clin North Am* **37**, 245–75.

Fischer SP, Fox JM, Del Pizzo W, *et al.* (1991) Accuracy of diagnosis from magnetic resonance imaging of the knee. A multi-center analysis of one thousand and fourteen patients. *J Bone Joint Surg Am* **73**, 2–10.

Fowkes LA and Andoni AP (2010) Bone marrow oedema of the knee. *Knee* **17**, 1–6.

Gillquist J, Hagber G and Oretorp N (1977) Arthroscopy in acute injuries of the knee joint. *Acta Orthop Scand* **48**, 190–6.

Hodler J and Resnick D (1992) Chondromalacia patellae: commentary. *Am J Roentgenol* **158**, 106–7.

Hughston JC (1968) Subluxation of the patella. *J Bone Joint Surg Am* **50**, 1003–26.

Ireland J, Trickey EL and Stoker DJ (1980) Arthroscopy and arthrography of the knee. A critical review. *J Bone Joint Surg Br* **62**, 3–6.

Kuroki H, Nakagawa Y, Mori K, *et al.* (2008) Ultrasound properties of articular cartilage in the tibio-femoral joint in knee osteoarthritis: relation to clinical assessment (International Cartilage Repair Society grade). *Arthritis Res Ther* **10,** R78.

Laurin CA, Dussault R and Levesque HP (1979) The tangential investigation of the patellofemoral joint. *Clin Orthop Rel Res* **144**, 16–26.

Lisbona R and Rosenthal L (1977) Observations on the sequential use of ^{99m}Tc-phosphate complex and ^{67}Ga imaging in osteomyelitis, cellulitis and septic arthritis. *Radiology* **123**, 123–9.

McCauley TR. Kier R, Lynch RJ, *et al.* (1992) Chondromalacia patellae: diagnosis with MR imaging. *Am J Roetngenol* **158**, 101–5.

McGinty JB and Matza RA (1978) Arthroscopy of the knee. Evaluation of an out-patient procedure under local anaesthetic. *J Bone Joint Surg Am* **60**, 787–9.

McQueen FM (2007) A vital clue to deciphering bone pathology: MRI bone oedema in rheumatoid arthritis and osteoarthritis. *Ann Rheum Dis* **66**, 1549–52.

Merchant AC, Mercer RL, Jacobsen RH and Cool CR (1974) Roentgenographic analysis of patellofemoral congruence. *J Bone Joint Surg Am* **56**, 1391–6.

Murray IPC, Dixon J and Kohan L (1990) SPECT for acute knee pain. *Clin Nucl Med* **15**, 828–40.

Negendank WG, Fernandez FR, Heilbrun LK and Tietge RA (1990) Magnetic resonance imaging of meniscal degeneration in asymptomatic knees. *J Orthop Res* **8**, 311–20.

Nicholas JA, Freiberger RH and Killeran PJ (1970) Double-contrast arthrography of the knee. Its value in the management of two hundred and twenty-five knee derangements. *J Bone Joint Surg Am* **52**, 203–20.

Pal CR, Tasker AD, Ostlere SJ and Watson MS (1999) Heterogeneous signal in bone marrow on MRI of children's feet: a normal finding? *Skeletal Radiol* **28**, 274–8.

Patel D (1978) Arthroscopy of the plica – synovial folds and their significance. *Am J Sports Med* **6**, 217–25.

Quinn SF and Brown TF (1991) Meniscal tears diagnosed with MR imaging versus arthroscopy: how reliable a standard is arthroscopy. *Radiology* **818**, 843–7.

Raunest J, Oberle K, Leonhert J, *et al.* (1991) The clinical value of magnetic resonance image in the evaluation of meniscal disorders. *J Bone Joint Surg Am* **73**, 11–16.

Recht M, Bobic V, Burstein D, *et al.* (2001) Magnetic resonance imaging of articular cartilage. *Clin Orthop Relat Res* **391S**, 379–96.

Reinig JW, McDevitt ER and Ove PN (1991) Progression of meniscal degenerative changes in college football players: evaluation with MR imaging. *Radiology* **181**, 255–7.

Ritchie JFS, Al-Sarawan M, Worth R, *et al.* (2004) A parallel approach: the impact of Schuss radiography of the degenerate knee on clinical management. *Knee* **11**, 283–7.

Simon MA and Kirchner PT (1980) Scintigraphic evaluation of primary bone tumours. Comparison of technetium-99m phosphonate and gallium citrate imaging. *J Bone Joint Surg Am* **62**, 758–64.

Slattery T and Major N (2010) Magnetic resonance imaging pitfalls and normal variations: the knee. *Magn Reson Imaging Clin N Am* **18**, 675–89.

Small NC (1988) Complications in arthroscopic surgery performed by experienced arthroscopists. *Arthroscopy* **4**, 215–21.

Smillie IS (1980) *Diseases of the Knee Joint*, 4th edn. Edinburgh: Churchill Livingstone.

Speer KP, Spritzer CE, Goldner JL and Garrett WE Jr (1991) Magnetic resonance imaging of traumatic knee articular cartilage injuries. *Am J Sports Med* **19**, 396–402.

Spiers ASC, Meagher T, Ostlere M, *et al.* (1993) Can MRI of the knee affect arthroscopic practice? *J Bone Joint Surg Br* **75**, 49–52.

Stoker DJ (1980) *Knee Arthrography*. London: Chapman and Hall.

Vahey TN, Broome DR, Kayes KJ, *et al.* (1991) Acute and chronic tears of the anterior cruciate ligament: differential features at MR imaging. *Radiology* **181**, 251–3.

Yulish BS, Montanez J, Goodfellow DB, *et al.* (1987) Chondromalacia patellae: assessment with MR imaging. *Radiology* **164**, 763–6.

4

Paediatric conditions

Characteristics

Trauma produces the same types of injury in the child as in the adult (Backx *et al.* 1989) but the patterns are age-related. The 5-year-old is more likely to experience the exacerbating effects of malalignment or torsional abnormalities affecting the patellofemoral mechanism (Figure 4.1 and see Figure 7.1, p. 147) and the growth plate, whereas the 15-year-old is prone to ligament tears and avulsions. Overuse syndromes and 'growing pains' more typically affect the older child.

Joint laxity is associated with a number of inherited conditions (Box 4.1) and may result in symptoms without an obvious precipitating injury. Similarly, familial hypermobility and persistent femoral anteversion adversely affect patellar tracking, yet it is often this very group of children who are adept athletically and thus promote patellar instability. Ligament sprains and osteochondral lesions occur with greater stress and will recur if muscle tone is not restored. During maturation, the problems associated with malalignment and laxity may reduce, although a proportion of patients continue to experience difficulties involving the patella or the medial (tibial) collateral ligament.

The last important characteristic is the fact that the symptomatic knee acts as a conduit for lumbar spine and particularly hip pathology in the growing child, and may also be the target organ in a child with emotional problems, including the individual who finds that the pressures of a competitive sport have become too great. Mild spastic hemiplegia, spinal cord lesions, limb length discrepancy and hip disorders such as transient synovitis, Perthes' disease, development dysplasia and slipped upper femoral epiphysis must be excluded by careful clinical examination, radiographic review and imaging, as appropriate.

Table 4.1 shows the symptoms which presented in 1000 consecutive children referred with knee complaints to a clinic in Edinburgh (Macnicol 1995). In a proportion with patellar pain and those with non-specific synovitis the term 'irritable knee' is appropriate, provided that referred pain has been ruled out, the joint feels warm and intermittent swelling is reported. The onset of symptoms could be attributed to sports in 60 per cent (Box 4.2).

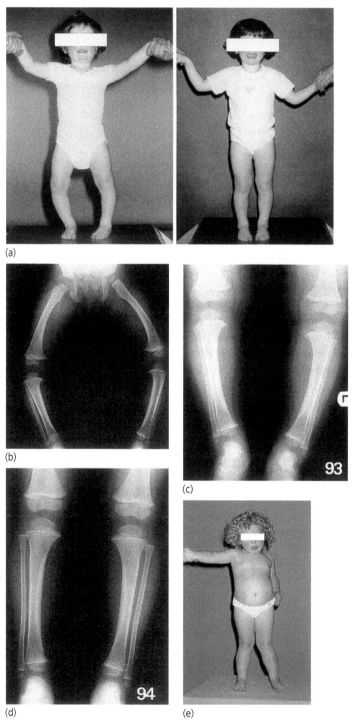

(a)

(b)

(c)

(d)

(e)

Figure 4.1a–d Constitutional genu varum and valgum, both of which resolve (e).

Arthroscopic intervention is required in a relatively small proportion, and is rarely indicated for the anterior knee pain and patellar instability groups. However, since magnetic resonance imaging (MRI) may be poorly tolerated, and chronic synovitis and anxiety may retard progress with physiotherapy, arthroscopic review is recommended in some children with patellar pain and apparent restriction of the passive range of movement (Table 4.2; Figure 4.2). As in the adult, the procedure reduces the synovitis and the aching pain. The child and parents are reassured that no major pathology is present and the symptoms often disappear once physiotherapy has been reinstituted. Only in the smaller child is the use of small-diameter arthroscopes or needlescopes necessary (see Figure 3.18c, p. 50) and distension of the paediatric knee is usually sufficient to allow safe use of the adult arthroscope and sheath.

Functional anatomy of the patellofemoral joint

The anatomical relationship of the patella to the femoral sulcus or trochlea is complex, extension producing contact between the lower pole of the patella and the trochlea, which may be flattened and deficient proximally. Flexion results in a progressively deeper engagement with the upper patellar pole. Static soft tissue restraints include the medial patellofemoral ligament (Figure 4.3), which contributes 60 per cent of medial stability (Amis *et al.* 2003), the lateral fascial superficial oblique and deep transverse (lateral patellar ligament) components of the retinaculum, and the inferior pull of the patellar tendon, which may be compromised by patella alta and lateral condylar 'conflict' or abnormal impingement. Medial patellomeniscal and lateral patellotibial ligaments are also recognized.

Dynamic control is achieved by the vastus medialis obliquus, which works in tandem with the medial patellofemoral ligament and further contributions from the remaining components of the quadriceps mechanism. If a patient has a history of recurrent patellar subluxation or dislocation, there is at least a 50 per cent risk of further episodes of instability. After acute lateral dislocation the risk of repeated dislocation is approximately 20 per cent. Ligament laxity, lower limb angular and torsional deformities, an increased Q-angle or genu recurvatum, a shallow sulcus (possibly with a 'crossing sign' on the true lateral radiograph), and patella alta (Figure 4.4 and also see Figure 7.4, p. 150) worsen the prognosis. The tibial tubercle–trochlear (femoral sulcus) 'offset' can be obtained by axial CT scans and may merit operative reduction if it measures more than 15 mm (Mulford 2007). Maltracking, patellar tilt (Figure 3.5, p. 40) and apprehension are features of this skeletal, torsional deformity, which is commonly encountered but difficult to treat surgically (see Chapter 7).

Box 4.1 Conditions associated with ligament laxity

- Down's syndrome
- Achondroplasia
- Ehlers–Danlos syndrome
- Nail–patella syndrome
- Marfan's syndrome
- Ellis–van Creveld syndrome
- Turner's syndrome
- Osteogenesis imperfecta
- Rubinstein–Taybi syndrome

Table 4.1 Knee disorders in 1000 consecutive cases

Patellar pain	61%
Osgood–Schlatter's disease	17%
Patellar dislocation	11%
Synovitis	4%
Meniscal lesion	2%
Other	5%

Box 4.2 Sports producing knee symptoms, in decreasing order of frequency

- Soccer*
- Rugby*
- Athletics
- Gymnastics*
- Skiing*
- Swimming
- (Highland) dancing
- Other (mountain biking, etc.)

*More likely to cause avulsion injuries.

Angular deformities

Patellar instability is often associated with a short quadriceps mechanism, the most extreme manifestation of this being congenital dislocation of the knee (Jacobsen and Vopalecky 1985) with hyperextension of the knee. The various angular deformities of the paediatric knee will therefore be discussed at this stage, followed by patellofemoral joint malfunction in a later section of this chapter when anterior knee pain will also be briefly discussed. Chapter 7 deals more fully with the unstable patella and its management in adolescence and early adult life.

■ Congenital dislocation of the knee

This condition is much rarer that developmental dysplasia and dislocation of the hip (DDH), with an incidence of approximately 1–2 per 100 000 live births. It is clinically obvious (Figure 4.5) and should be distinguished from benign hyperextension of the knee where knee flexion is full. The condition is a continuum of worsening hyperextension deformity and limited flexion (Curtis and Fisher 1969) (Figure 4.6), the knee appearing 'back to front' with an obvious transverse anterior skin crease. Ultrasound scans portray the relationship of the femoral and tibial condyles, defining the extent of the subluxation/dislocation. The femoral condyles are prominent because the tibia is displaced anteriorly and proximally. If the hamstring tendons subluxate forwards they potentiate the deformity.

Hyperextension with slight subluxation is probably an intrauterine moulding deformity, analogous to neonatal hip instability. In these normal infants the knee often reduces with a clunk as it is flexed, the hamstrings and iliotibial band shifting to the flexor side of the joint axis. If the knee can be flexed to 30–40°, splintage with increasingly flexed anterior casts and physiotherapy is usually effective. Splintage can be discontinued at 6–8 weeks, the knee eventually returning to a normal shape, with minimal residual hyperextension and slight loss of flexion. More severe knee dislocation is recalcitrant to conservative measures. Other abnormalities are present, including a dysplastic patella tethered proximally by a shortened, fibrotic quadriceps tendon and obliteration of the suprapatellar pouch. Anomalous or absent cruciate ligaments may be

Table 4.2 Knee disorders encountered in 100 consecutive arthroscopies

Meniscal lesions	27
Osteochondritis dissecans	26
Synovitis	20
Normal	18
Cruciate pathology	5
Chondromalacia patellae	4

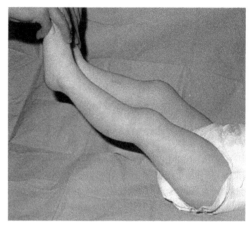

Figure 4.2 Loss of right knee extension when compared with the normal knee.

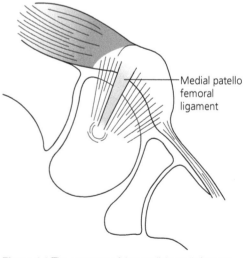

Figure 4.3 The anatomy of the medial patellofemoral ligament, which tightens on knee extension.

Medial patello femoral ligament

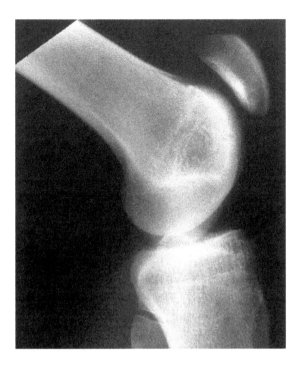

Figure 4.4 A lateral radiograph showing patella alta.

seen at exploration (Katz *et al.* 1967). Associated conditions include DDH, clubfoot, calcaneovalgus, dislocation of the elbow and syndromes such as arthrogryposis.

Skeletal traction is contraindicated so a sequential surgical release is undertaken, including the fascia lata and vastus lateralis, a V–Y lengthening of the distal quadriceps and any tethering adhesions. The operation is best undertaken by 6 months of age so that secondary changes are minimized. Delay leads to a progressive, sloping deformity of the upper tibia, where its posterior surface abuts against the distal, anterior femur, an alteration that makes stable open reduction difficult. Failure to elongate the lateral structures leads to a worsening valgus angulation.

An extremely rare form of congenital snapping knee has been described (Ferris and Jackson 1990). The tibia subluxes anteriorly in extension and reduces with a pronounced clunk at 30° of

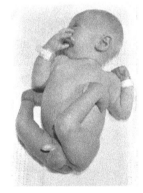

Figure 4.5 Bilateral congenital dislocation of the knee in a newborn infant.

flexion. The condition is associated with laxity syndromes such as Larsen's, the Catel–Manzke or congenital short tibia. Dysmorphism of the joints worsens as the child grows. Division and possibly re-routing of the iliotibial band, with suturing of the biceps tendon to the vastus lateralis, may control the subluxation.

■ Neurological hyperextension

The hyperextended knee (genu recurvatum) is a common feature of several neurological conditions. The usual mechanism is muscle imbalance, in which a strong or spastic quadriceps overcomes the action of weak hamstrings. Iatrogenically, the hamstring deficit may be due to excessive or inappropriate soft-tissue release in patients with cerebral palsy.

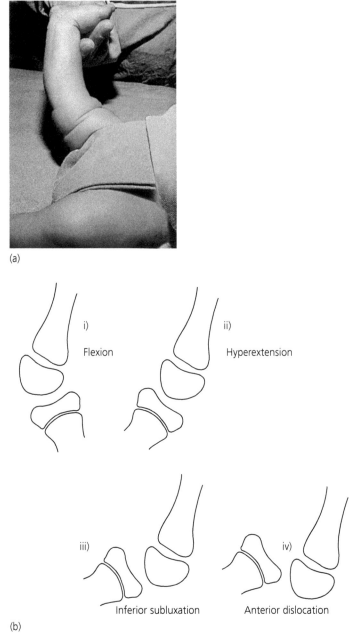

(a)

(b)

Figure 4.6 Hyperextension deformity of the knee (a) is part of a continuum of increasing abnormality (b).

Poliomyelitic hamstring paralysis in the presence of an active quadriceps group results in the stretching of the posterior tissues of the knee. Gross recurvatum may develop, difficult to control without a calliper. Posterior soft-tissue reefing is not successful and probably the best surgical option at maturity is the anterior patellar bone block procedure, fixing the patella to the upper, anterior tibia so that it acts as a 'doorstop' in extension. When the knee is totally flail, slight hyperextension tensions the posterior tissues, enabling the patient to lock out the joint so that is stable when weightbearing.

A second cause of neurological recurvatum arises when the knee is forced into hyperextension by an equinus foot. The patient may have cerebral palsy or have suffered the effects of a head injury. Achilles' tendon lengthening prevents progressive knee deformity.

■ Post-traumatic tibial recurvatum

Compression or fracture of the proximal tibial growth plate and the apophysis of the tibial tuberosity (see Figure 8.10, p. 178) may produce a progressive recurvatum if there is sufficient growth remaining (Pappas *et al.* 1984). The Salter–Harris type V fracture, with or without a splitting of the physis, results from forced hyperextension and may be associated with cruciate ligament tears. Moroni *et al.* (1992) described the role of proximal tibial osteotomy at skeletal maturity when the sloping upper tibial deformity and knee hyperextension (Figure 4.7) are maximal. If the injury is recognized earlier than this, an epiphysiodesis or posterior stapling of the upper tibia will prevent the inexorable progress towards recurvatum. A contralateral proximal tibial epiphysiodesis should be considered if leg-length discrepancy is developing.

The osteotomy should be supratubercular (Figure 4.8), as close to the deformity as possible. An anterior opening wedge using bone bank is effective, without osteotomy of the fibula. A posterior closing wedge osteotomy (Bowen *et al.* 1983) may be more risky and further shortens the tibia. Choi *et al.* (1999) have described the successful use of the Taylor spatial frame to produce gradual correction of the proximal tibial slope. The osteotomy should start below the

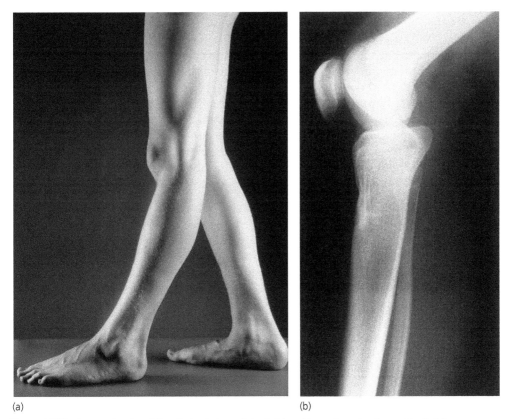

(a) (b)

Figure 4.7 The hyperextension deformity is obvious clinically (a) and is confirmed radiographically (b).

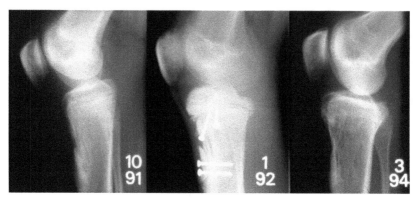

Figure 4.8 A supratubercular anterior opening wedge osteotomy allows immediate correction.

tibial tuberosity if patellar positioning is acceptable, although in most cases the lack of anterior tibial growth produces a relative patella alta.

Tibial recurvatum also develops in certain of the skeletal dysplasias. The associated ligament laxity counteracts successful correction and the subchondral plate may be softened and unreliable. Iatrogenic recurvatum is now rare but used to complicate prolonged traction of the leg with the knee in extension ('frame knee'), cast immobilization, proximal tibial traction wire or pin fixation, and tibial tuberosity transfer before skeletal maturity.

▪ Flexion deformity

During the first few days of life a mild physiological flexion deformity of the knee is commonplace and rapidly resolves. More obvious and permanent fixed flexion may be seen at birth in arthrogryposis and spina bifida, whereas in cerebral palsy, myopathic and infective conditions, and juvenile idiopathic arthritis the deformity appears later. Serial plaster splints or backslabs applied during the first few weeks of life may be used to augment simple stretching but attention needs to be paid to the skin, especially in children with impaired sensation. The chief shortcoming of serial splintage is that, although the knee may indeed straighten, the correction is often spurious. The knee joint hinges open posteriorly and the proximal anterior tibia impacts against the femoral condyles, failing to glide forwards in a normal and congruous fashion. To overcome this problem, reverse dynamic slings (Stein and Dickson 1975) have been used in haemophilia and are certainly applicable in the older child.

The surgical correction of the paediatric deformity is by an extensive soft tissue release since the effects of supracondylar extension osteotomy alone will reverse with further skeletal growth (Figure 4.9). The posterior exposure is achieved by medial and lateral longitudinal incisions or a transverse 'lazy S' incision, provided that the skin is allowed to heal postoperatively before stretching casts are applied. The hamstring tendons and posterior cruciate ligament are divided after careful identification of the popliteal vessels and the common peroneal and posterior tibial nerves. The posterior capsule should be released fully after opening into the joint space posteriorly.

Nerves and vessels must be protected from the deleterious effects of rapid stretching, the same principle applying during correction of severe valgus of the knee. In younger patients serial casts work well but they lose their effectiveness after puberty. Arthrogrypotic deformity corrects reasonably well with soft tissue release combined with corrective osteotomy (Del Bello and Watts 1996; Murray and Fixsen 1997) or circular frame distraction (Brunner *et al.* 1997).

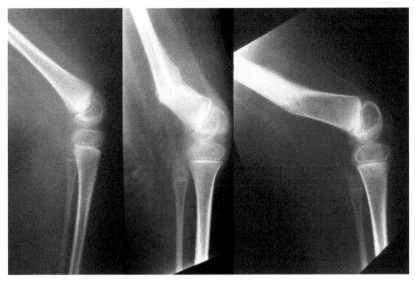

Figure 4.9 The effects of a supracondylar extension femoral osteotomy will reverse with time owing to further skeletal growth, unless it is combined with a posterior soft tissue release.

Genu varum

Babies are usually born with bow legs which persist through the toddler stage (Figure 4.10). The appearances may be accentuated by internal tibial torsion and these 'late correctors' may be a source of great anxiety for the parents. Resolution or progression of the varus can be monitored photographically as well as by measuring the intergenicular distance when the child is standing. If the bowing progresses, asymmetry of the legs may indicate a local cause; short stature suggests a skeletal dysplasia, and there may be a family history such as in familial hypophosphataemic rickets. Progression after 3 years rules out the benign physiological form. Metabolic, dietary and other factors should be investigated in addition to an orthopaedic assessment.

Blount's disease

Tibia vara or Blount's disease (Blount 1937) was first recognized by Erlacher in 1922, before an extensive review of the condition by Blount. Repetitive, compressive injury of the proximal tibia posteromedially leads on to progressive varus and internal tibial torsion. Overgrowth of the lateral tibial proximal physis and the medial femoral distal epiphysis occurs with time.

Figure 4.10 The mean tibiofemoral angle changes from varus to valgus during normal early childhood.

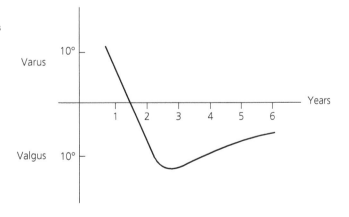

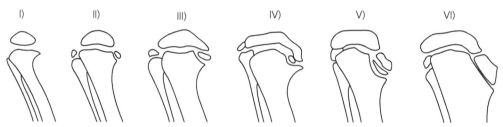

Figure 4.11 Grading the severity of Blount's disease (I–VI) (after Langenskiold 1952).

Langenskiold (1952) classified infantile tibia vara, dividing the condition into grades of worsening severity (Figure 4.11). Grades I and II can be expected to resolve as they are consistent with normal skeletal growth. The radiographic tibiofemoral (Salenius and Vankka 1975) and metaphyseal–diaphyseal angle (Levine and Drennan 1982) are monitored, Drennan's angle (Figure 4.12) being abnormal when it exceeds 15°. Arthrography of the knee is also of investigative value in any condition that is causing progressive deformity (Figure 4.13).

The aetiology of Blount's disease includes obesity, racial type and possibly early walking age. The incidence is estimated at 0.05 per 1000 live births with variations between different populations. Satisfactory correction from a single tibial osteotomy is more certain if undertaken by the age of 4 years (Ferriter and Shapiro 1987) although the Scandinavian experience is of a more benign condition that can be surgically treated effectively up to the age of 8 years (Langenskiold 1981). The internal rotation should also be corrected and weight reduction ensured if the child is obese.

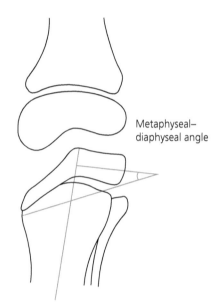

Figure 4.12 The metaphyseal–diaphyseal angle (Levine and Drennan 1982).

Recurrence is likely when a bone bar or tether is missed. These can be mapped with MRI and should be excised in patients under 10 years of age, at the time of osteotomy. After this age corrective osteotomy can be combined with a proximal tibial epiphysiodesis. In unilateral Blount's disease, a contralateral proximal tibial epiphysiodesis will prevent worsening leg-length discrepancy. For severe, or late neglected, cases, elevation of the medial tibial plateau (Siffert 1982; Van Huyssteen et al. 2005) is achieved by an osteotomy, in this case incorporating a segment of proximal fibula (Figure 4.14), or a distraction frame.

Adolescent Blount's disease is usually unilateral and less severe than the infantile form. Pain may precede the deformity and shortening of up to 2 cm develops. Internal tibial rotation is less obvious and the shape of the tibial epiphysis is relatively normal with no 'beaking' of the medial tibial metaphysis. The proximal lateral and tibial distal femoral growth plates are widened.

Corrective osteotomy combined with lateral, proximal tibial epiphysiodesis (Macnicol and Gupta 1997) is a reliable means of improving alignment. Leg-length discrepancy is prevented by appropriately timed epiphysiodesis above and below the opposite, normal knee joint. Distraction osteogenesis offers an alternative approach (Monticelli and Spinelli 1984) with

Figure 4.13 Arthrography defines the unossified proximal tibia.

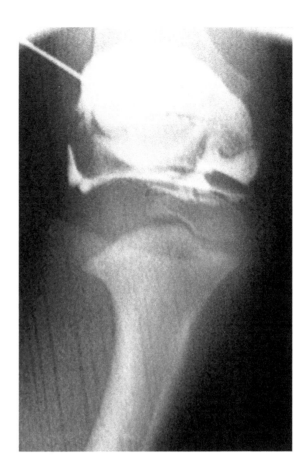

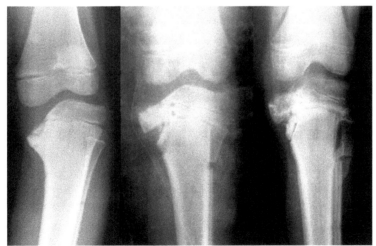

Figure 4.14 Elevating medial tibial osteotomy utilizing a transferred, proximal segment of fibula.

further refinements described by Coogan *et al.* (1996). A recent experience with the multiaxial correction using the Ilizarov fixator has been described by Clarke *et al.* (2009).

Corrective osteotomies described in the orthopaedic literature are illustrated in Figure 4.15. The dome osteotomy is popular and reasonably easy to perform (Macnicol 2002). Correction of combined coronal, sagittal and axial (rotational) deformities is not possible with transverse,

Figure 4.15a–f The different proximal tibial osteotomies described in the literature (Macnicol 2002).

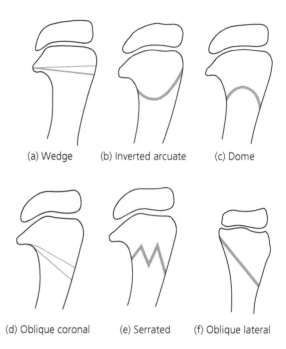

(a) Wedge (b) Inverted arcuate (c) Dome

(d) Oblique coronal (e) Serrated (f) Oblique lateral

spike, oblique and serrated osteotomies, as they are more constrained. Conventional fixation of the fragments with Steinmann pins, screws or plates requires precision. External fixation may therefore be preferred, allowing alignment and rotation to be adjusted postoperatively.

Complications of proximal tibial osteotomy (Steel *et al.* 1971) include common peroneal and other nerve deficits, compartment syndrome, laceration of the anterior tibial artery, inaccurate correction, failure of fixation causing recurrent deformity, pin site and wound infection, and limb-length discrepancy. Correction of the internal rotation of Blount's disease may imperil arterial supply at the level of the proximal tibial diaphysis.

Varus deformity may also follow infection, trauma, nutritional and renal rickets or skeletal dysplasia, including focal fibrocartilaginous dysplasia, which affects the tibia and very rarely the femur (Figure 4.16) (Macnicol 1997). Leg-lengthening procedures may also exaggerate or produce angulation of the knee, usually a varus deformity.

Valgus deformity

Physiological valgus of the knee ceases to be a functional or cosmetic problem in most children by the age of 6 years (Figure 4.10, p. 65). An intermalleolar distance of greater than 5 cm when standing may merit review in mid-childhood but there is no evidence that osteoarthritis will develop prematurely in the valgus knee. The angulation may predispose to patellar problems, however.

It is invidious to state that a definite (standing) intermalleolar distance at the age of 12 years should be surgically corrected but concern about function is legitimate if the distance exceeds 15 cm, allied to knee valgus angulation of 15°. Medial ligament pain, limp and the onset of patellar subluxation reinforce the decision to operate although muscle strengthening, weight reduction, when appropriate, and medial shoe wedges may prove sufficient.

When valgus appears to be increasing, medial stapling (Fraser *et al.* 1995), '8 plating' (Stevens *et al.* 1999) or epiphysiodesis (Bowen *et al.* 1985; Volpon 1997) are effective when properly timed. A standing anteroposterior radiograph will demonstrate any obliquity of the knee joint and confirm whether the procedure should be above or below the knee. Strong implants are

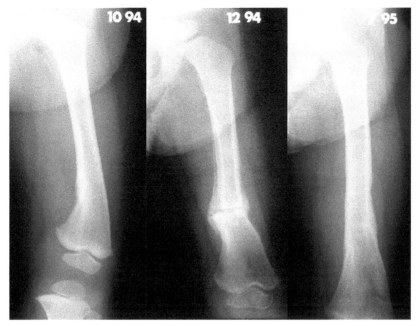

Figure 4.16 Focal fibrocartilaginous dysplasia of the femur producing a varus angulation.

required and experience has shown that a 10 cm intermalleolar gap will close in approximately 1 year. Obviously, there must be sufficient potential growth to effect the correction and the implants must be removed as soon as physiological alignment is achieved. Failure to time removal accurately will convert a knock-knee to a bow-leg deformity, causing immense dissatisfaction. Staples or plates should be inserted extraperiosteally but, even with all due care, overcorrection may occur, so regular monitoring is essential until skeletal maturity. Limb-length discrepancy must also be assessed when unilateral correction is undertaken (Macnicol 1999).

A distal femoral osteotomy is the only option at the end of growth (Healy *et al.* 1983; Edgerton *et al.* 1993). Valgus deformity may be secondary to loss of ipsilateral hip abduction in conditions such as DDH and Perthes' disease, or may present as a complex deformity in skeletal dysplasia (Figure 4.17). In these cases, abduction (valgus) osteotomy of the proximal femur may have to be combined with corrective osteotomies above and below the knee.

Figure 4.17 A varus hip deformity may produce a secondary knee valgus alignment.

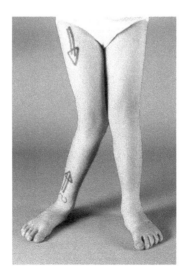

■ Post-fracture genu valgum

Unilateral and, initially, progressive genu valgum may follow a proximal metaphyseal tibial fracture (Skak *et al.* 1987; Ogden *et al.* 1995) (Figure 4.18) particularly if there is comminution or associated fibular fracturing. Many theories have been advanced to explain the asymmetrical physeal growth (Figure 4.19), including inadequate reduction and splintage, differential vascular stimulation of the growth plate, abnormal loading through the proximal tibial growth plate, interposition of soft tissue (pes anserinus, medial collateral ligament, periosteum) in the fracture site medially, and tethering by the united fibula if it has shortened. It is wise to await the spontaneous correction of the deformity although this is not always assured (Figure 4.20).

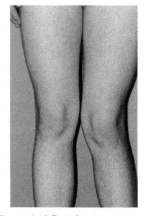

Figure 4.18 Post-fracture genu valgum.

Anterior knee pain

This common complaint is discussed more fully in Chapter 7. The aetiology is usually considered to be compression of the retropatellar surface during later childhood and adolescence, ascribed to muscle imbalance brought on by a period of skeletal growth with rapid leg elongation. The hamstrings are almost invariably tight, reducing straight-leg raising to 50° or less. The quadriceps may appear wasted and lack normal tone. Calf tightness may also be present, foot dorsiflexion being reduced to 0° when the knee is straight. Similar compression pain may afflict the calcaneum (Sever's disease of the heel).

Provided that the history is consistent with this chronic 'stress' syndrome and examination of the spine, hips and knees is within normal limits, hamstring stretching exercises from a physiotherapist are effective and reassuring. Should the patellar pain persist, follow-up and investigations are required. Table 7.1 (p. 147) details the various sites of conditions that may produce patellar pain – at the patella itself, in the peripatellar region, along the quadriceps

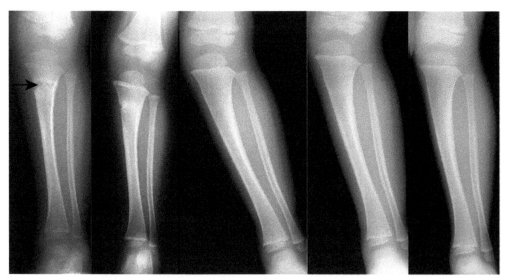

Figure 4.19 This sequence of radiographs of the knee and shin shows how the proximal tibial and fibular valgus worsens initially after fracturing (arrows), before gradually correcting in most cases.

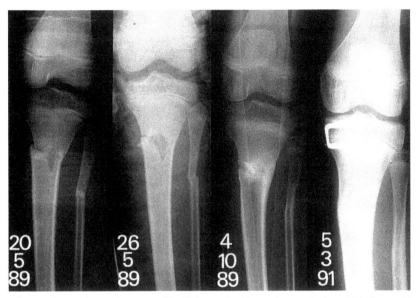

Figure 4.20 Proximal metaphyseal fractures of the tibia may lead to a valgus malunion which does not invariably correct. Comminuted fractures of both the tibia and the fibula are most likely to angulate, and occasionally a medial stapling is required to correct the valgus deformity.

and patellar tendon mechanism, superficial to the patella, and referred pain. The patella may also act as a conduit for the anxieties of the human condition, being a site for psychosomatic complaints (Figure 1.14, p. 11). Overt malfunction and injury to the patellofemoral mechanism are discussed in Chapters 7 and 8.

Osteochondritis dissecans

Osteochondritis dissecans (OCD) is a condition of unknown aetiology although trauma, possibly repeated impaction, has been implicated. This does not explain why most athletic children and adolescents do not develop OCD, so predisposing vascular and congenital ossification abnormalities have been proposed. In some families OCD may affect several joints and is associated with short stature, as is the case in many of the skeletal dysplasias.

Alexander Munro (primus), Professor of Anatomy in Edinburgh, first described the characteristics of the cadaveric lesion in 1738. Paget (1870) recognized that the clinical abnormality, which he described as the 'quiet necrosis', led on to the formation of a loose body. The condition was differentiated from knee infection, particularly tuberculosis, and in that sense is analogous to Perthes' disease. The term 'osteochondritis dissecans' was used by Konig in 1888, progressive separation of the osteochondral fragment being recognized. This may also happen in Perthes' disease (Steenbrugge and Macnicol 2002). The condition is relatively rare (approximately 2 per 1000 of the population) and affects males two or three times more commonly than females. The knee joint is the usual site for OCD but it may also afflict the elbow and ankle. A familial form is recognized and may be associated with short stature among the other relatives.

The impact of OCD on knee function, and the chances of successful surgical treatment, relate to the size and position of the lesion (Figure 4.21) as well as the health of the overlying articular cartilage and the stability of the separating fragment. The most important predictor is the age of the patient as healing is more likely before the growth plates start to close. In the juvenile

71

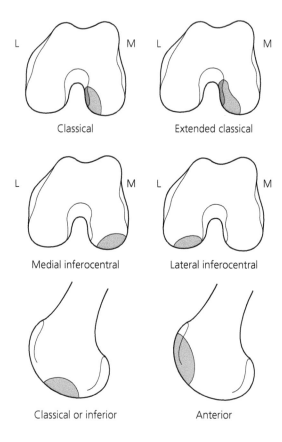

Figure 4.21 The usual sites of osteochondritis dissecans.

Classical

Extended classical

Medial inferocentral

Lateral inferocentral

Classical or inferior

Anterior

form the lesion should be differentiated from benign abnormalities of ossification which account for a proportion of 'healing' cases. Yoshida *et al.* (1998) reported that restriction of sports resulted in an 81 per cent healing rate in the juvenile group, especially if the overlying cartilage was intact. MR scanning has offered a better portrayal of the lesion than the classical radiographic 'four views', and avoids invasive arthroscopy in providing both diagnosis and prognostication, as scans can be repeated as required.

Arthroscopic appearances have been graded as follows (Figure 4.22) (Guhl 1982):

I – irregularity and softening of the articular surface but no fissures or definable fragment
II – articular cartilage breached but not displaceable
III – definable fragment but still attached by some cartilage (flap lesion)
IV – loose body with defect in the articular surface (see Figure 4.24, p. 74).

The magnetic resonance imaging (MRI) characteristics have been described as a similar continuum (Dipaola *et al.* 1991):

I – no break in the articular cartilage which may look thickened
II – low T_2 signal behind the fragment that may have a fibrous tissue attachment
III – articular cartilage presents with a high T_2 signal suggesting fluid behind the lesion (loosening)
IV – loose body with defect in the articular surface.

De Smet *et al.* (1997) recommend that the grade I lesion is present when a line of T_2 high signal <5 mm in length lies deep to the OCD lesion. Grade II is likely when the line changes to a homogeneous signal of similar length, while grade III is present when a T_1 focal defect

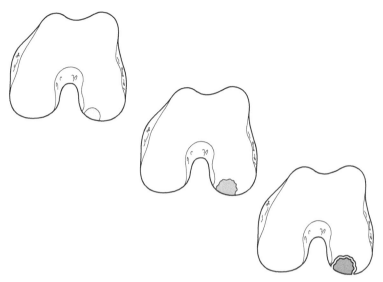

Figure 4.22 Stages in the formation of a loose body secondary to osteochondritis dissecans.

of similar dimension involves the articular surface. Grade IV is represented by a line of T_2 high signal crossing the subchondral plate into the lesion (Figure 4.23). A grade V lesion is suggested, namely when the loosening fragment no longer fits the osteochondral crater. On occasion the synovium may adhere to the surface of the mobile lesion if it is adjacent to the intercondylar region.

The goals of treatment are to stimulate healing whenever possible (Wall *et al.* 2008) and to minimize the effects of the osteochondral defect upon joint function, if separation of the OCD fragment has occurred. A conservative approach is more likely to be successful in the juvenile

Figure 4.23 The magnetic resonance appearances of separating osteochondritis dissecans.

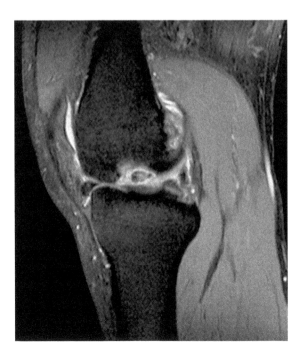

form, diagnosed before the teenage years. Healing by protection of the knee is still possible up to the age of 15 years, but after closure of the growth plates and epiphyseal fusion some form of surgical intervention becomes increasingly likely. Three to six-monthly MRI monitoring of the lesion allows a change in therapy if mechanical symptoms develop and loosening is suggested by imaging.

Weight reduction and an avoidance of games or sports are advised for a minimum of 3 months if symptoms and effusions develop. It is debatable whether splintage or bracing are helpful but they may reduce shearing forces at the site of the lesion. Physiotherapy, combining stretching, proprioception and strengthening isometric exercises, is appropriate and ensures that the patient is kept under regular, professional review over the next 6–9 months. If healing does not occur but an intact lesion is evident on the MRI, the base of the osseous crater can be drilled (Edmonds *et al.* 2010), either antegrade or retrograde arthroscopically. Over 80 per cent of these stable lesions respond to this stimulus in the local blood supply.

When the fragment appears to be loosening but is not yet displaced it should be stabilized by Herbert screws (Figure 4.24) or other headless implants that will not leave a major defect in the articular cartilage surface. Bone pegs and biodegradable implants have also been recommended (Tabaddor *et al.* 2010), but may cause a local inflammatory reaction. The historical use of Smillie pins sometimes led to loss of implant fixation (Figure 4.25) and removal of the pins proved technically difficult. When the lesion is detaching with only a hinge of articular cartilage, or is separated, the size of the fragment decides management. If the diameter is less than 1.5 cm it may be removed arthroscopically, particularly when relatively distant from a weightbearing surface. In time, the defect will fill with fibrocartilage and joint mechanics do not appear to be adversely affected in the longer term.

For fragments larger than 1.5 cm in diameter the osseous base should be curetted and drilled in order to encourage vascularity. The loose fragment may have increased in size by accretion so replacement may make it stand proud of the joint surface unless the crater is enlarged and deepened appropriately. Every effort should be made to accommodate the fragment in its rightful place, countersinking the osteochondral body and then securing it with one or more screws. However, the fragment should be discarded if it remains a poor fit (Figure 4.26).

Figure 4.24 An osteochondritic fragment stabilized with Herbert screws.

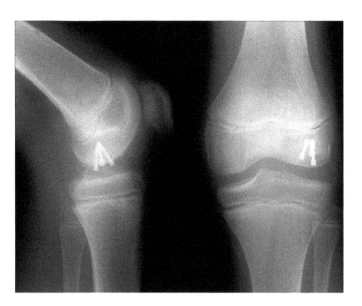

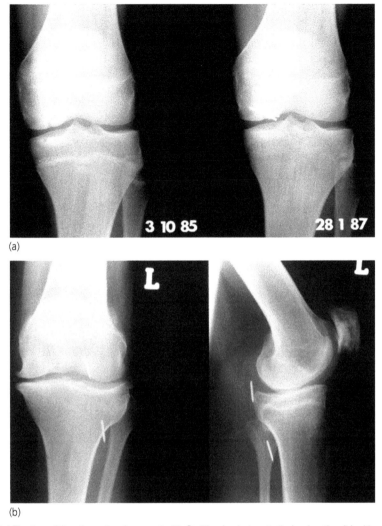

3 10 85   28 1 87

(a)

(b)

Figure 4.25 (a) Fixation of the dissecting fragment with Smillie pins led on to their migration (b) with potentially serious complications. Note the development of lateral compartment osteoarthritis.

Autologous osteochondral plug insertions and osteochondral allografts are also being used as a means of filling the femoral defect (Emmerson *et al.* 2007). As an alternative, autologous bone grafts have been combined with matrix-supported autologous chondrocytes (Khan *et al.* 2010). Only time will tell how effectively these newer techniques improve on the loss of a significant osteochondritic fragment.

Protected weightbearing and the early use of continuous passive motion improve outcome following fragment fixation, with rehabilitation being slow and graduated, over a period of 9 months. The natural history of OCD is poorly reported but, in general, the adolescent condition promotes degenerative

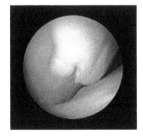

Figure 4.26 An osteochondritic loose body has enlarged by accretion and will no longer fit anatomically in the distal femoral crater.

75

changes if it fails to heal. In contrast, the juvenile form that heals without complication in the classical position runs a minimal risk of osteoarthritis 30 years later. Degenerative change is more likely when OCD develops in other areas of the knee, including the extended classical site which affects a significant weightbearing area of the medial femoral condyle. The adult form of OCD often heals poorly (Linden 1997), the onset of osteoarthritis being hastened by approximately 10 years.

Loose body formation

The patient may present either *de novo* or some time after primary treatment of a known OCD lesion, which has failed to heal back in position. The classic complaint is of intermittent locking, sometimes producing acute stabs of articular pain as the loose body becomes entrapped between weightbearing surfaces. Effusions are produced by the resulting synovitis. The fragment may be palpated intermittently if it is large enough to feel but not so large as to anchor it in the intercondylar space, in the suprapatellar pouch or posteriorly within a recess. With time the loose body may become attached to a mesentery of the synovial membrane, then ceasing to move around the knee joint.

Radiographs (four views) and MR scanning (Figure 4.27) for the smaller, radiolucent fragment should be requested in order to assess the size and number of loose bodies, the degree to which degenerative changes have developed and the presence or absence of other pathology.

Arthroscopic removal of loose bodies is usually successful provided one ensures the rule of correct 'Ps':

* Positioning of the knee
* Portal placement
* Probing
* Pinching off the fluid irrigation when necessary
* Percutaneous needle stabilization of the loose body
* Pushing the fragment when grasped with forceps (rather than pulling at it)
* Patience.

With time a loose body enlarges (Figure 4.26, p. 75) and ceases to fit into the osteochondritic crater as it rounds off and is covered by fibrocartilage. Reattachment is then harmful, particularly if the anchored loose body is left 'proud' of the articular surface.

Patellar instability

Although the patellofemoral mechanism is the major site of problems in childhood, most of the symptoms do not develop as a result of sports alone. The exceptions to this rule are those children where repetitive exercises induce overuse syndromes: gymnastics, swimming and athletics are most likely to produce problems. The extensor mechanism is vulnerable along its full length and avulsion injuries are relatively common, including Sinding–Larsen–Johansson syndrome, avulsion marginal fractures and tibial apophyseal fracture (see Chapters 7 and 8). Harris growth arrest lines may be seen on skyline radiographs (Figure 4.28) and indicate a past history of traumatic episodes of patellar subluxation (Abrahams and Macnicol 2001). Most of these injuries settle with rest from the sport, coupled with physiotherapy and supportive strapping. Splintage with casts should be avoided, even for the painful and persistent Osgood–Schlatter condition (Figure 7.20, p. 163). In approximately a third of children, the sport will no longer be pursued, and only a further third will return to the same level of competitive activity.

Figure 4.27a,b MR scanning often defines small loose bodies more accurately than radiographs.

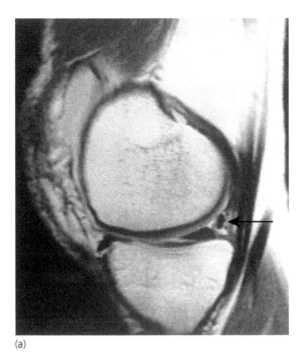

(a)

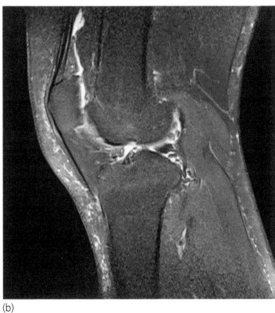

(b)

Patellar instability is often associated with a relatively short quadriceps mechanism, and the degree to which this is present may be classified in terms of diminishing severity from congenital dislocation (see Figure 4.6, p. 62), to habitual dislocation and finally to the recurrent or intermittent dislocation and subluxation which affect the adolescent (Macnicol and Turner 1994). Relevant skeletal abnormalities are shown in Figure 7.1 (p. 147), but as these usually cannot be altered, at least during a particular stage in childhood, therapy consists of stretching the quadriceps and hamstring muscle groups, and improving inner range (vastus medialis) power. If quadriceps elongation is not achieved, relative patella alta persists (see Figure 4.4,

77

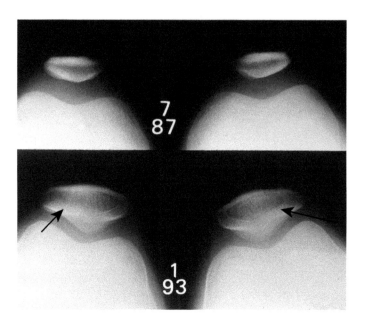

Figure 4.28 Growth arrest lines within the patella developed when it was traumatized by earlier dislocations.

p. 61) (Micheli *et al.* 1986) and may be worsened by lateral release (Hughston and Deese 1988). Hence realignment must only be considered after a careful assessment of the mechanics of the paediatric patellofemoral mechanism (Goa *et al.* 1990).

In the athletic child lateral patellar release may be all that is necessary when physiotherapy fails (Dandy and Griffiths 1989). More extensive procedures are rarely indicated and should be avoided when there is gross ligament laxity and when the patella dislocates in a sinusoidal manner, both in extension and flexion (see Figure 7.8, p. 151). Pain at rest is another relative contraindication to patellar realignment, which must always be preceded by a diagnostic arthroscopy so that the state of the chondral surfaces is known.

For acute patellar dislocation the knee is usually treated conservatively. Later medial retinacular reefing and possible repair of the medial patellofemoral ligament (see Chapter 7) is combined with lateral release. Habitual and recurrent patellar dislocations in children may merit surgery when:

- A prolonged period of conservative management has failed to stabilize the patella
- Swelling and pain accompany the dislocation, indicating chondral damage
- Gross and possibly syndromic laxity is present.

Surgical options are discussed in Chapter 7 and should be advised only if the surgeon is experienced in this demanding form of orthopaedic treatment.

Soft tissue swellings

These are discussed in Chapter 9. The popliteal cyst presents before the age of 10 years and is more common in boys. The swelling is most obvious when the knee is fully extended (Figure 4.29) and lies in relation to the semimembranosus posteromedially, rather than centrally like the 'Baker's cyst' of the degenerate knee that forms because of repeated effusions. Transillumination with a torch or pen light will confirm the cystic nature of the swelling. If there is any concern about the diagnosis (villonodular synovitis, synovial chondromatosis) then an ultrasound and/ or MR scan is justifiable. Dinham (1975) confirmed that popliteal cysts disappear in a few years and that their excision was therefore quite unnecessary. Parental reassurance is important.

The lateral meniscal cyst (see Figure 2.4, p. 16) forms as a result of a tear which allows synovial fluid to track peripherally through the body of the meniscus. The tear is chronic but may not be symptomatic of itself. As the cyst enlarges pressure builds up beneath the fascia lata distally, causing an ache which varies in intensity during the day. The lateral swelling of the cyst is best seen with the knee flexed to 90° and MR scanning defines the abnormality well.

Excising the cyst may disappoint as the swelling often recurs, the primary pathology being unaltered. Arthroscopic 'saucerization' of the tear and decompression of the cyst by opening up the passage through the lateral meniscus is often successful. Recurrence may still occur, so the patient should be warned of this. The medial meniscal cyst or ganglion (see Figure 3.12, p. 44) is rare and can be excised directly if preliminary MR scans reveal no significant meniscal tear. As these cysts are multiloculate aspiration is of no value.

Acute haemarthrosis

Sudden swelling of the traumatized knee is relatively rare in children playing sports, and usually indicates the formation of a haemarthrosis secondary to patellar dislocation (with or without osteochondral fracture), more major intra-articular fractures (Chapter 8), ligament avulsions and tears, and other rare pathologies (Figure 4.30). Injuries to the cruciate and medial ligaments were also found to account for half the cases of haemarthrosis reported by Eiskjaer *et al.* (1988). Arthroscopy reveals that haemorrhage occurs from the synovial invaginations and peripheral folds as well as from the cruciate ligament stump or from osteochondral fractures. Young children are not immune to significant ligament ruptures. Waldrop and Broussard (1984) reported a mophead (isolated) anterior cruciate ligament tear in a child of 3 years, and Joseph and Pogrund (1978) encountered a medial collateral ligament tear in a 4-year-old child after a road traffic collision.

Severe ligament disruption is more likely in later childhood and adolescence, the younger child

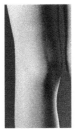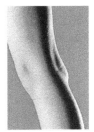

Figure 4.29 The popliteal cyst in childhood usually disappears.

CAUSES OF HAEMARTHROSIS
(55 cases over 10 years)

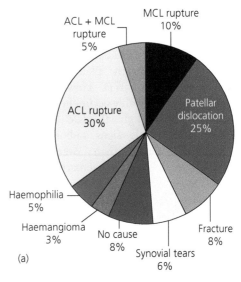

- MCL rupture 10%
- ACL + MCL rupture 5%
- Patellar dislocation 25%
- ACL rupture 30%
- Haemophilia 5%
- Haemangioma 3%
- No cause 8%
- Synovial tears 6%
- Fracture 8%

(a)

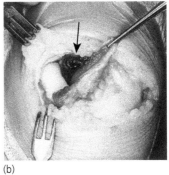

(b)

Figure 4.30 (a) Causes of haemarthrosis of the knee in 55 children over a 10-year period. The yellow segment indicates synovial tears with no obvious associated pathology; (b) Haemangioma of the fat pad producing repeated haemarthroses.

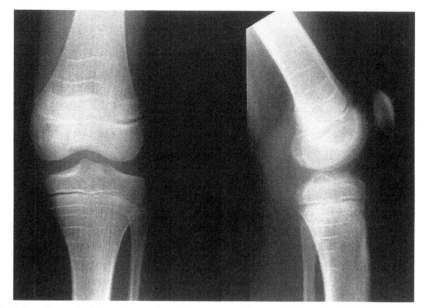

Figure 4.31 Growth arrest (Harris) lines produced by the stress of skiing every winter.

experiencing metaphyseal fractures, ligament avulsions and growth plate disturbance (see Figure 8.8, p. 177). However, occult ligament injury probably occurs in all cases of avulsion injury, and growth plate disturbance may produce subtle signs radiographically (Figure 4.31), rather than overt physeal arrest (Figure 4.32). The haemarthrosis may promote a persisting synovitis or a mild form of complex regional pain syndrome (reflex sympathetic dystrophy), both of which will prolong morbidity. Direct synovial injury from a blow over the anteromedial aspect of the knee during games or an accident occasionally results in a symptomatic medial shelf syndrome, or patellar tendonitis.

The other causes of swelling of the knee tend to be slower and more chronic (see Chapter 9) or represent one of the signs of soft tissue or skeletal injury, discussed in Chapters 5–8.

Ligament injuries

◾ Medial collateral ligament

Medial collateral ligament sprains and tears are managed conservatively, as described by

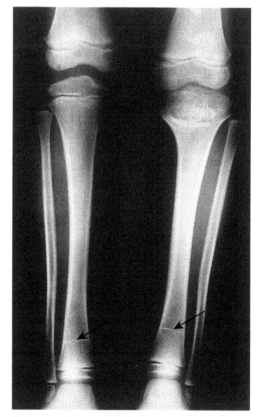

Figure 4.32 Proximal tibial growth arrest produced by an injury when mountain biking. Note associated temporary growth arrest lines.

Indelicato (1983) in the adult. It is wise to take an MR scan to rule out concomitant injury, looking particularly for anterior cruciate ligament rupture, meniscal lesions, bone bruising or osteochondral fractures. Splintage is best avoided, but if examination under anaesthesia reveals significant medial gapping and an appreciable suction sign, a moulded backshell or a hinged brace may be appropriate, together with protected weightbearing for approximately 4 weeks. Commercially available canvas backshells are best avoided as they are poorly tolerated by the child, and often ill-fitting.

Anterior cruciate ligament

Avulsion of the tibial eminence by the anterior cruciate ligament has attracted much attention since Meyers and McKeever (1970) reported a series of 47 cases. Their grades I (12 per cent of the total) and II (44 per cent of the total) injuries (Figure 4.33) did well with conservative treatment in 80 per cent of those two groups. They recommended open reduction for the type III, fully avulsed fragment which is often irreducible (44 per cent of the total). This was recognized by Zaricznyj (1977), who graded the type III injury as follows: (a) complete fragment pull off but no rotation; (b) complete displacement with rotation. A type IV avulsion was also described, consisting of a larger, comminuted fracture extending into the medial and lateral tibial plateaux.

Accurate reduction involves the replacement of one or both 'wings' of the fragment below the anterior meniscal horns and the intermeniscal ligament, It is suggested that internal fixation may then be unnecessary, but the risk of leaving the fragment proud, and the anterior cruciate ligament unacceptably lax is a real one.

If splintage is felt to be appropriate the knee should not be extended fully as this may lift the fragment upwards by tightening the ligament. However, there is a view that extension (but not hyperextension) will allow the femoral condyles to push the tibial fragment into place (Robinson and Driscoll 1981; Hallam *et al.* 2002). Splintage for 8 weeks is sufficient to ensure union of the fragment if it has been anatomically replaced and a lateral radiograph has confirmed the reduction. Rehabilitation is slow, with restriction of full extension and flexion for up to a year. Residual laxity is often apparent later, and Grove *et al.* (1983) considered the results of non-operative treatment to be unsatisfactory.

Open reduction and fixation, often possible by an arthroscopically assisted technique, should ensure the best outcome. Lateral and medial meniscal tears have been reported in association with the avulsion, but tend to heal without suturing. Medial collateral ligament tears are also a possibility. Insertion of an intra-epiphyseal, cannulated screw is usually safe if it is inserted obliquely (Figures 4.34, 4.35). This alignment is usually necessary if the knee is being held in only partial flexion in order to relax the anterior cruciate ligament injury. The screw should be counter-sunk to prevent residual prominence of the secured fragment. The knee should then be flexed and extended to ensure fixation is secure, especially if

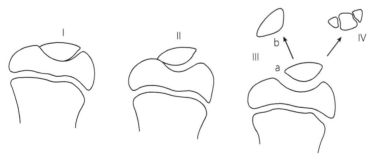

Figure 4.33 The grading of intercondylar eminence avulsion fractures.

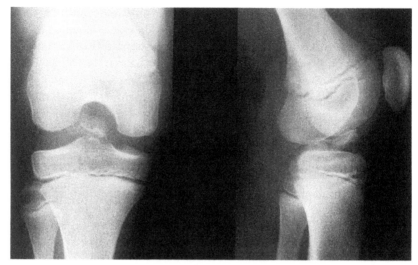

Figure 4.34 A type III B fracture which was irreducible.

Figure 4.35 Reduction and
fixation of the fragment with an
intra-epiphyseal screw.

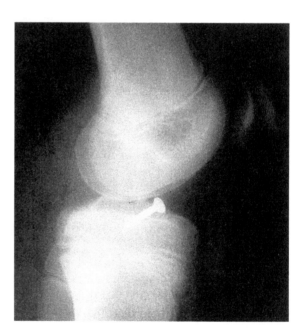

comminution is present. Operative treatment is also advisable if collateral ligament tears and meniscal detachment are revealed on preliminary MR scans (Lisser and Weiner 1991). Late cases are still worth exploring, reattaching the displaced fragment anatomically as it may otherwise block full extension. Mid-substance tears are probably underdiagnosed, and it is likely that some degree of ligament disruption coexists with all avulsion fractures, whether tibial or femoral.

Ligament reconstruction is indicated for complete, intra-substance ruptures, because it has been realized that conservative treatment or acute repair is as fruitless as it is in the adult. However, early diagnosis of anterior cruciate ligament rupture may allow a substantial portion of the natural ligament to be incorporated in any reconstruction. The damaged ligament is sutured alongside a two- or four-strand semitendinosus autogenous graft. This is left attached distally and is only placed in a bone tunnel through the proximal tibial growth plate if the patient is within 2 years of maturity. In the relatively rare case involving a younger child, reinforcement of the natural ligament is possible by routing the graft over the upper surface of the tibial epiphysis, tunnelling proximal to the physis (Henning 1992). Femoral attachment at the isometric point is achieved by screw or staple fixation, avoiding implant damage to the growth plate, and filling the bone tunnel fully with the graft. The 'over the top' route is preferred by some surgeons, and reduces concern about distal femoral growth plate damage.

Graft protection is ensured for a minimum of 3 months, with limited weightbearing and supervised movement of the knee, allowing virtually full extension from the outset but controlling the power applied through the quadriceps group. There is a natural tendency towards a 'quadriceps-avoidance gait' (see Chapter 10) so that bracing is of limited value. Proprioception and confidence are built up progressively and full sporting activity is usually allowed at the anniversary of the operation. The results of treatment for tibial eminence avulsion are often disappointing. Smith (1984) found that half the patients in his series had pain or instability on average 7 years later, and Gronqvist *et al.* (1984) considered that late instability was proportional to the age of the child when injured. A recent review by Lafrance *et al.* (2010) confirms the importance of precise surgical technique. The results of anterior cruciate ligament reconstruction have been reported as favourable in both short-term review (McCarroll *et al.* 1988) and in the longer term (Frosch *et al.* 2010) so it is to be hoped that the depressing natural history of chronic anterior cruciate deficiency will be altered favourably.

■ Posterior cruciate ligament

This injury is rare (Mayer and Micheli 1979), approximately 10 per cent of the frequency of anterior cruciate ligament rupture. It is important to recognize the significance of posterior cruciate ligament rupture, for the long-term disability is persistent and virtually impossible to overcome later. The mechanism is usually a blow over the upper shin when playing football or impacts from mountain biking or skiing. If bone has been avulsed from the distal femur or proximal tibia (Figure 4.36), reattachment of the anchor point is achieved

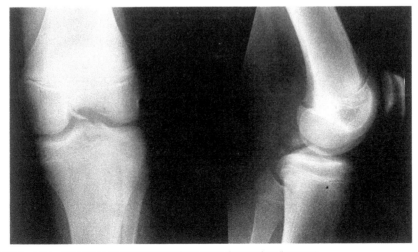

Figure 4.36 Avulsion of the femoral attachment of the posterior cruciate ligament.

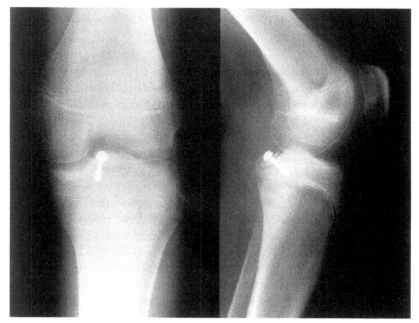

Figure 4.37 Internal fixation of the fragment with a lag screw and washer.

with an intra-epiphyseal screw (Figure 4.37) and rehabilitation is reasonably rapid, provided that there has been no delay in treatment. Mild residual laxity is likely to persist but further skeletal growth tends to lessen this. Associated knee injuries are rare; occasionally the posterolateral structures may be damaged.

Although a conservative approach to the adolescent or adult injury offers acceptable results in knees with isolated mild or moderate posterior laxity, significant laxity and combined ligament tears merit operative ligament reconstruction. Arthroscopic technique with a trans-tibial tunnel for the graft may lead to angulatory graft failure so there is now greater interest in the inlay method whereby the bone block left attached to the graft is punched into a closely-fitting trench in the upper tibia posteriorly (Noyes *et al.* 2003; Stannard *et al.* 2003; Kim *et al.* 2009). The evidence available clinically and in the literature does not allow a definite recommendation for which technique to use and most surgeons will confine themselves to a surgical method that is relatively familiar, and safe. The management of this injury is further discussed in Chapter 5.

Lateral complex avulsion

Avulsion of the biceps and popliteus tendons results from major varus stress and is fortunately rare. In children the proximal fibular epiphysis may separate so its reattachment is essential to preserve biceps femoris function. The iliotibial tract is usually spared, but repair is always advised when there is significant gapping and a suction sign over the posterolateral joint line, since the tendons quickly retract and become irreparable. Peroneal nerve traction lesions may coexist in the adult but are unusual in the child.

After surgery the knee is protected in slight flexion using a cast in the younger child or a brace in the adolescent. Residual laxity is common but may lessen if the child has several years of skeletal growth ahead.

Meniscal tears

The presentation and management of meniscal lesions will be discussed fully in Chapter 6 but certain paediatric aspects will be considered in this section. The discoid anomaly (Kramer and Micheli 2009) is relatively common in the younger child, causing one form of the snapping knee. However, it is uncommon to encounter it as an acute meniscal problem, tears developing slowly over a period of months. The classic, and reasonably normal discoid meniscus, covering much of the lateral tibial condyle (Figures 4.38, 4.39), may develop a tear in its medial edge. Partial excision of the damaged segment is achieved arthroscopically or through a mini-arthrotomy, allowing the rim to function relatively normally. However, it should be remembered that the dynamic attachments of the classical discoid meniscus are also abnormal so that mild symptoms are likely to persist. If the Wrisberg form of anomaly is encountered (Figure 4.40), complete excision may be necessary, although this decision should be deferred for as long as possible. Preservation of meniscal tissue remains the goal, particularly in the growing child. Meniscal repair is appropriate for displacing 'bucket handle' tears and peripheral splits, although healing of menisci undoubtedly occurs as a natural process without surgical intervention if a peripheral separation or longitudinal split is stable and the knee is protected. Radial tears are rare in childhood, although they may affect the lateral meniscus in the adolescent. The lesion should be saucerized in an attempt to prevent the tear from spreading peripherally, and if a peripheral cyst develops this can be decompressed through the line of cleavage of the tear.

Figure 4.38 (a) The types of lateral discoid meniscus. Excision of the central portion of the classical discoid meniscus may preserve its function (left), but the Wrisberg type usually merits complex incision. (b) Reduction in the lateral femoral condylar angle may predispose towards the formation of a discoid lateral meniscus. (From Fujikawa *et al.* 1978).

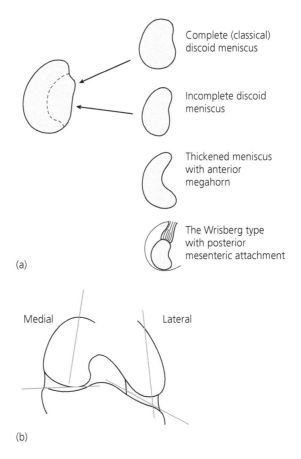

Complete (classical) discoid meniscus

Incomplete discoid meniscus

Thickened meniscus with anterior megahorn

The Wrisberg type with posterior mesenteric attachment

(a)

Medial   Lateral

(b)

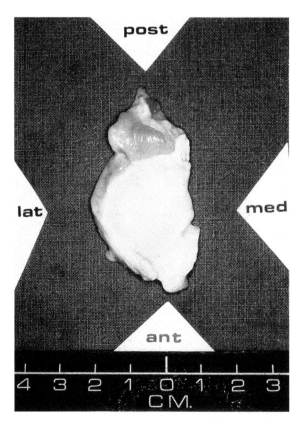

Figure 4.39 The classical, Watanabe discoid meniscus covers most of the lateral tibial condyle.

Minor lesions of the meniscus are produced by impingement or subluxation. This is a product of meniscal mobility and the lax mesentery of the meniscotibial ligament is akin to the recognized problem of patellar hypermobility. A blush of inflammatory tissue similar to early pannus is seen overlying the anterior meniscal horn (Figure 4.41) and there is a concurrent articular cartilage lesion. These meniscal impingements are seen in sports demanding repetitive stresses, such as gymnastics or dancing, and may be associated with articular cartilage debris from overuse.

Meniscectomy in childhood is known to produce significant later problems in a high proportion of cases (Zaman and Leonard 1981; Menzione *et al.* 1983; Abdon *et al.* 1990). The same is true for the adolescent (McNicholas *et al.* 2000). Partial meniscectomy and successful meniscal repair should improve the prognosis, although there are no long-term reports of the outcome after these procedures as yet. An analysis of the literature dealing with the effects of discoid meniscal partial excision also confirms that there are no grounds for complacency (Ikeuchi 1982; Hayashi *et al.* 1988; Vandermeer and Cunningham 1989; Aichroth *et al.* 1991; Okazaki *et al.* 2006;).

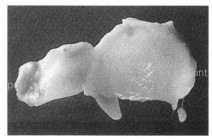

Figure 4.40 The Wrisberg type of discoid lateral meniscus.

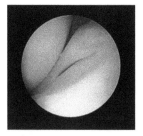

Figure 4.41 The medial meniscus in a 4-year-old child's knee. Early pannus is present over the anterior and peripheral portion of the meniscus.

Osteochondral fractures

True osteochondral fractures occur in association with patellar dislocation; these are differentiated from osteochondritis dissecans by their bleeding base (Figure 4.42) and acute onset. Cartilaginous flaps and small separated fragments do not usually merit replacement, but osteochondral fragments over 1 cm in diameter should be fixed in place and usually unite. Zaidi *et al.* (2006) reviewed MR scans in children following acute, traumatic patellar lateral dislocation. Approximately 80 per cent sustained tears of the medial restraints, avulsion of medial patellar fragments and bone bruising. Half of the osteochondral avulsions are extra-articular (medial patellar border) and half are intra-articular from the lateral sulcus or patella as it relocates (Nietos *et al.* 1994) (see Figure 7.8, p. 151).

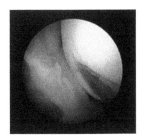

Figure 4.42 41 An osteochondral fracture of the medial femoral condyle.

If the lesion fails to unite after fixation, the fragment should be removed before adaptive changes occur within the patellofemoral joint. Even the loss of large osteochondral fragments may be consistent with satisfactory function since the defect fills slowly with fibrocartilage. Long-term reviews suggest that arthritic changes are advanced by 10 years, but there is no convincing evidence that replacement of the fragment significantly alters the natural history unless a very large fragment is lost and affects patellar stability. As with osteochondritis dissecans, there is a role for osteochondral grafting and autologous chondrocyte transplants when a defect cannot be replaced in the acute stage of this lesion.

Miscellaneous conditions

When a child with a symptomatic knee following injury is assessed, generalized and local pathology should always be considered, in addition to the typical injuries described earlier. Developmental conditions, bleeding disorders, atopy (asthma, hay fever and eczema) and synovial lesions must all be considered. Injuries to the growth plate may be subtle or overt, and in some cases the symptoms coincide with a sporting injury but are primarily acquired from a different disease process. Therefore it is vital to take a full history and examine the child completely, even after the most obvious sporting injury. An underlying congenital condition such as a skeletal dysplasia or congenital insensitivity to pain (Figure 4.43) (Macnicol and Kuo

Figure 4.43 Radiographs showing destruction of a knee affected by congenital insensitivity to pain.

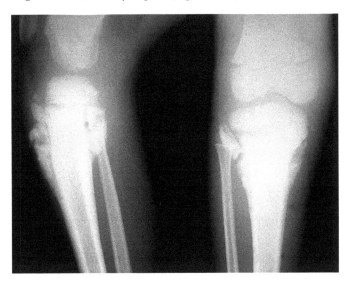

1996) may first present as a knee problem in mid-childhood. Proximal tibiofibular subluxation (Figure 4.44) and referred pain from the hip are two conditions which may also confound the inexperienced. Finally, benign and malignant neoplasms must always be included in the differential diagnosis (Chapter 9).

Pain syndromes

Reflex sympathetic dystrophy (RSD) is now known as complex regional pain syndrome (CRPS type I) while causalgia or neurogenic pain is CRPS type II (Stanton-Hicks *et al.* 1995).

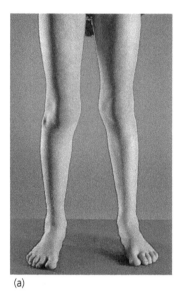

(a)

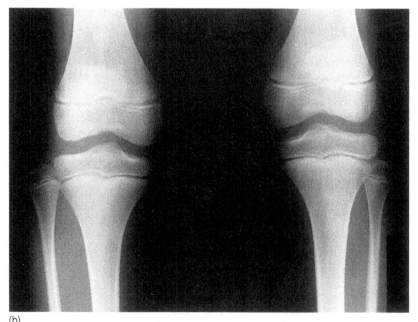

(b)

Figure 4.44 (a) Anterolateral subluxation of the right proximal tibiofibular joint with overgrowth of the fibula. (b) Chronic subluxation of the right fibular head. Surgery is rarely appropriate.

The condition is characterized by spontaneous pain, burning sensations, hypersensitivity and paraesthesiae, type II differing in that peripheral nerve injury is also evident. Scar neuroma, nerve tumour or glomus tumour should always be considered. Muscle wasting and stiffness develop and the skin is cold, mottled and bluish with a waxy or swollen feeling when touched.

Children under 6 years of age are not affected. Girls present six times as commonly as boys and the condition usually affects the leg. Recovery is more likely in children for whom physiotherapy and cognitive behavioural therapy are effective, without recourse to pharmacological medication or sympathetic block (Wilder *et al.* 1992). The child under psychological pressure from the parents, the coach or the sport, may suffer emotionally. In these instances the knee may become the target organ of complaint and minor malfunctions may be much exaggerated. Counselling or cessation of the sport may be the only means of resolving the conflict. Remember also that every active child is 'sporting' in the sense that regular and repetitive exercise occurs with play. When the demands of skeletal growth combine with an active lifestyle and the pressures of organized sport, the knee is frequently the site of first complaint.

References

Abdon P, Turner MS, Pettersson H, *et al.* (1990) A long-term follow-up study of total meniscectomy in children. *Clin Orthop* **257**, 166–70.

Abrahams A and Macnicol MF (2001) Growth arrest and recurrent patellar dislocation: a new sign. *Knee* **8**, 163–5.

Aichroth PM, Patel DV and Marx CL (1991) Congenital discoid lateral meniscus in children; a follow-up study and evolution of management. *J Bone Joint Surg Br* **73**, 932–6.

Amis AA, Firer P, Mountney J, *et al.* (2003) Anatomy and biomechanics of the medial patellofemoral ligament. *Knee* **10**, 215–20.

Backx FJG, Erich WBM, Kemper ABA and Verbeek ALM (1989) Sports injuries in school-aged children: an epidemiologic study. *Am J Sports Med* **17**, 239–40.

Blount WP (1937) Tibia vara. Osteochondrosis deformans tibiae. *J Bone Joint Surg Am* **19**, 1–10.

Bowen JR, Morley DC, McInverny V and MacEwen GD (1983) Treatment of genu recurvatum by proximal tibial closing-wedge anterior displacement osteotomy. *Clin Orthop* **179**, 194–9.

Bowen JR, Leahy JL, Zheng Z and MacEwen GD (1985) Partial epiphysiodesis at the knee to correct angular deformity. *Clin Orthop* **198**, 184–5.

Brunner R, Hefti F and Tgetgel JD (1997) Arthrogrypotic joint contracture at the knee and foot: correction with a circular frame. *J Paediatr Orthop B* **6**, 192–7.

Choi JH, Chung CY, Cho TJ and Park SS (1999) Correction of genu recurvatum by the Ilizarov metehod. *J Bone Joint Surg Br* **81**, 769–74.

Clarke SE, McCarthy JJ and Davidson RS (2009) Treatment of Blount disease: a comparison between the multiaxial correction system and other external fixators. *J Pediatr Orthop* **29**, 103–9.

Coogan PG, Fox JA and Fitch RD (1996) Treatment of adolescent Blount's disease with the circular external fixation device and distraction osteogenesis. *J Pediatr Orthop* **16**, 450–4.

Curtis BH and Fisher RL (1969) Congenital hyperextension with anterior subluxation of the knee: surgical treatment and long-term observations. *J Bone Joint Surg Am* **51**, 255–8.

Dandy DJ and Griffiths D (1989) Lateral release for recurrent dislocation of the patella. *J Bone Joint Surg Br* **71**, 121–5.

De Smet AA, Ilahi OA and Graf BK (1997) Untreated osteochondritis of the femoral condyles: prediction of patient outcome using radiographic and MR findings. *Skeletal Radiol* **26**, 463–7.

Del Bello DA and Watts HG (1996) Distal femoral extension osteotomy for knee flexion contracture in patients with arthrogryposis. *J Pediatr Orthop* **16**, 122–6.

Dinham JM (1975) Popliteal cysts in children. *J Bone Joint Surg Br* **57**, 69–71.

Dipaola J, Nelson DW and Colville MR (1991) Characterising osteochondral lesions by magnetic resonance imaging. *Arthroscopy* **7**, 101–4.

Edgerton BC, Mariani EM and Morrey BF (1993) Distal femoral varus osteotomy for painful genu valgum. A five-to-12 year follow-up study. *Clin Orthop* **288**, 261–9.

Edmonds EW, Albright J, Bastrom T and Chambers HG (2010) Outcomes of extra-articular, intra-epiphyseael drilling for osteochondritis dissecans of the knee. *J Paediatr Orthop* **30**, 870–8.

Eiskjaer S, Larsen ST and Schmidt MB (1988) The significance of hemarthrosis of the knee in children. *Arch Orthop Trauma Surg* **107**, 96–8.

Emmerson BC, Gortz S, Jamali AA, *et al.* (2007) Fresh osteochondral allografting in the treatment of osteochondritis dissecans of the femoral condyle. *Am J Sports Med* **35**, 907–14.

Erlacher P (1922) Deformierende Prozesse de Epiphysengenend bei Kindern. *Arch Orthop Unfallchir* **20**, 81–4.

Ferris BD and Jackson AM (1990) Congenital snapping knee (habitual anterior subluxation of the tibia in extension). *J Bone Joint Surg Br* **72**, 453–6.

Ferriter P and Shapiro F (1987) Infantile tibia vara: factors affecting outcome following proximal tibial osteotomy. *J Pediatr Orthop* **7**, 1–7.

Fraser RK, Dickens DR and Cole WG (1995) Medial physeal stapling for primary and secondary genu valgum in late childhood and adolescence. *J Bone Joint Surg Br* **77**, 733–5.

Frosch KH, Stengel G, Brodhun T, *et al.* (2010) Outcomes and risks of operative treatment of rupture of the anterior cruciate ligament in children and adolescents. *Arthroscopy* **26**, 1539–50.

Fujikawa K, Tomatsu T and Malso K (1978) Morphological analysis of meniscus and articular cartilage in the knee joint by means of arthrogram. *J Jpn Orthop Assoc* **52**, 203–15.

Goa GX, Lee EH and Bose K (1990) Surgical management of congenital and habitual dislocation of the patellae. *J Pediatr Orthop* **10**, 255–60.

Gronqvist H, Hirsch G and Johansson L (1984) Fractures of the anterior tibial spine in children. *J Pediatr Orthop* **4**, 465–7.

Grove TP, Miller SJ III, Kent BE, *et al.* (1983) Non-operative treatment of the torn anterior cruciate ligament. *J Bone joint Surg Am* **65**, 184–8.

Guhl JL (1982) Arthroscopic treatment of osteochondritis dissecans. *Clin Orthop* **167**, 65–74.

Hallam PJB, Fazal MA, Ashwood N, *et al.* (2002) An alternative to fixation of displaced fractures of the anterior intercondylar eminence in children. *J Bone Joint Surg Br* **84**, 579–82.

Hayashi LK, Yamaga H, Ida K, *et al.* (1988) Arthroscopic meniscectomy for discoid lateral meniscus in children. *J Bone Joint Surg Am* **70**, 1495–500.

Healy WL, Anglen JO, Wasilewski SA and Krackow KA (1983) Distal femoral varus osteotomy. *J Bone Joint Surg Am* **70**, 102–9.

Henning CE (1992) Anterior cruciate ligament reconstruction with open epiphyses. In: Aichroth PM and Cannon WD (eds) *Knee Surgery Current Practice*. London: Martin Dunitz, pp. 181–5.

Hughston JC and Deese M (1988) Medial subluxation of the patellae as a complication of lateral retinacular release. *Am J Sports Med* **16**, 383–8.

Ikeuchi H (1982) Arthroscopic treatment of discoid lateral meniscus: technique and long-term results. *Clin Orthop* **167**, 19–28.

Indelicato PA (1983) Non-operative treatment of complete tears of the medial collaeral ligament of the knee. *J Bone Joint Surg Am* **65**, 323–9.

Jacobsen K and Vopalecky F (1985) Congenital dislocation of the knee. *Acta Orthop Scand* **7**, 194–9.

Joseph K and Pogrund H (1978) Traumatic rupture of the medial ligament of the knee in a four year old child: case report and review of the literature. *J Bone Joint Surg Am* **60**, 402–3.

Katz MP, Grogono BJS and Soper KC (1967) The aetiology and treatment of congenital dislocation of the knee. *J Bone Joint Surg Br* **49**, 112–20.

Khan WS, Johnson DS and Hardingham TE (2010) The potential of stem cells in the treatment of knee cartilage defects. *Knee* **17**, 369–74.

Kim SJ, Kim TE, Jo SB and Kung YP (2009) Comparison of the clinical results of three posterior cruciate ligament reconstruction techniques. *J Bone Joint Surg Am* **91**, 2543–9.

Kramer DE and Micheli LJ (2009) Meniscal tears and discoid meniscus in children: diagnosis and treatment. *J Am Acad Orthop Surg* **17**, 698–707.

Lafrance RM, Giordano B, Goldblatt J, *et al.* (2010) Pediatric tibial eminence fractures: evaluation and management. *J Am Acad Orthop Surg* **18**, 395–405.

Langenskiold A (1952) Tibia vara. *Acta Chir* **103**, 9–14.

Langenskiold A (1981) Tibia vara: osteochondrosis deformans tibiae. Blount's disease. *Clin Orthop* **158**, 77–81.

Levine AM and Drennan JC (1982) Physiological bowing and tibia vara: the metaphyseal-diaphyseal angle in the measurement of bow-leg deformities. *J Bone Joint Surg Am* **64**, 1158–63.

Linden B (1997) Osteochondritis dissecans of the femoral condyles: a long term follow-up study. *J Bone Joint Surg Am* **53**, 769–76.

Lisser S and Weiner LS (1991) Ligament injuries in children. In: Scott WN (ed.) *Ligament and Extensor Mechanism Injuries of the Knee; Diagnosis and Treatment.* St Louis: Mosby.

Macnicol MF (1995) Sports injuries of the knee in children. *Orthop Int Ed* **3**, 27–36.

Macnicol MF (1997) Focal fibrocartilaginous dysplasia of the femur. *J Pediatr Orthop B* **8**, 661–3.

Macnicol MF (1999) The correction of lesser leg length inequalities. *Curr Orthop* **288**, 212–17.

Macnicol MF (2002) Realignment osteotomy for knee deformity in childhood. *Knee* **4**, 113–20.

Macnicol MF and Gupta MS (1997) Epiphysiodesis using a cannulated tube saw. *J Bone Joint Surg Br* **79**, 307–9.

Macnicol MF and Kuo RS (1996) Congenital insensitivity to pain: orthopaedic implications. *J Pediatr Orthop B* **5**, 292–5.

Macnicol MF and Turner MS (1994) The knee. In: Benson MKD, Fixsen JA, Macnicol MF (eds) *Children's Orthopaedics and Fractures.* Edinburgh: Churchill Livingstone, pp. 484–5.

Mayer PJ and Micheli LJ (1979) Avulsion of the femoral attachment of the posterior cruciate ligament in an 11-year-old boy: case report and review of the literature. *J Bone Joint Surg Am* **61**, 431–2.

McCarroll JR, Retting AC and Shelbourne DK (1988) Anterior cruciate ligament injuries in the young athlete with open physes. *Am J Sports Med* **16**, 44–9.

McNicholas MJ, Rowley DI, McGurty D, *et al.* (2000) Total meniscectomy in adolescence. A 30-year follow-up. *J Bone Joint Surg Br* **82**, 217–21.

Menzione M, Pizzutillo PD, Peoples AB, *et al.* (1983) Meniscectomy in children: a long-term follow-up study. *Am J Sports Med* **11**, 111–15.

Meyers MH and McKeever FM (1970) Fracture of the intercondylar eminence of the tibia. *J Bone Joint Surg Am* **41**, 209–22.

Micheli LJ, Slater JA, Woods E, *et al.* (1986) Patella alta and the adolescent growth spurt. *Clin Orthop* **213**, 159–62.

Monticelli G and Spinelli R (1984) A new method of treating the advanced stages of tibia vara (Blount's disease). *Ital J Orthop Traumatol* **10**, 245–303.

Moroni A, Pezzuto V, Pompili M and Zinghi G (1992) Proximal osteotomy of the tibia for the treatment of genu recurvatum in adults. *J Bone Joint Surg Am* **74**, 577–86.

Mulford JS (2007) Assessment and management of chronic patellofemoral instability. *J Bone Joint Surg Br* **89**, 709–16.

Murray C and Fixsen JA (1997) Management of knee deformity in clinical arthrogryposis multiplex congenital (amyoplasia congenita). *J Pediatr Orthop B* **6**, 186–91.

Nietos N, Nietosvaara Y, Aalto K, *et al.* (1994) Acute patellar dislocation in children: incidence and associated osteochondral fractures. *J Pediatr Orthop* **14**, 513–15.

Noyes FR, Medvecky MJ and Bhargava M (2003) Arthroscopically assisted quadriceps double-bundle tibial inlay posterior cruciate reconstruction: an analysis of techniques and a safe operative approach to the popliteal fossa. *Arthroscopy* **19**, 894–905.

Ogden JA, Ogden RN, Pugh L, *et al.* (1995) Tibia valga after proximal metaphyseal fractures in childhood: a normal biological response. *J Pediatr Orthop* **15**, 489–93.

Okazaki K, Miura H, Matsuda S, *et al.* (2006) Arthroscopic resection of the discoid lateral meniscus: long-term follow-up for 16 years. *Arthroscopy* **22**, 967–71.

Paget J (1870) On the production of some of the loose bodies in joints. *St Bartholomew's Hosp Rep* **6**, 1–4.

Pappas AM, Anas P and Toczylowski HM (1984) Asymmetrical arrest of the proximal tibial physis and genu recurvatum deformity. *J Bone Joint Surg Am* **66**, 575–81.

Robinson SC and Driscoll SE (1981) Simultaneous osteochondral avulsion of the femoral and tibial insertions of the anterior cruciate ligament. *J Bone Joint Surg Am* **63**, 1342–3.

Salenius P and Vankka E (1975) The development of the tibiofemoral angle in children. *J Bone Joint Surg Am* **57**, 259–61.

Siffert RS (1982) Intra-epiphyseal osteotomy for progressive tibia vara: a case report and rationale of management. *J Pediatr Orhtop* **2**, 81–3.

Skak SV, Jensen TT, Poulsen TD, *et al.* (1987) Epidemiology of knee injuries in children. *Acta Orthop Scand* **58**, 78–81.

Smith JB (1984) Knee instability after fractures of the intercondylar eminence of the tibia. *J Pediatr Orthop* **4**, 462–6.

Stannard JP, Riley RS, Sheils TM, *et al.* (2003) Anatomic reconstruction of the posterior cruciate ligament after multiligament knee injuries. A combination of the tibial-inlay and two-femoral-tunnel techniques. *Am J Sports Med* **31**, 196–202.

Stanton-Hicks M, Janig W, Hassenbuch S, *et al.* (1995) Reflex sympathetic dystrophy: changing concepts and taxonomy. *Pain* **63**, 127–33.

Steel HH, Sandrow RE and Sullivan PD (1971) Complications of tibial osteotomy in children for genu varum or valgum. *J Bone Joint Surg Am* **53**, 1629–35.

Steenbrugge F and Macnicol MF (2002) Osteochondritis dissecans of the femoral head in Perthes' disease: a cause for concern? *Acta Orthop Belgica* **68**, 485–9.

Stein H and Dickson RA (1975) Reversed dynamic slings for knee flexion contractures in the haemophiliac. *J Bone Joint Surg Br* **57**, 282–3.

Stevens PM, Maguire M, Dales MD and Robins AJ (1999) Physeal stapling for idiopathic genu valgum. *J Paediatr Orthop* **19**, 645–9.

Tabaddor RR, Banffy MB, Andersen JS, *et al.* (2010) Fixation of juvenile osteochondritis dissecans lesions of the knee using poly96L/4D-lactide copolymer bioabsorbable implants. *J Paediatr Orthop* **30**, 14–20.

Van Huyssteen AL, Hastings CJ, Olesak M and Hoffman EB (2005) Double elevating osteotomy for late-presenting infantile Blount's disease: the importance of concomitant lateral epiphysiodesis. *J Bone Joint Surg Br* **87**, 710–15.

Vandermeer RD and Cunningham FK (1989) Arthroscopic treatment of the discoid lateral meniscus: results of long-term follow-up. *Arthroscopy* **5**, 101–9.

Volpon JB (1997) Idiopathic genu valgum treated by epiphysiodesis in adolescence. *Int Orthop* **21**, 228–31.

Waldrop JI and Broussard TS (1984) Disruption of the anterior cruciate ligament in a three-year-old child. *J Bone Joint Surg Am* **66**, 1113–14.

Wall EJ, Vourazeris J, Myer GD, *et al.* (2008) The healing potential of stable juvenile osteochondritis dissecans knee lesions. *J Bone Joint Surg Am* **90**, 2655–64.

Wilder RT, Berde CB, Wolohan M, *et al.* (1992) Reflex sympathetic dystrophy in children. Characteristics and follow up of 70 patients. *J Bone Joint Surg Am* **74**, 910–19.

Yoshida S, Ikata T, Takai H, *et al.* (1998) Osteochondritis dissecans of the femoral condyle in the growth stage. *Clin Orthop Relat Res* **346**, 162–70.

Zaidi A, Babyn P, Astori I, *et al.* (2006) MRI of traumatic patellar dislocation in children. *Pediatr Radiol* **36**, 1163–70.

Zaman M and Leonard MA (1981) Meniscectomy in children: results in 59 knees. *Injury* **12**, 425–8.

Zaricznyj B (1977) Avulsion fracture of the tibial eminence: treatment by open reduction and pinning. *J Bone Joint Surg Am* **59**, 1111–14.

5

Ligamentous injuries

Introduction

Over the last few decades no topic in orthopaedic management has evoked greater interest than knee ligament tears and their management. The knee is vulnerable to soft tissue injury because it is an unconstrained hinge placed at a site where collisions and twisting stresses are readily sustained at sport and during everyday activity.

The integrity of the normal knee is maintained by the two cruciate ligaments centrally and a succession of structures around the periphery of the joint. Medially, the two laminae of the tibial collateral ligament and the posteromedial capsular corner of the knee are reinforced by the pes anserinus muscle group (sartorius, gracilis and semitendinosus) and the semimembranosus (see Figures 1.4 and 1.5, p. 5). On the lateral side, the fibular collateral ligament and arcuate ligament posteriorly are augmented by the tendons of popliteus and biceps femoris. Further forward the anterolateral femorotibial ligament and iliotibial band (see Figure 1.2, p. 3, Figure 1.6, p. 6) reinforce the capsule.

Anteriorly the quadriceps mechanism is a vital, dynamic stabilizer while the sturdy posterior capsule, including its oblique popliteal ligament, is reinforced by the semimembranosus, popliteus and gastrocnemius tendons (see Figure 1.7, p. 6). The joint surfaces and menisci impart little stability to the joint which is therefore highly dependent on the passive and dynamic supports described.

In the child, avulsion of the skeletal attachment of the ligament is more likely until the age when the growth plate is fusing. Low-velocity trauma in the adult usually results in a mid-substance rupture, but it is also clear that the ligament avulsion produced by greater force inevitably causes a varying degree of soft tissue disruption. Noyes *et al.* (1974) assessed the pathological changes in stressed ligaments during experiments in primates and found that ligament failure often preceded tibial eminence avulsion by the anterior cruciate ligament (ACL), with a 57 per cent incidence at a slow loading rate and a 28 per cent incidence at a faster loading rate. Tearing of the ligament is usually more substantial when assessed throughout its length microscopically, involving the neural network as well as collagen fibres, elastin and capillaries. An intact synovial sheath may disguise the extent to which the ligament is ruptured.

The bone–ligament junction is an important structure, allowing a controlled gradient between hard and soft tissue. Bone, with a matrix of principally chondroitin sulphate, blends with a layer of calcified fibrocartilage (detectable histologically as a basophilic blue line of mineralization) and then a wider zone of fibrocartilage (Panni *et al.* 1993). The type I collagen

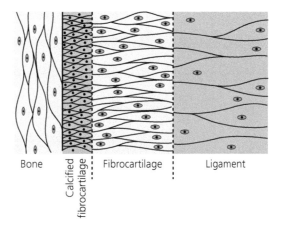

Figure 5.1 The bone–ligament junction forms a resilient gradient of progressively more elastic tissue from bone (left) to calcified fibrocartilage, unmineralized fibrocartilage and then ligament (right).

Bone   Calcified fibrocartilage   Fibrocartilage   Ligament

fibrils of 25–300 mm diameter are anchored in this resilient zone of fibrocartilage which acts as a 'stretching brake' (Figure 5.1). The bone–ligament junction is three to four times as strong as the central part of the ligament, and in the normal situation it is unlikely to yield. However, fibrous tissue replaces the fibrocartilage layer when artificial ligament replacements are used. This envelope, similar to the fibrous tissue layer around the cement mantle of an arthroplasty, has relatively poor tensile properties so that the attachment of Dacron directly to bone is physiologically unsatisfactory. Panni *et al.* (1993) found that the Kennedy ligament augmentation device (LAD), wrapped in tendinous connective tissue, produced less fibrous tissue than an uncovered artificial ligament, although the layer was always thicker than that seen with the bone–patellar tendon–bone autograft bedded into bone tunnels.

Ligament injuries are arbitrarily divided into three grades:

First-degree sprain – in which there may be micro-tears within the structure of the ligament, but the strength of the ligament is clinically unimpaired.
Second-degree sprain – in which there is a partial tear of the fibres composing the ligament, such that some lengthening and subsequent laxity is evident (5–10 mm more than the opposite side).
Third-degree sprain – in which the ligament is torn across completely and offers no stability to the knee (more than 10 mm of excess laxity, and with no feeling of an 'end point').

Avulsion injuries occur between bone and the zone of calcified fibrocartilage. This junction is more vulnerable in the child and adolescent, and is somewhat akin to the growth plate.

Although a great deal has been written about the passive, restraining action of the ligaments (Figure 5.2), this is only one part of their function. It is clear that all ligaments are supplied with sensory nerve endings, and these mechanoreceptors can be identified on the surfaces of the ligament (Table 5.1, Figure 5.3). Thus, the ligaments provide a very important sensory or proprioceptive role, feeding afferent impulses to the central nervous system and thereby setting up reflexes which inhibit potentially injurious movements of the knee (see Figure 1.1, p. 2).

Medial ligament tears

The medial ligament not only prevents valgus deviation of the tibia below the femur, but also prevents the tibia from rotating externally under the femoral condyles. A knowledge of this second function is important, as the tests used to assess the medial ligament and associated supporting structures are devised to show any pathological forward and outward movement of the medial tibial condyle. There will therefore not only be an increased tilting of the knee, but also a rotation, which is termed anteromedial laxity if in excess of that found in the other knee.

Figure 5.2 If a force (newtons) is progressively applied to a ligament, as shown on the ordinate, the slack is first taken up before the ligament stretches under load in a way that is dictated by its modulus of elasticity. As long as the yield point is not exceeded, the ligament will return to its prestressed state. When deformation (irreversible elongation) occurs, by definition the ligament is beginning to tear. The extent of this plastic change is proportional to the load (strain) applied. The mean maximum failure load (yield point) is approximately 1500 N for the anterior cruciate ligament, double this for the posterior cruciate ligament and never more than half this for autogenous grafts.

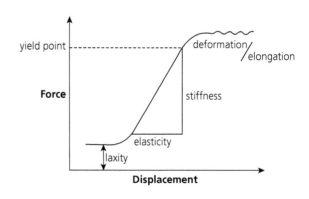

Table 5.1 Proprioception is provided by a variety of intra-articular sensors

Type	Location	Function
Golgi tendon organ (fusiform corpuscle)	Ligaments, meniscal horns	Dynamic mechanoreceptor (high threshold)
Ruffini (globular corpuscle)	Ligaments, menisci, capsule, fat pad	Static and dynamic mechanoreceptor
Pacinian (conical corpuscle)	Ligaments, menisci, capsule, fat pad	Dynamic mechanoreceptor (low threshold)
Free nerve endings: thinly myelinated and unmyelinated*	All articular tissues except cartilage	Nociceptors or non-nociceptive mechanoreceptors

* Neuropeptide release causes inflammation (and later osteoarthritis) by stimulating the proliferation of synoviocytes.

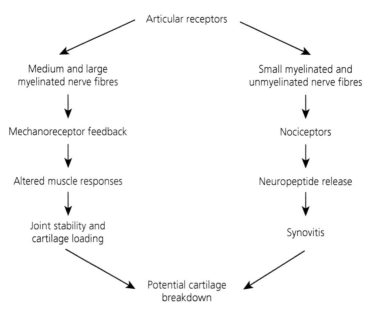

Figure 5.3 Classification of articular receptors.

It has already been mentioned that the knee should be assessed in extension and in a little over 10° of flexion, the latter affording a more precise assessment of the medial structures alone, whereas the former tests the integrity also of the posterior capsule and the cruciate ligaments. A further assessment is carried out with the knee in 90° of flexion. Not only should an abnormal degree of external tibial rotation be noted when performing the anterior drawer test, but also an increase in forward glide of the medial plateau of the tibia will occur if the foot is externally rotated after an initial assessment with the tibia and foot in the neutral position (see Chapter 2).

Pathology

The site of the medial ligament tear can often be identified by palpation and there may be associated bruising after 12–24 hours. Significant disruption of the medial collateral ligament will result in tearing of not only the more superficial tibial collateral portion, but also the deeper, capsular component (Figures 5.4, 5.5). This will allow a suction sign to develop, whereby the increased tilting of the tibia on the femur draws in the soft tissues as the joint opens up abnormally on the medial side (Figure 2.13, p. 22). The leaking of blood from the disrupted capsule will be manifest by loss of the normal haemarthrosis after such injuries. Instead, there will be a boggy ecchymosis medially and valgus stress will cause the inner side to hinge open if the patient is anaesthetized (Figure 5.6).

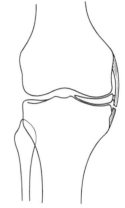

Figure 5.4 The medial ligaments are closely linked anatomically with the medial meniscus.

Treatment

First-degree sprains are treated by the local application of ice, compression and occasionally strapping. Early movement is encouraged by physiotherapy, although pain will prevent a normal range of movement or full weightbearing initially. Associated tears of the medial meniscus or ACL are unlikely, yet it is occasionally necessary to investigate the knee further by means of magnetic resonance (MR) scanning and possibly arthroscopy if an obstructive lesion

Figure 5.5 Magnetic resonance image of a medial collateral ligament tear.

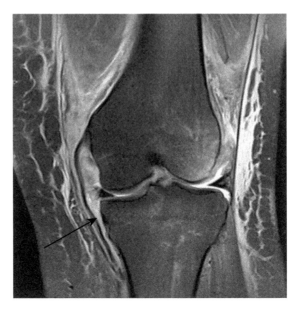

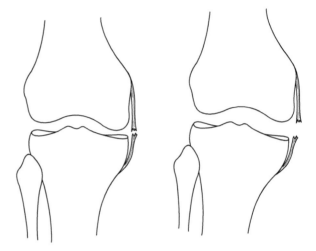

Figure 5.6 Valgus stress will open up the medial side of the knee, dependent on the extent of the soft tissue injury and the degree of protective muscle spasm.

appears to be present. Meniscal tears, chondral flaps and osteoarthritis may impede recovery, and intermittent symptoms may persist for over a year (Azar 2006).

Second-degree tears are treated in similar fashion, although there is a greater incidence of associated injury. Investigation includes the standard biplanar radiographs and MR scanning. An examination under anaesthesia including arthroscopy is often advised in order to assess the pathological valgus laxity and concurrent injuries more accurately. Strapping and protected weightbearing may be helpful for up to 6 weeks, and quadriceps and hamstring drill should be supervised for several months. With time the abnormal laxity should reduce as interstitial healing proceeds; however, a mild degree of residual laxity is common and splintage of the knee in flexion is sometimes advisable during the first 2–4 weeks.

Complete or third-degree tears can be managed conservatively since surgical intervention does not appear to hasten recovery (Indelicato 1983). This applies particularly to tears above the joint line, unless avulsion of the adductor tubercle is present, when reattachment is a relatively simple procedure. In the acute phase, pain limits activity and a 2–4-week period of backshell splintage and protected weightbearing is necessary (Miyamoto *et al.* 2009).

Mid-portion tears of the ligament are more disruptive since the meniscotibial ligament is involved. Magnetic resonance scans and possibly arthroscopy will allow an assessment of the meniscal rim and posteromedial capsule. If the meniscus is stable there is no advantage from surgical repair, but if the meniscus is dislocated a peripheral repair should be attempted (see Chapter 6). Direct suture of the middle or lower thirds of the tibial collateral ligament is ineffectual, although reefing and augmentation with the pes anserinus or a medial strip of patellar tendon has been advocated when associated tears of the ACL merit intervention. In general, medial collateral injury is now managed conservatively unless specific features make surgery advisable. In particular, combined ACL and medial ligament tears provide a relative indication to repair or reconstruct both structures, particularly when valgus laxity in extension persists after ACL reconstruction. However, in women or less athletic individuals there is an increased risk of postoperative stiffness so that medial ligament repair should not be considered (Shelbourne and Basle 1988).

Anterior cruciate ligament tears

Anterior cruciate ligament tears present acutely or chronically, and in the acute lesion the other knee ligaments may be clinically normal. Amis and Scammell (1993) found that anterior displacement of the tibia sufficient to disrupt the ACL leaves the collateral ligaments unstretched, although the posteromedial and posterolateral structures are stretched. Non-contact deceleration and sudden, inward twisting of the knee may also cause 'isolated' ACL rupture, the patient experiencing a popping sensation in approximately half the cases. Hyperflexion with the tibia internally rotated may rupture either or both cruciate ligaments, and forced hyperextension will cause varying degrees of ACL tear (Figure 5.7). Combined injuries occur from impact over the side of the knee; the medial collateral structures are torn, followed by the ACL, which angulates against the lateral femoral condyle. There may be associated meniscal injuries, patellar subluxation, bone bruising and osteochondral fractures.

Immediate examination will reveal anterolateral laxity but later swelling and spasm will obscure this. The Ritchey–Lachman test (see Chapter 2) identifies this laxity more readily than the 90° drawer test since the restraining effect of the posterior meniscal horns is reduced and the collateral structures are relatively lax. In time, the secondary restraints slacken under the increased load, although the knee may compensate so that disabling instability and a positive pivot shift are not invariable. The patient will adapt by using a 'quadriceps-avoidance' gait (Berchuck et al. 1990), reducing anterior movement of the proximal tibia and the magnitude of knee flexion and extension. Kinematic studies show these changes during walking or jogging, but activities employing greater flexion of the knee, such as climbing or descending stairs, are not appreciably affected. Even after surgical reconstruction this altered pattern may persist, similar to the altered gait adopted after the historic operation of pes anserinus transfer (Perry et al. 1980).

Undoubtedly the most disabling symptom experienced by the individual convalescing after ACL rupture is the sense of giving way or buckling, induced unexpectedly when the weightbearing knee is rotated. Concordance between this symptom of instability and a positive pivot shift test is high, although the test may be pronounced negative by the inexperienced examiner and is often difficult to elicit in the conscious patient who actively guards against the subluxation.

The long-term prognosis after ACL rupture is difficult to predict, partly because each patient represents a different combination of aspirations, secondary laxity and morphological features such as leg alignment, lateral tibial contour and muscle tone (Macnicol 1989), and

Figure 5.7 Magnetic resonance image of a torn anterior cruciate ligament.

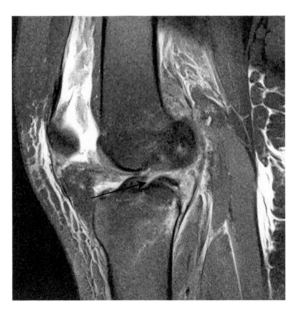

partly because the orthopaedic literature on the subject is conflicting. Most studies are retrospective, including a mix of different patient groups and varying patterns of associated injury. Furthermore, there is still a lack of uniform, preoperative and postoperative grading. If the knee fails to compensate, chronic anterolateral laxity may initiate a remorseless train of events leading to meniscal tears, articular cartilage wear and progressive osteoarthritis (Figures 5.8, 5.9). The radiographic changes include:

- Avulsion, prominence or spurring of the intercondylar spines
- Narrowing of the intercondylar notch
- The Segond fracture (lateral capsular sign) (see Figure 3.3b, p. 39)
- Notching of the lateral femoral condyle posterior to Blumensaat's line (similar to the glenohumeral Hill–Sachs lesion)
- Arthritic change, initially in the lateral compartment.

Although the osteoarthritic process may stabilize the knee, lateral meniscal tears and chondral lesions generally conspire to produce symptoms. If pain persists at times other than when the knee suddenly subluxes, it may be inadvisable to consider surgical reconstruction of the ligament. Arthroscopic intervention should then be limited to meniscal and articular cartilage pathology. However, when pain and effusions are short lived, occurring immediately after the episode of buckling, stabilization of the knee is recommended. Reconstruction has been shown to decrease the incidence of later meniscal tears from approximately 60 per cent to 10 per cent (Balkfors 1982). Meniscal repair is also more likely to succeed although it is still less effective than in the otherwise normal knee (Cannon and Vittori 1992).

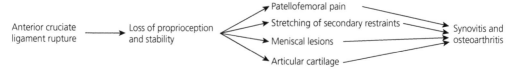

Figure 5.8 Rupture of the anterior cruciate ligament may initiate a remorseless train of events leading to osteoarthritis.

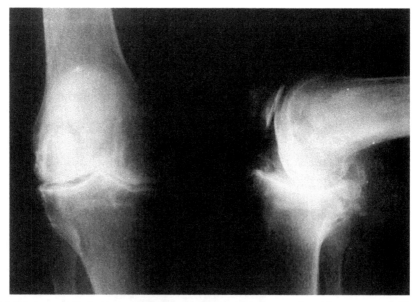

Figure 5.9 A documented anterior cruciate ligament tear 20 years before produced these gross arthritic changes.

The evolution of ACL reconstruction

During the nineteenth century, a number of surgeons recognized the features of ACL rupture and attempted to brace the knee. Bonnet of Lyon published a book in 1845 which described proximal ACL avulsion, haemarthrosis and tibial subluxation, and both he and Stark of Edinburgh (Stark 1850) used hinged braces for the unstable knee. Georges Noulis, a Greek surgeon, published a description of the Lachman test in 1875 and Segond, a French surgeon, published in 1879 the pain, pop and swelling characteristic of ACL rupture, together with the fracture that bears his name (Pässler 1993). Annandale (1885) was the first to record a successful meniscal repair, while Hey-Groves (1917) wrote extensively on the subject of cruciate ligament repair. Attempts with tendon substitutes, fascia lata, the meniscus and black silk were usually only partially satisfactory and the reconstructions tended to stretch with time.

Palmer (1938) and Smillie (1978) published seminal work on the soft tissue injuries involving the knee, and now knee reconstructive surgery is widely practised throughout the world. In 1963, Kenneth Jones published his method of ACL reconstruction using the central third of the patellar ligament. This operation, using tibial and femoral tunnels, has become established as the 'gold standard' procedure. Kurosaka et al. (1987) then reported his technique of graft fixation using screws, allowing the procedure to be undertaken arthroscopically. Fu et al. (2008) developed the principle of anatomical graft placement, whether single bundle or double bundle reconstruction, which provides greater rotational stability.

A bewildering number of retrospective reports dealing with the proposed advantages of ACL repair and reconstruction are only gradually leading to any consensus about the management of this condition, and many of the recommendations remain controversial and poorly researched. However, some of the principal issues will be addressed:

* Is there a convincing reason to repair or reconstruct all acute injuries?
* How does the knee joint function shortly after rupture of the ACL?
* What are the long-term sequelae of an untreated rupture?
* What are the relative indications for chronic reconstruction?
* Is there any evidence to show which form of reconstruction is more likely to succeed?
* What happens to autografts in the long term, and will the knee continue to benefit from surgery after 10 years?
* Is there a place for artificial ligaments and allografts?
* Should extra-articular reinforcement be used to augment the intra-articular graft?
* Is there evidence to suggest that the intra-articular graft should ever be supported with a ligament augmentation device?

These questions raise the issue of the natural history of an untreated ACL rupture. A review of previously published data and reports allows a comparison of the results of non-operative treatment based on physiotherapy, or lack of treatment in undiagnosed cases, with surgical intervention (Engebretsen et al. 1990). Untreated rupture of the ACL causes a subjective feeling of instability that is manifest by episodes of giving way, a sudden buckling of the knee due to pathological translation of the tibia upon the femur and a momentary loss of proprioceptive coordination. This deficiency is less likely in cases of partial rupture or when skeletal alignment and tibial condylar contours contribute to greater intrinsic stability. Abnormally large peak loading and shear stresses act on the articular cartilage, menisci, and the peripheral capsule and ligaments when the pivotal ACL is deficient. Stretching of these secondary restraints leads to the 'ACL syndrome' with cartilage erosion, meniscal tears and anterolateral or complex laxity. Late sequelae include post-meniscectomy or obstructive meniscal degeneration, pathological laxity and progressive osteoarthritis (Woo et al. 2004).

It has also been observed that the absence of the ACL restraint is well tolerated by some patients, who can continue to perform their normal activities and even engage in sports without external support for 20–30 years (Woo *et al.* 2004, 2006a). As already mentioned, this may be due to a less convex lateral tibial condyle, varus alignment, stronger secondary restraints, quadriceps avoidance gait and additional, poorly understood musculoskeletal factors. Other patients remain asymptomatic by modifying their activities and changing to less strenuous forms of recreation. Finally there are patients who do very well with a knee brace and experience no instability problems. It remains unclear whether this asymptomatic, or minimally symptomatic, 'conservative' group will remain free of symptoms or whether subtle pathological translations and rotations will lead to accelerated degenerative articular changes. Classic studies, of which there are still far too few, provide some insight into this question (Frobell *et al.* 2010). Patient selection would be of most value if it was possible to select as surgical candidates the 'at-risk' group that will suffer objectively and subjectively from cruciate ligament insufficiency. Surgery, and its potential complications, could be avoided in those individuals who will enjoy normal knee function despite an ACL-deficient knee (Drogset *et al.* 2006; Woo *et al.* 2006a). Progression is more likely to occur when the following criteria are present (Roos *et al.* 1995; Woo *et al.* 2006b):

* Younger patient
* Heavy manual employment or strenuous sports activity with high demands in terms of joint performance, and an inability or refusal to modify activities
* Pre-existing meniscal and cartilage lesions exacerbating instability episodes
* Continuing difficulties with activities of normal living, recurrent swelling, and instability after 6 months of intensive rehabilitation
* Previous ACL rupture in the opposite knee with the same decompensation.

Conservative treatment is more applicable in:

* Patients over 45 years of age
* Less active patients with a sedentary job.

If both patient and physician are initially reluctant to proceed with surgery, the development of a meniscal tear will promote the need for combined meniscal repair and joint stabilization (Macnicol 1992).

Acute intervention

Acute ACL rupture is usually associated with a varying degree of injury to other ligaments of the knee, the menisci, or both structures. In combination with collateral ligament ruptures it further compromises stability (Laprade *et al.* 2004). Consequently, a direct correlation has been suggested between the complexity of the injuries associated with ACL rupture and the need for surgical repair or reconstruction. In contrast, patients without associated ligamentous or meniscal injuries (those having 'isolated' ACL ruptures) are assumed to have a better prognosis since the secondary restraints protect autogenous or allogenic grafts which inevitably weaken in the early postoperative period due to tissue necrosis, revascularization, and remodelling. The ultimate load to failure of patellar tendon autograft has been shown to be 53 per cent of the original insertion strength at 3 months following implantation, 52 per cent at 6 months, 81 per cent at 9 months and 81 per cent at 12 months (Woo *et al.* 2006a).

In children and adolescents, reattachment of the ACL is sometimes appropriate (see Chapter 4), particularly those cases of intercondylar eminence avulsion where the fragment is otherwise irreducible (see Figure 4.34, p. 82). If the growth plate is open, surgical procedures through the physis should be avoided unless the child is within a year or two of maturity, when carefully drilled tunnels, filled completely with the autogenous graft, and an avoidance of metal implants crossing the physes, reduce the risk of premature growth arrest (Gaulrapp and Haus 2006).

Acute ACL reconstruction is also indicated in patients with an associated grade III collateral ligament rupture or with a repairable meniscal tear. Where osteochondral fracture or major, multidirectional laxity is encountered, early surgical intervention may be justifiable but an increased risk of stiffness from fibrosis has been reported (Sgaghone *et al.* 1993) so that there is a strong case for waiting a few weeks until the acute haemarthrosis has resorbed (Shelbourne *et al.* 1991). Partial ACL ruptures are generally more significantly torn than may appear on the MR scan or arthroscopic probing, but a conservative approach with surgical follow-up is appropriate as a trial period in all but the top-level athlete. The morbidity from surgery should never be minimized (Sandberg *et al.* 1987).

Indications for chronic reconstruction

A conservative approach is justifiable initially after arthroscopy or MR scanning has confirmed the presence of a chronic ACL deficiency. However, the therapeutic effect of exercise and of bracing is often short lived or unacceptable (see Chapter 10) so the patient returns later, stating that the knee is still troublesome. Motivation and general fitness are important attributes if the reconstruction is to succeed in the chronic situation. The physiotherapist who has been treating the patient is therefore an important and perceptive ally in reaching the correct decision about late surgical intervention.

Timing of surgery

Meniscal repair is known to be more effective when undertaken within a few weeks of the injury (Meunier *et al.* 2007; Steenbrugge *et al.* 2004). If a non-operative approach is elected at the initial consultation, early arthroscopy should be considered to exclude a meniscal detachment and to confirm the findings on MR scanning.

If a meniscal repair is deemed to be necessary, cruciate ligament reconstruction is obligatory since residual instability reduces the prospect for successful healing and salvage of the meniscus. In the acute stage, when the articular cartilage is still intact, the result of ACL reconstruction and meniscal repair, in term of joint function and stability, is better than in the chronic stage, although acute cases may require later manipulation under anaesthesia and arthroscopy to release adhesions (DeHaven *et al.* 2003).

This reinforces the decision to postpone surgery for an acute cruciate tear combined with a medial collateral ligament rupture by 4–6 weeks. The patient then recovers from the post-traumatic knee inflammatory reaction and stiffness, lowering the risk of adhesions and postoperative manipulation (Woo *et al.* 2006b). The patient whose knee still feels unstable after a conservative trial and is unhappy with athletic restrictions will generally request surgery, although this decision may be delayed for some time by the unconvinced patient. The perceived instability is most likely with activities that involve deceleration, acceleration, and cutting or side-stepping, so the decision belongs to the patient. A more compelling indication is the patient whose knee gives way unexpectedly during everyday activities such as crossing a road or negotiating stairs. Some authors are also concerned that vigorous strengthening programmes run the risk, with time, of damaging other structures in the knee (Li *et al.* 1996; Halinen *et al.* 2006).

■ Indications for surgery

In addressing this question, all the structures that contribute to stability of the joint have to be considered: the ACL itself, the menisci, and the peripheral restraints (Woo *et al.* 2006b). There is no question about the need to preserve meniscal tissue, which forms both a stabilizing wedge interposed between the femoral condyle and tibial plateau posteriorly (Laprade *et al.* 2007) and an additional 'hoop restraint' effect circumferentially. The preservation of this peripheral fibrous ring also supports the collateral structures. Laxity from rupture of the collateral ligament and capsule is minimized in the acute stage if the ACL is reconstructed, permitting postoperative physiotherapy. Cast immobilization can then be avoided (Halinen *et al.* 2006).

In addition, any coexisting meniscal tear (part of the 'unhappy triad' pattern) is repaired. A lateral-posterolateral complex ligamentous tear merits a meticulous apposition of all stabilizing structures although chronic global anterior laxity, with pronounced anteromedial and anterolateral displacement of the tibial plateau, is a very difficult surgical proposition. It is unlikely that reconstruction of the ACL (central pivot) alone, an extra-articular repair alone, or even their combination, will correct the complex laxity fully, so the debate continues (Woo *et al.* 2006a).

■ Method of reconstruction

Probably the key issue here is what provides adequate structural stabilization following an ACL reconstruction: is it the graft, is it the augmentation if present, or is it the overall mass of scar tissue that occupies the intercondylar notch? It is common during follow-up arthroscopy at about 1 year to find a scar that starts anterosuperiorly, where the synovial plica normally attaches. This is not the expected, gleaming cruciate ligament with its constituent bundles. More deeply, the graft may indeed be attached at the anatomically correct 'isometric' sites corresponding to surgical intention, but the functionally important scar fibres influence the traditional concept of isometry (DeHaven *et al.* 2003). It is reasonable to assume that a strong, accurately placed graft offers the best prospect for the development of a sound substitute ligament. Bathed by synovial fluid, the autograft becomes revascularized at a variable rate. A graft attached by bone blocks inserted into osseous tunnels revascularizes in 6–10 months, which is more rapid than the synovialization and revascularization of a graft that has been sutured directly to the bone or anchored within a tunnel (Woo *et al.* 2006b; Poolman *et al.* 2007).

In acute reconstruction a double semitendinosus graft appears to give as much stability as the patellar tendon central one third, despite its relative initial weakness (Figure 5.10). In chronic reconstruction the bone-patellar tendon-bone autograft is looked on as the gold standard, although its advantage over hamstring grafting is not clear cut (Marder *et al.* 1991; Aglietti *et al.* 1992). The 2-year results are similar apart from greater donor site morbidity with patellar tendon harvesting. Patellar symptoms complicate the use of the patellar graft more frequently than with semitendinosus (Sachs *et al.* 1989), although the strength of fixation of the former may be greater. By 8 weeks in the goat model, failure of the graft shifts from its site of attachment to the mid-substance of the tissue (Holden *et al.* 1988). Clancy *et al.* (1981) showed in rhesus monkeys that the graft remained weak for at least a year, and recent clinical studies confirm that laxity usually persists to some degree. Double bundle grafts provide superior rotational stability compared with single bundle reconstruction techniques and quadruple hamstring grafts are increasingly promoted (Fu *et al.* 2008). Whatever graft is chosen, it is essential that the placement of the tendons is as isometric as possible, paying particular attention to the tibial and femoral attachments of the natural ACL (Figure 5.11).

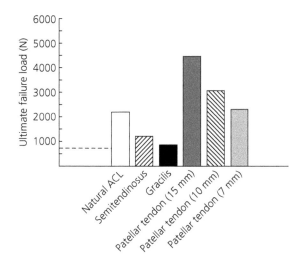

Figure 5.10 The strength of anterior cruciate ligament (ACL) substitutes. The dotted line indicates the maximum strength of graft fixation initially.

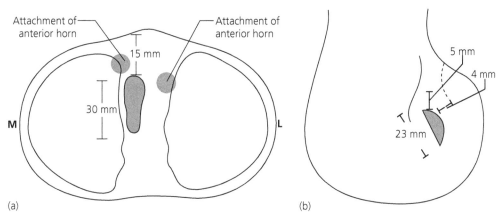

(a)　　　　　　　　　　　　　　　　(b)

Figure 5.11 Placement of the substitute ligament can never be entirely isometric, but anatomical insertion should be mimicked as closely as possible. (a) The 'footprint' attachment of the anterior cruciate ligament to the proximal tibia viewed from above. (b) The equally broad attachment of the ligament to the medial surface of the lateral femoral condyle anteroinferior to the posterior femoral notch (right knee).

■ Operative details

Systematic arthroscopic examination of the knee allows careful inspection of the status of all intra-articular structures. A high-flow superomedial inflow cannula is established, followed by placement of the arthroscope through a standard inferolateral portal. Both inferomedial and inferolateral portals may be placed within the margins of an existing skin incision. The articular surfaces, patellar mechanism, and both menisci should be visualized, probed and their integrity documented in the operative note. The ACL and posterior cruciate ligament (PCL) are inspected and probed both at resting length and under tension (Figure 5.12). Associated

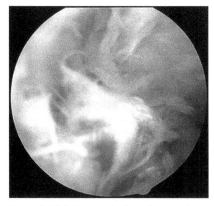

Figure 5.12 Arthroscopic view of a completely torn anterior cruciate ligament.

injuries amenable to arthroscopic treatment are treated before addressing the ligamentous reconstruction (DeHaven *et al.* 2003). The MR scan details are carefully compared to the arthroscopic findings. Intra-articular meniscal suture placement (see Chapter 6) is easier while the knee is unstable, and before notchplasty and osseous tunnel drilling cause significant intra-articular bleeding. Likewise, damage to the articular cartilage is documented and treated prior to insertion of the ACL graft (Meunier *et al.* 2007).

The stump of the ACL is debrided with a full-radius shaver and the ligamentum mucosum excised to provide enhanced visualization. The fat pad and synovium overlying the PCL are protected as they will offer nutritional support for the inserted graft. The notchplasty begins with debridement of the soft tissue and periosteum from the lateral wall of the notch. The entire surface of the lateral wall is uniformly debrided. Some bleeding may be encountered at this point and should be controlled with electrocautery, inflation of the tourniquet or both. Sufficient hydrostatic pressure via gravity inflow irrigation or infusion pump minimizes undesired intra-articular bleeding. Once the notch is visualized, the surgeon can identify the extent of osseous notchplasty that will be necessary. There is no consensus as to what constitutes an indication for the notchplasty size (Pässler and Höher 2004). However, notchplasty is indicated where there is difficulty visualizing the femoral attachment and when graft impingement occurs against either the lateral femoral condyle or the roof of the notch.

An osseous notchplasty is more frequently needed in the chronic ACL-deficient knee when osteophyte formation and encroachment are evident at the articular margin of the anterior notch. If the notch requires significant widening, a curved osteotome may be introduced through the medial portal to remove the anterior-inferior bone. Large bone fragments should be removed with a grasper. Minimal articular cartilage removal is desirable. Additional bone resection can often be carried out with the full-radius shaver or burr. Regardless of the technique used, the surgeon should not mistake the so-called 'resident's ridge' for the posterior margins of the notch. This slightly more stenotic region of the intercondylar notch often deceives the less experienced surgeon into believing the over-the-top position has been reached. The error in landmark selection may cause the femoral tunnel to be placed more anteriorly than desired (Garofalo *et al.* 2007).

In the selection of ideal osseous tunnels the relationship of the intercondylar notch to the ACL graft is critical. Proper graft positioning will allow full extension and prevent impingement. The normal ACL is composed of a large number of fibres. Each fibre differs in length, has a different origin and insertion, and is under varying tension during the full range of motion of the knee. In contrast, the graft replacing the ACL will have parallel fibres. Even with optimal positioning of the osseous tunnels, the fibres of the graft will undergo length and tension changes throughout the range of motion. Although the ACL replacement will therefore not duplicate the original ligament, placing the centre of the osseous tunnels at the most isometric points will maximize efficiency (Figure 5.13).

The selection point for the centre of the osseous tunnel requires an accurate view of the over-the-top position and superolateral aspect of the intercondylar notch (Musahl *et al.* 2005). Flexing the knee to 70° or more enhances the visualization of both these landmarks and aids in preparation of the femoral osseous tunnel. If femoral interference screw fixation is desired, the selection of the femoral tunnel site should reproducibly result in an osseous tunnel with a 1–2 mm thick posterior cortical wall. This provides a posterior buttress for interference screw fixation and protects the posterior vessels and nerves. A placement guide keys off the over-the-top position but the surgeon must still adjust the rotation of the drill guide to place it in the axilla of the notch. The centre of the selected femoral tunnel site is then marked with a guidewire. This point is verified visually and with a probe to confirm the correct distance from the over-the-top position. Selecting the correct tibial tunnel site is important for appropriate

Figure 5.13 A schematic drawing of the ideal tunnel placements, viewed from the side (a), from the front (b) and with the anterior cruciate ligament graft being introduced (c).

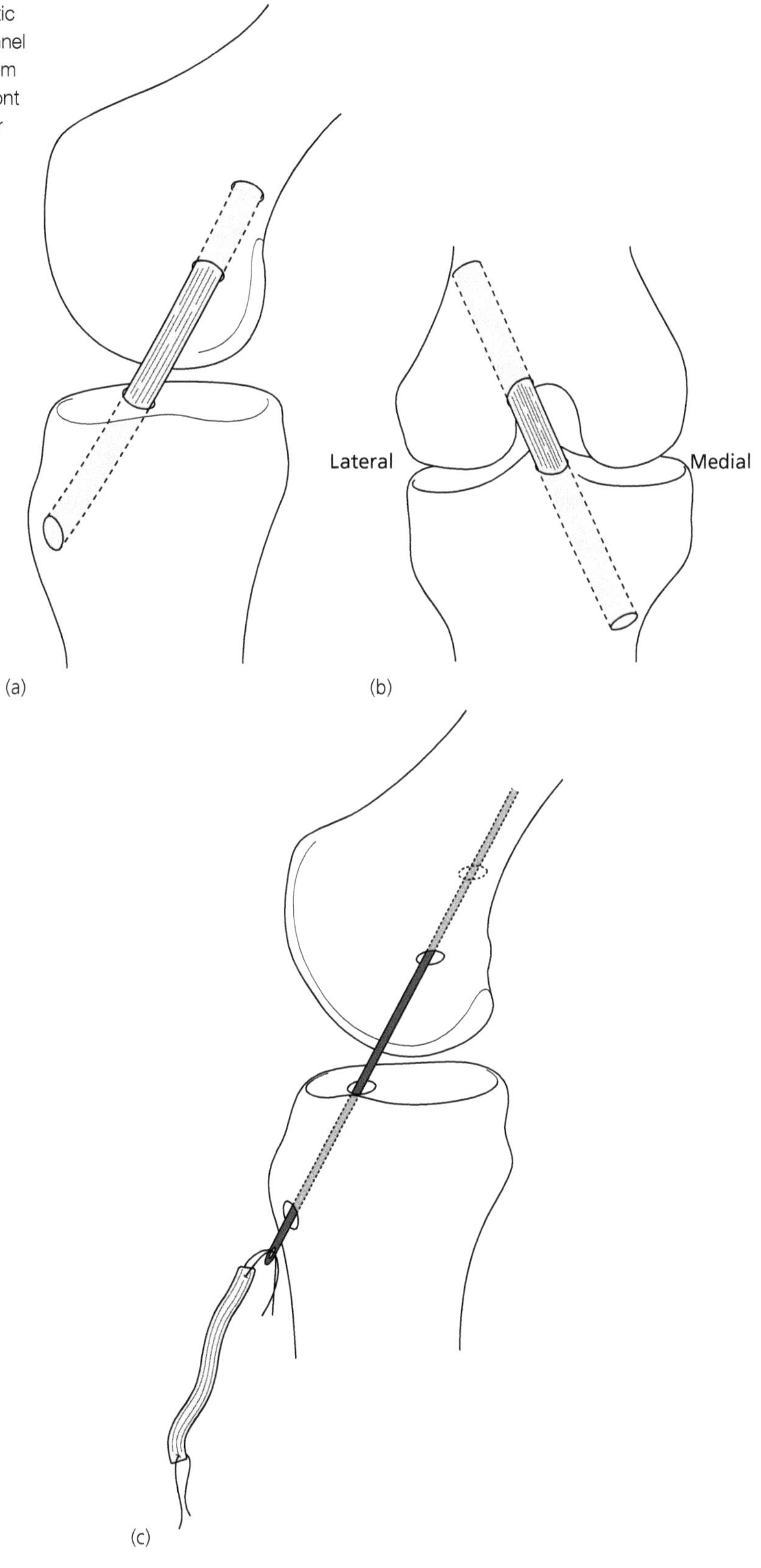

Lateral

Medial

(a)

(b)

(c)

tunnel length and angulation, which in turn affects graft fixation and potential impingement and abrasion. The recommended position for graft placement has moved posteriorly as ACL reconstructive surgery has evolved (Pässler and Höher 2004; Fu *et al.* 2008). The current recommendation is to locate the centre of the tibial tunnel just posterior to the anatomical centre of the ACL tibial footprint. Four consistent anatomical landmarks are used to locate the tibial tunnel centre: the anterior horn of the lateral meniscus, the medial tibial spine, the PCL, and the ACL stump. The anteroposterior centre of the tibial tunnel is located by extending a line in continuity with the inner edge of the anterior horn of the lateral meniscus. This point is consistently located 6–7 mm anterior to the anterior border of the PCL attachment (Musahl *et al.* 2005).

The mediolateral (coronal plane) placement of the tunnel centre should correspond to the depression medial to the medial tibial spine in the centre of the ACL stump. This tunnel placement should allow the ACL graft, once in place, to touch the lateral aspect of the PCL but not be significantly angulated by it. Similarly, it should neither abrade nor impinge against the medial aspect of the lateral femoral condyle or the roof of the intercondylar notch in extension. With the tunnel centre chosen, the knee is flexed 90°, and the tip of the tibial drill guide is placed into position through the medial infrapatellar portal. The skin incision is retracted medially and distally while the drill sleeve is placed against the tibial cortex, medial to the tubercle. The drill guide length is set to the calculated length, and a guidewire is drilled into place. Visualization of the tip of the guidewire as it enters the joint allows adjustments in pin location. It is important to realize that the residual ACL stump may deceive the surgeon into believing the guidewire is more posterior than it actually is. Because of the 50° to 60° angle with which the wire penetrates the plateau, the entry point is actually 2–3 mm anterior to where the tip is first visualized. Careful confirmation as the pin enters the joint or removal of an adequate amount of the ACL remnant helps minimize this source of error.

As the drill is advanced, a curette or curved artery forceps may be used to prevent proximal migration of the guidewire, as well as accidental plunging of the drill bit into the joint. The tibial tunnel is then plugged to preserve joint distension while a shaver is used to remove any debris and to chamfer the tunnel edges. Residual tissue anterior to the graft exit site or roof impingement is believed to contribute to formation of a postoperative 'cyclops lesion' (DeHaven *et al.* 2003). Thus, it is important to remove debris from the tunnel edges anteriorly as well as posteriorly. If the tibial tunnel ends up too far anteriorly, a femoral drill bit or a burr placed through the tibial tunnel can be used to move the entrance posteriorly. With the tibial tunnel drilled and posterior edge chamfered, the femoral tunnel can be prepared. The knee is flexed 70°, the guidewire placed in the pre-marked position through the tibial tunnel and then advanced only 10–15 mm. A calibrated cannulated drill is inserted over the wire by hand until it engages the lateral wall of the intercondylar notch. Care should be taken to prevent damage to the PCL while the drill is being advanced. The power reamer is attached, and the tunnel is reamed to the desired depth.

Next, a pin is advanced through both tunnels with the knee flexed to between 90° and 110°. The pin contains an eyelet that will be threaded with the graft's sutures for passage. It is drilled out from the anterolateral thigh under power. To assist the drill's emergence, the flat edge of a metallic instrument can be placed just proximal to the exit point as the drill bit tents the skin. A drill puller may then be placed over the tip to stabilize the drill, cover the sharp tip and pass the sutures across the joint. Care must be taken to maintain knee flexion at the same angle to prevent bending or breaking the pin.

The surgeon threads the patellar bone plug suture through the eyelet of the pin. One assistant must hold the graft and the remaining tibial plug sutures, while also preventing the nylon suture from being pulled out of the patellar plug. This is easily achieved by pinching together both sides of the nylon suture as it emerges from the drill hole for the patellar plug. The drill puller is drawn proximally until the nylon suture exits the skin over the anterolateral thigh. A haemostat is attached to both free ends of the suture to pull the graft into the tibial tunnel.

Under arthroscopic visualization, the graft is passed into the femoral tunnel with cephalad traction on the proximal suture. The cancellous surface is placed anterolaterally so that the collagen fibres of the new ligament are posterior in the femoral tunnel. A haemostat may be placed through the inferomedial portal to help the proximal plug past the PCL and properly orientate the graft in the femoral tunnel. The graft is fully seated when the junction of the bone plug and ligament, marked earlier with a pen, is visualized at the tunnel mouth (Figure 5.14). The distal plug is rotated 90° externally so that the cancellous bone surface is posterior in the tibial tunnel. However, if the graft should impinge, the tibial bone plug may be rotated, a larger notchplasty performed or the tibial tunnel shifted posteriorly (Poolman *et al.* 2007).

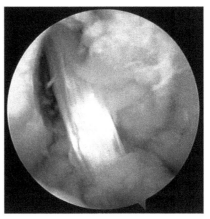

Figure 5.14 Anterior cruciate ligament graft in place.

Cannulated interference screws have the advantages of providing one of the highest initial fixation strengths attainable. They do not require additional drilling nor do they depend upon potentially weak sutures or knots. The screws are completely contained within bone (Kaeding *et al.* 2005), which reduces the incidence of local irritation due to prominent implants. The femoral interference screw is placed first. The guidewire is inserted into the anterolateral notch created earlier in the femoral tunnel. This will position the screw against the cancellous side of the plug, away from the collagen fibres. The guidewire is placed during graft passage and advanced as the femoral plug is seated. Once the screwdriver and wire have been removed, distal traction of approximately 18 kg (40 lb) is applied to the three sutures in the tibial bone plug to test the femoral fixation under arthroscopic visualization. Should anchorage prove inadequate, another screw placement may be attempted. If stable fixation cannot be obtained or if the posterior cortex has been violated, proximal fixation may be obtained with additional sutures placed in the bone plug and tied to the lateral femoral screw. This requires a lateral femoral incision and femoral tunnel drilling using a rear entry drill guide.

An alternative is to use an endoscopic button, which may be placed arthroscopically over the lateral femoral cortex through a small diameter drill hole (Oh *et al.* 2006). This is similar to the endoscopic fixation used for hamstring tendon ACL reconstructions. The knee is then cycled 5–10 times through a full range of motion with the graft under tension. This will confirm the femoral fixation and allows an estimation of the excursion of the tibial bone plug within the tibial tunnel. Although true isometry is not possible with a linear, cylindrical graft, less than 2 mm excursion of the tibial plug is usual (Yonetani *et al.* 2005). More than 2 mm excursion suggests inadequate proximal fixation, injury to the graft, or poor selection of the femoral tunnel site. As the length of the graft is greatest during extension, the tibial interference screw is placed when the knee is positioned between near-extension and 20° of flexion (Kaeding *et al.* 2005).

Both autografts and allografts go through a predictable sequence of stages after implantation. Initially, a fairly rapid loss of cellularity occurs, before the graft is repopulated with cells from local and distant sources. This response is poorly understood but may be related to loss of vascularity, innervation or both. Allograft acellularity may, in addition, be due to an immunological reaction. After a period of cellular decline, the graft enters a healing phase, a process referred to as 'ligamentization'. Since such grafts are abnormal mechanically, they are not truly ligamentized in a functional sense. Four stages of ligamentization of autografts have been described. Repopulation with fibroblasts occurs over the first 2 months, with the graft being viable as early as 3 weeks after implantation. Over the next 10 months rapid remodelling occurs, with more fibroblasts, neovascularity and a reduction in mature collagen. Over the next 2 years the collagen matures so that by 3 years the graft appears to be ligamentous histologically (Woo *et al.* 2006a).

■ Principles of rehabilitation

Progression of the rehabilitation should be based on careful monitoring of functional status. Early emphasis is placed on achieving full hyperextension, equal to the opposite side. Passive and active ranges of motion are allowed as tolerated. Full weightbearing can occur as soon as tolerated and controlled exercises may be performed without the use of a brace. The patient should be made aware that healing and tissue maturation continue to take place for a year after surgery, usually once the skin scar changes from pink to white. For further information about rehabilitation, see Chapters 10 and 11.

■ Long-term benefits of reconstruction

Any improvement in knee stability must be set against the complications and failures of ligament reconstruction. In addition to graft rupture (partial or complete), loss of movement, effusions, wound infection and septic arthritis, patellar symptoms, tenderness at tunnel sites and over metal implants, and muscle hernia are recognized problems. Reviews of the results of ACL reconstruction are rarely sufficiently extensive in time and detail (Johnson *et al.* 1984) since remodelling of the graft is very slow. The inserted tissue is known to remain mechanically inferior for several years (Ballock *et al.* 1989) and is dependent on the avoidance of impingement by ensuring correct placement (Figure 5.15), physiological loading and adequate revascularization for its survival. Impingement between the graft and the femur in extension (Howell and Taylor 1993), loss of fixation and an inadequate return of proprioception imperil the graft throughout the first few years of function. Thereafter, a low grade synovitis, particularly from breakdown products, may promote the very degenerative changes that the procedure is designed to prevent.

As yet there is no clear answer to the question about long-term benefits. Stability may be gained effectively in the short to medium term, with a return to sport at high level, but the eventual outcome is unknown compared with the natural history. Proprioception never recovers to the level of the normal knee before injury. It is to be hoped that clinical reviews in the next few years will address these issues, although comparative prospective, longitudinal studies are likely to be rare. Osteoarthritis progresses with time and later meniscal or graft malfunction require recognition and responsible management (Aït *et al.* 2006).

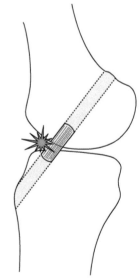

Figure 5.15 If the graft is placed too anteriorly, with the tibial tunnel anterior to the slope of the intercondylar roof, impingement during extension will lead to restricted movement and possible rupture of the graft.

Alternatives to autografting

The interest in artificial ligaments has waned as longer-term results have revealed that rupture of the prosthesis is relatively common, if not inevitable. Artificial fibres that have been used include:

- A ligament in its own right (prostheses such as the Stryker Dacron polyester, or ABC ligament, a composite of Dacron and carbon fibre yarns)
- An augmentation device offering temporary support (Kennedy polypropylene LAD)
- A scaffold to encourage a neoligament to form (Leeds-Keio open weave polyester device) (Figure 5.16a).

The advantages of prosthetic replacement were obvious. The operation was relatively quick and the grafts were easy to handle, no morbidity from graft harvesting accrued (unless the ligament augmentation device was used) and contamination was not a concern. Acceptable results at a mean of 3 years were reported (Dahlstedt *et al.* 1990; Macnicol *et al.* 1991) and over a longer period (Murray and Macnicol 2004), although the presence of synovitis locally in relation to breakdown products and exposed polyester was a concern (Figure 5.16b). Nearly all of these artificial substitutes have been withdrawn from the market. At present, synthetic ligaments should be restricted to further reconstruction for failed autogenous grafts, and perhaps as a primary procedure in the patient who is unlikely to place much demand on the knee.

Allograft replacement offers many advantages if the graft can be harvested and stored safely (Kuhn and Ross 2007; West and Harner 2005). Ethylene oxide sterilization is now avoided since the ethylene glycol elicits a foreign body response. So contamination must be prevented, avoiding donors who have had viral infection such as hepatitis, acquired immune deficiency syndrome, multiple sclerosis or Creutzfeldt–Jakob disease. The Achilles, tibialis anterior, peroneal and toe flexor tendons are appropriate and should be stored at −80 °C. Fresh frozen grafts are preferred to freeze-dried tissue which may be more antigenic. Secondary sterilization by gamma irradiation (25 000 Gy) is also recommended (Henson *et al.* 2009; Lattermann and Romine 2009). Both this and freezing cause the allograft to stretch under load, perhaps to a greater degree than with autografts, although both types are subjected to the same biological process of necrosis, revascularization and remodelling (Cabaud *et al.* 1980; Shino *et al.* 1984).

Biological artificial ligaments, perhaps made of processed collagen, or allografts may achieve a more defined role in knee ligament surgery in the future. They are indicated when there is a lack of available autogenous tissue, particularly in revisions, and possibly in the older patient. Where harvesting a strip of patellar tendon appears unwise owing to patellofemoral pathology, or malalignment, then there may again be a relative indication to avoid autogenous grafting.

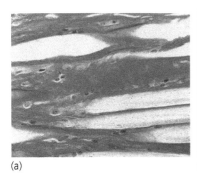 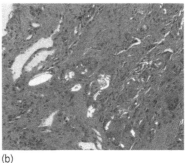

(a)   (b)

Figure 5.16 Although collagen fibres may form along the strands of the artificial ligament (a), wear particles within the knee initiate an inflammatory response and the release of injurious enzymes (b).

◼ Additional extra-articular grafting

Noyes and Barber (1991) considered that a combined intra-articular and lateral iliotibial band extra-articular procedure produced better functional results in chronic anterior cruciate deficiency than an intra-articular procedure alone. This was using allografts, but with autografts the consensus is that the addition of an extra-articular reconstruction, even in chronic and marked laxity, confers no definite benefit (Larson 1993). A biomechanical study in human cadavers confirmed this impression (Amis and Scammell 1993) and there is a risk that associated posterolateral laxity may become symptomatic.

Extra-articular procedures alone tend to slacken unacceptably and there seems to be little difference clinically between proximal (MacIntosh and Darby 1976) or distal (Ellison 1979) substitutions (Carson 1988). However, in patients with relatively low athletic demands, the lateral sling may be sufficient and avoids the risks associated with intra-articular surgery. Symptoms from the unphysiological positioning of the lateral band are, however, common (O'Brien *et al.* 1991) and may outweigh the stabilizing effect. Where chronic laxity is multidirectional, the procedure may also worsen the component of posterolateral laxity which may not be fully appreciated preoperatively.

Posterior cruciate ligament tears

Rupture of the PCL may occur in isolation or in combination with other components of the knee (Figure 5.17). In chronic laxity the arcuate complex will stretch and posterolateral laxity becomes more obvious, followed by eventual laxity of the medial restraints. The mechanisms of injury include:

- A blow to the front of the flexed knee which drives the proximal tibia backwards, a relatively common occurrence in road traffic collisions and football tackles (the foot is usually fixed)
- Forced flexion of the knee, particularly if a load is applied to the body from above or the foot is plantar flexed

Figure 5.17 Magnetic resonance image of a posterior cruciate ligament rupture.

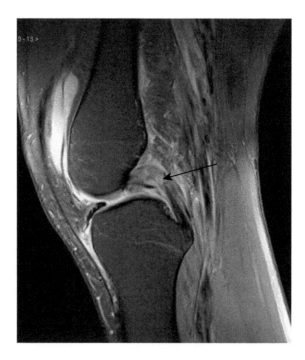

- Hyperextension of the knee which, after tearing the ACL, will disrupt the PCL
- Major angulatory, rotational or distraction forces which effectively produce dislocation of the joint.

Trickey (1968) reported that the ligament was most commonly avulsed from the tibial attachment, and certainly this is both the more likely site of the injury in the child and adolescent, and the most amenable to repair. However, so many cases of PCL rupture are neither diagnosed nor fully investigated that the incidence of tears at different levels is not accurately known; Insall (1984) suggests that upper, middle and lower third tears or avulsions occur in equal frequency. The PCL is ruptured relatively infrequently in sports injuries, and is more likely in soccer or rugby players than in skiers (Jakob 1992). Since ACL rupture is 5–10 times more common it constitutes a reason for surgical intervention much more regularly. The tests for cruciate and posterolateral laxity have been presented in Chapter 2 and further modifications have been described (Jakob 1992). The problem relates to the daunting extent of the subsequent surgery, if that is felt to be indicated.

■ Surgical treatment

After acute rupture the clinical tests of a posterior drawer sign, tibial drop-back and posterior shift (active and passive) of the lateral plateau are usually evident. Sometimes the signs may be hard to elicit (Hughston 1988), possibly because the arcuate complex is intact, and popliteal tenderness is not always evident, particularly in cases of femoral avulsion. A haemarthrosis, and restricted and painful flexion, should alert the examiner to the possibility of PCL injury which can be confirmed by MR scan or arthroscopy using the 70° telescope. The posterior and mid-portions of the PCL are readily visualized, particularly through a central portal, although synovitis and haemorrhage may obscure the view. A posterolateral portal affords good access to all but the femoral attachment of the ligament (Stannard *et al.* 2005).

Surgical reattachment of the ligament is advisable for ruptures less than 4–6 weeks old, particularly tibial bone avulsions (Trickey 1968, 1980). The ligament should heal well in its vascular, retrosynovial site, whether there is bone avulsion or not (see Chapter 4). With mid-substance tears, reconstruction with semitendinosus or a strip of patellar tendon should be considered if posterior laxity exceeds the contralateral knee by more than 10 mm in association with persistent symptoms. Partial tears of the PCL, with intact ligaments of Wrisberg and Humphry, may allow the knee to compensate by quadriceps tone, so that acute intervention is unwarranted (Fanelli 2008).

Access to the femoral attachment is through an anteromedial or longitudinal anterior incision. By means of a special tibial guide and a front-to-back bone tunnel the posterior insertion can be reached. Equally, the tibial end can be reached through a popliteal incision, carefully reflecting one or other head of the gastrocnemius and incising the oblique popliteal ligament and capsule. Complex laxity, involving the posterolateral and posteromedial corners of the knee, may require reattachment of the popliteus and the biceps tendons, since these retract. The arcuate complex should be reefed proximally (Trillat 1978) and the posteromedial capsule tightened distally. It is important to correct varus laxity as much as possible, and the knee should be splinted in extension to prevent tibial sag postoperatively.

Unfortunately bracing of the knee fails to control posterior subluxation so that when fixed splintage is discontinued at 3–6 weeks, laxity may rapidly recur. Ligament augmentation with artificial fibres is therefore recommended, although this does not guarantee protection of the graft and breakdown products may produce a local synovitis later. The use of a patello-tibial Steinmann pin to prevent postoperative tibial dropback ('olecranization') is not recommended as it cannot be left safely *in situ*.

The late results of posterior cruciate reconstruction are relatively disappointing for acute mid-substance, complex and late-diagnosed tears. But the principle of early restoration of ligament integrity should not be forgotten, confirmed by the satisfactory results of early intervention (Clancy *et al.* 1983). Degenerative changes correlate with the degree of residual laxity (Torg *et al.* 1989) and, in the athlete particularly, surgical intervention is warranted. Many surgeons, however, remain unconvinced that the PCL tear should be managed operatively. More recent opinion about arthroscopic versus the inlay method of posterior cruciate reconstruction is briefly discussed towards the end of Chapter 4.

Lateral ligament complex injuries

The lateral structures of the knee which work together to stabilize the joint include the fibular collateral ligament, fascia lata, the popliteus muscle and tendon, the biceps femoris muscle, the lateral head of gastrocnemius, and the arcuate ligament. If the structures are disrupted, it is usual for the common peroneal nerve to be injured as it will also be stretched, and unfortunately the recovery after this traction injury to the nerve is minimal. It is difficult to distinguish which of the various lateral structures are principally injured, but in addition to varus laxity the knee may hyperextend and externally rotate if the leg is held by the toe or heel with the patient lying supine (see also Chapter 2; Figure 2.23 p. 29).

This posterolateral instability can occur with an intact fascia lata, and the usual structures injured primarily are the fibular collateral ligament (Figure 5.18), the popliteus tendon and the arcuate complex (Figures 1.16 and 1.17, p. 6). It is difficult clinically to distinguish posterolateral laxity from the hyperextension that occurs after the PCL, and possibly the posterior capsule, have torn. If all posterior structures are ruptured, the medial tibial condyle, in addition to the lateral tibial condyle, subluxes posteriorly and radio-opaque markers on both medial and lateral sides of the joint may help to differentiate between posterior and posterolateral laxity (Levy *et al.* 2010).

Posterolateral laxity is best detected with the knee in 30° of flexion. If there is posterior subluxation of the tibia when the knee is 90° flexed, then the PCL is probably also compromised. The reverse pivot shift test (Jakob *et al.* 1981) is more likely to be positive than Hughston's

Figure 5.18 Magnetic resonance image of a lateral collateral ligament rupture.

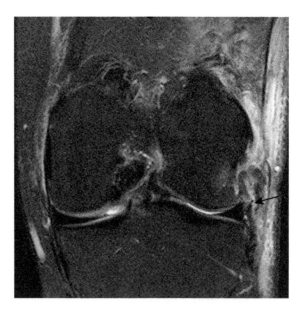

external rotation recurvatum test (Hughston and Norwood 1980), the posteriorly subluxed lateral tibial condyle reducing as the flexed knee is extended with the tibia externally rotated. Anterolateral and posterolateral laxity may coexist and are not necessarily symptomatic.

■ Treatment

Lateral ligament complex tears are symptomatic, the patient experiencing both instability and pain when standing. It is essential to repair or reattach the biceps tendon and the fascia lata as they will retract rapidly after injury. The fibular collateral ligament and the popliteus tendon attachment to the femoral condyle can be advanced anterosuperiorly, using a segment of bone incorporating their insertion to ensure an adequate reattachment. If the arcuate ligament is well defined, this can be reefed additionally. Therefore, early repair is usually advisable and should secure a satisfactory result.

The complexities of surgical reconstruction for chronic posterolateral instability are beyond the scope of this book. Conservative management, emphasizing biceps and popliteus exercises, are more likely to succeed in the knee that presents with valgus alignment. When the laxity coexists with varus, surgical reefing of the posterolateral structures (Trillat 1978; Hughston and Jacobson 1985) may have to be combined with a proximal tibial valgising osteotomy. A ligament augmentation device or free autogenous graft may be necessary to bolster the reconstruction, and the extent of posterior cruciate insufficiency should be judged at surgery, although cruciate reconstruction is usually unnecessary.

Iiotibial band friction syndrome

A less devastating but chronically troublesome injury affecting the lateral side of the knee is the iliotibial band friction syndrome. The fascia lata inserts into the patella, the proximal tibia at Gerdy's tubercle and the biceps femoris tendon (see Figure 10.5, p. 218). The trailing posterior edge of the fascia lata may rub over the lateral femoral condyle producing pain and tenderness a finger's breadth proximal to the lateral joint line. Runners and cyclists describe how the

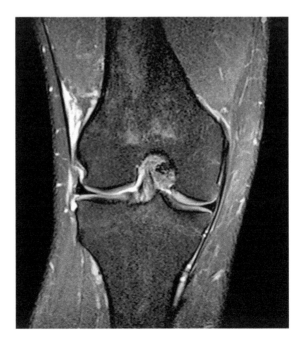

Figure 5.19 The bright signal on magnetic resonance scanning is located at the lateral femoral condylar surface and overlying fascia lata in the iliotibial band friction syndrome.

symptoms develop after perhaps 30 minutes of exercise, initially wearing off as the leg is rested. An MR scan is diagnostic (Figure 5.19) although an ultrasound may be all that is necessary.

A period of rest from sport, coupled with stretching of the fascia lata and hip abductor muscle strengthening, may prove effective. If the affected leg is the longer one, an insole in the contralateral shoe may reduce loading through the symptomatic limb. Local swelling and persistent symptoms may be a reason for the injection of a local steroid preparation into the site of friction, augmented by a short course of oral anti-inflammatory analgesia. In a few cases a limited surgical release of the tight edge of the fascia lata is indicated and is almost invariably successful if the diagnosis is correct. The differential diagnosis includes sciatica, popliteus or biceps femoris tendinopathy, lateral knee compartment pathology and malfunction of the proximal tibiofibular joint.

References

Aglietti P, Buzzi R and Zaccherotti G (1992) Patellar tendon versus semitendinosus and gracilis in ACL reconstruction. In: *Meeting Abstracts and Outlines of the 18th Annual Meeting of the American Orthopaedic Society for Sports Medicine.* San Diego, CA: American Orthopaedic Society for Sports Medicine, pp. 29–30.

Aït Si Selmi T, Fithian S and Neyret P (2006) The evolution of osteoarthritis in 103 patients with ACL reconstruction at 17 years follow-up. *Knee* 13, 353–8.

Amis AA and Scammell BE (1993) Biomechanics of intra-articular and extra-articular reconstruction of the anterior cruciate ligament. *J Bone Joint Surg Br* 75, 812–17.

Annandale T (1885) An operation for displaced semilunar cartilage. *Br Med J* i, 779–81.

Azar FM (2006) Evaluation and treatment of chronic medial collateral ligament injuries of the knee. *Sports Med Arthrosc* 14, 84–90.

Balkfors B (1982) The course of knee ligament injuries. *Acta Orthop Scand* 198, 1–91.

Ballock RT, Woo SLY, Lyon RM, *et al.* (1989) Use of patellar tendon autograft for anterior cruciate ligament reconstruction in the rabbit: a long-term histologic and biomechanical study. *J Orth Res* 7, 474–85.

Berchuck M, Andriacchi TP, Bach BR, *et al.* (1990) Gait adaptations by patients who have a deficient anterior cruciate ligament. *J Bone Joint Surg Am* 72, 8871–7.

Bonnet A (1845) *Traité des maladies des articulations.* Paris: Baillière.

Cabaud HE, Feagin JA and Rodkey WG (1980) Acute anterior cruciate ligament injury and augmented repair. Experimental studies. *Am J Sports Med* 8, 395–401.

Cannon WD Jr and Vittori JM (1992) The incidence of healing in arthroscopic meniscal repairs in anterior cruciate ligament-reconstructed knees versus stable knees. *Am. J Sports Med* 20, 176–81.

Carson WG (1988) The role of lateral extra-articular procedures for anterolateral rotatory instability. *Clin Sports Med* 7, 751–72.

Clancy WG Jr, Narechamia RG, Rosenberg TD, *et al.* (1981) Anterior and posterior cruciate ligament reconstruction in Rhesus monkeys: a histological, micro-angiographic and biomechanical analysis. *J Bone Joint Surg Am* 63, 1270–84.

Clancy WG Jr, Shelbourne KD, Zoellner GB, *et al.* (1983) Treatment of the knee joint instability secondary to rupture of the posterior cruciate ligament: report of a new procedure. *J Bone Joint Surg Am* 65, 310–22.

Dahlstedt L, Dalen N and Jonsson V (1990) Gore-tex prosthetic ligament versus Kennedy ligament augmentation device in anterior cruciate ligament reconstruction: a prospective randomised 3-year follow-up of 41 cases. *Acta Orthop Scand* 61, 217–24.

DeHaven KE, Cosgarea AJ and Sebastianelli WJ (2003) Arthrofibrosis of the knee following ligament surgery. *Instr Course Lect* 52, 369–81.

Drogset JO, Grondtvedt T and Robak OR (2006) A sixteen-year follow-up of three operative techniques for the treatment of acute ruptures of the anterior cruciate ligament. *J Bone Joint Surg Am* **88**, 944–52.

Ellison AE (1979) Distal iliotibial-band transfer for anterolateral rotatory instability of the knee. *J Bone Joint Surg Am* **61**, 330–7.

Engebretsen L, Benum P, Fasting O, *et al.* (1990) A prospective randomised study of three surgical techniques for treatment of acute ruptures of the anterior cruciate ligament. *Am J Sports Med* **18**, 585–90.

Fanelli GC (2008) Posterior cruciate ligament rehabilitation: how slow should we go? *Arthroscopy* **24,** 234–5.

Frobell RB, Roos EM, Roos HP, *et al.* (2010) A randomized trial of treatment for acute anterior cruciate ligament tears. *N Engl J Med* **363**: 331–42.

Fu FH, Shen W, Starman JS, *et al.* (2008) Primary anatomic double-bundle anterior cruciate ligament reconstruction: a preliminary 2-year prospective study. *Am J Sports Med* **36,** 1263–74.

Garofalo R, Moretti B, Kombot C and Moretti L (2007) Femoral tunnel placement in anterior cruciate ligament reconstruction: rationale of the two incision technique. *J Orthop Surg* **21**, 2–10.

Gaulrapp HM and Haus J (2006) Intraarticular stabilization after anterior cruciate ligament tear in children and adolescents: results 6 years after surgery. *Knee Surg Sports Traumatol Arthrosc* **14**, 417–24.

Halinen J, Lindahl J, Hirvensalo E and Santavirta S (2006) Operative and non-operative treatments of medial collateral ligament rupture with early anterior cruciate ligament reconstruction: a prospective randomized study. *Am J Sports Med* **34**, 1134–40.

Henson J, Nyland J, Chang HC, *et al.* (2009) Effect of cryoprotectant incubation time on handling properties of allogeneic tendons prepared for knee ligament reconstruction. *J Biomater Appl* **24**, 343–52.

Hey-Groves EW (1917) Operation for repair of the crucial ligaments. *Lancet* **ii**, 674–8.

Holden JP, Grood ES, Butler DL, *et al.* (1988) Biomechanics of fascia lata ligament replacements: early post-operative changes in the goat. *J Orth Res* **6**, 639–47.

Howell SM and Taylor MA (1993) Failure of reconstruction of the anterior cruciate ligament due to impingement by the intercondylar roof. *J Bone Joint Surg Am* **75**, 1044–55.

Hughston JC (1988) The absent posterior drawer test in some acute posterior cruciate ligament tears of the knee. *Am J Sports Med* **16**, 39–43.

Hughston JC and Jacobson KE (1985) Chronic posterolateral rotatory instability of the knee. *J Bone Joint Surg Am* **67**, 351–9.

Hughston JC and Norwood LA Jr (1980) The posterolateral drawer test and external rotation recurvatum test for posterolateral rotatory instability of the knee. *Clin Orthop* **147**, 82–7.

Indelicato PA (1983) Non-operative treatment of complete tears of the medial collateral ligament of the knee. *J Bone Joint Surg Am* **65**, 323–9.

Insall JN (1984) Chronic instability of the knee. In: Insall JN (ed.) *Surgery of the Knee*. New York, NY: Churchill Livingstone.

Jakob RP (1992) Acute posterior cruciate ligament tears – diagnosis and management. In: Aichroth PM and Cannon DW Jr (eds) *Knee Surgery: Current Practice*. London: Martin Dunitz, pp. 322–8.

Jakob RP, Hassler H and Säbli H-U (1981). Observations on the rotary instability of the lateral compartment of the knee: experimental studies on the functional anatomy and the pathomechanism of the true and reversed pivot shift sign. *Acta Orthop Scand* **52**(Suppl 191), 1–32.

Johnson RJ, Eriksson E, Haggmark T, *et al.* (1984) Five- to ten-year follow-up evaluation after reconstruction of the anterior cruciate ligament. *Clin Orthop Rel Res* **183**, 122–40.

Jones KG (1963) Reconstruction of the anterior cruciate ligament. A technique using the central one third of the patellar ligament. *J Bone Joint Surg Am* **45**, 925–32.

Kaeding C, Farr J, Kavanaugh T and Pedroza A (2005) A prospective randomized comparison of bioabsorbable and titanium anterior cruciate ligament interference screws. *Arthroscopy* **21**, 147–51.

Kuhn MA and Ross G (2007) Allografts in the treatment on anterior cruciate ligament injuries. *Sports Med Arthrosc* **15**, 133–8.

Kurosaka M, Yoshiya S and Andrish JT (1987) A biomechanical comparison of different surgical techniques of graft fixation in anterior cruciate ligament reconstruction. *Am J Sports Med* **15**, 225–9.

Laprade RF, Johansen S, Wentorf FA and Engebretsen L (2004) An analysis of an anatomical posterolateral knee reconstruction: an in vitro biomechanical study and development of a surgical technique. *Am J Sports Med* **32**, 1405–14.

Laprade RF, Morgan PM, Wentorf FA, *et al.* (2007) The anatomy of the posterior aspect of the knee. An anatomic study. *J Bone Joint Surg Am* **89**, 758–64.

Larson RL (1993) Principles of replacement and reinforcement. In: *Mini Symposium: Knee Ligament Injuries. Curr Orthop* **7**, 94–100.

Lattermann C and Romine SE (2009) Osteochondral allografts: state of the art. *Clin Sports Med* **28**, 285–301.

Levy BA, Stuart MJ and Whelan DB (2010) Posterolateral instability of the knee: evaluation, treatment, results. *Sports Med Arthrosc* **18**, 254–62.

Li RC, Maffulli N, Hsu YC and Chan KM (1996) Isokinetic strength of the quadriceps and hamstrings and functional ability of the anterior cruciate deficient knees in recreational athletes. *Br J Sports Med* **30**, 161–4.

MacIntosh DL and Darby TA (1976) Lateral substitution reconstruction. *J Bone Joint Surg Br* **58**, 142–6.

Macnicol MF (1989) The torn anterior cruciate ligament. *J R Coll Edinb* **34**(Suppl), 9–11.

Macnicol MF (1992) The conservative management of the anterior cruciate ligament-deficient knee. In: Aichroth PM and Cannon WD (eds) *Knee Surgery, Current Practice*. London: Martin Dunitz, pp. 217–21.

Macnicol MF, Penny ID and Sheppard L (1991) Early results of Leeds-Keio anterior cruciate ligament replacement. *J Bone Joint Surg Br* **73**, 377–80.

Marder RA, Raskind JR and Carroll M (1991) Prospective evaluation of arthroscopically assisted reconstruction. Patellar tendon vs semitendinosus and gracilis. *Am J Sports Med* **19**, 478–84.

Meunier A, Odensten M and Good L (2007) Long-term results after primary repair or non-surgical treatment of anterior cruciate ligament rupture: a randomized study with a 15-year follow-up. *Scand J Med Sci Sports* **17**, 320–7.

Miyamoto RG, Bosco JA and Sherman OH (2009) Treatment of medial collateral ligament injuries. *J Am Acad Orthop Surg* **17**, 1521–61.

Murray AW and Macnicol MF (2004) 10–16 year results of Leeds-Keio anterior cruciate ligament reconstruction. *Knee* **11**, 9–14.

Musahl V, Plakseychuk A, VanSyoc A and Fu FH (2005) Varying femoral tunnels between the anatomical footprint and isometric positions: effect on kinematics of the anterior cruciate ligament-reconstructed knee. *Am J Sports Med* **33**, 712–18.

Noyes FR and Barber SD (1991) The effect of an extra-articular procedure on allograft reconstructions for chronic ruptures of the anterior cruciate ligament. *J Bone Joint Surg Am* **73**, 822–32.

Noyes FR, Delucas JL and Torvik PJ (1974) Biomechanics of anterior cruciate ligament failure: an analysis of strain-rate sensitivity and mechanisms in primates. *J Bone Joint Surg Am* **56**, 236–53.

O'Brien SJ, Warren RF, Wickiewicz TL, *et al.* (1991) The iliotibial band lateral sling procedure and its effect on the results of anterior cruciate ligament reconstruction. *Am J Sports Med* **19**, 21–5.

Oh YH, Namkoong S, Strauss EJ, *et al.* (2006) Hybrid femoral fixation of soft-tissue grafts in anterior cruciate ligament reconstruction using the EndoButtol CL and bioabsorbable interference screws: a biomechanical study. *Arthroscopy* **22**, 1218–24.

Palmer I (1938) On the injuries to the ligaments of the knee joint. A clinical study. *Acta Chir Scand* **81**(Suppl.), 53.

Panni AS, Denti M, Franzese S and Montaleone M (1993) The bone-ligament junction: a comparison between biological and artificial ACL reconstruction. *Knee Surg Sports Traumatol Arthrosc* **1**, 9–12.

Pässler HH (1993) The history of the cruciate ligaments: some forgotten (or unknown) facts from Europe. *Knee Surg Sports Traumatol Arthrosc* **1**, 13–16.

Pässler HH and Höher J (2004) Intraoperative quality control of the placement of bone tunnels for the anterior cruciate ligament. *Unfallchirurg* **107**, 263–72.

Perry J, Fox JM, Boitano MA, *et al.* (1980) Functional evaluation of the pes anserinus transfer by electromyography and gait analysis. *J Bone Joint Surg Am* **62**, 973–80.

Poolman RW, Farrokhyar F and Bhandari M (2007) Hamstring tendon autograft better than bone-patellar-tendon bone autograft in ACL reconstruction. A cumulative meta-analysis and clinically relevant sensitivity analysis applied to a previously published analysis. *Acta Orthop* **78**, 350–4.

Roos H, Adalbrecht T, Dahlberg L and Lohmander LS (1995) Osteoarthritis of the knee after injury to the anterior cruciate ligament or meniscus: the influence of time and age. *Osteoarthritis Cartilage* **3**, 261–7.

Sachs RA, Daniel DM, Stone ML and Garfein RF (1989) Patellofemoral problems after anterior cruciate ligament reconstruction. *Am J Sports Med* **17**, 760–5.

Sandberg R, Balkfors B, Nilsson B, *et al.* (1987) Operative versus non-operative treatment of recent injuries to the ligaments of the knee. *J Bone Joint Surg Am* **69**, 1120–6.

Sgaghone NA, Del Pizzo W, Fox JM, *et al.* (1993) Arthroscopic-assisted anterior cruciate ligament reconstruction with the pes anserine tendons: comparison of results in acute and chronic ligament deficiency. *Am J Sports Med* **21**, 249–56.

Shelbourne KD and Basle JR (1988) Treatment of combined anterior cruciate ligament and medial collateral ligament injuries. *Am J Knee Surg* **1**, 56–8.

Shelbourne KD, Wilekens JH, Mollabashy A and Decarlo M (1991) Arthrofibrosis in acute cruciate ligament reconstruction. The effect of timing on reconstruction and rehabilitation. *Am J Sports Med* **19**, 332–6.

Shino K, Kawasaki T, Hirose H, *et al.* (1984) Replacement of the anterior cruciate ligament by an allogenic tendon graft. An experimental study in the dog. *J Bone Joint Surg Br* **66**, 672–81.

Smillie IS (1978) *Injuries of the Knee Joint*, 5th edn. Edinburgh: Churchill Livingstone.

Stannard JP, Brown SL, Farris RC, *et al.* (2005) The posterolateral corner of the knee: repair versus reconstruction. *Am J Sports Med* **33**, 881–8.

Stark J (1850) Two cases of rupture of the crucial ligaments of the knee joint. *Edin Med Surg* **74**, 267–71.

Steenbrugge F, Verdonk R and Verstraete K (2004) Magnetic resonance imaging of the surgically repaired meniscus: a 13-year follow-up study. *Acta Orthop Scand* **75**, 323–7.

Torg JS, Barton TM, Pavlov H, *et al.* (1989) Natural history of the posterior cruciate-deficient knee. *Clin Orthop* **246**, 208–16.

Trickey EL (1968) Rupture of the posterior cruciate ligament of the knee. *J Bone Joint Surg Br* **50**, 334–41.

Trickey EL (1980) Injuries to the posterior cruciate ligament: diagnosis and treatment of early injuries and reconstruction of late instability. *Clin Orthop Rel Res* **147**, 76–81.

Trillat A (1978) Posterolateral instability. In: Schulitz KP, Krahl H and Stein WH (eds) *Late Reconstruction of Injured Ligaments of the Knee.* Berlin: Springer-Verlag, pp. 99–105.

West RV and Harner CD (2005) Graft selection in anterior cruciate ligament reconstruction. *J Am Acad Orthop Surg* **13**, 197–207.

Woo SL, Thomas M and Chan Saw SS (2004) Contribution of biomechanics, orthopaedics and rehabilitation: the past present and future. *Surgeon* **2**, 125–36.

Woo SL, Abramowitch SD, Kilger R and Liang R (2006a) Biomechanics of knee ligaments: injury, healing and repair. *J Biomech* **39**, 1–20.

Woo SL, Wu C, Dede O, *et al.* (2006b) Biomechanics and anterior cruciate ligament reconstruction. *J Orthop Surg* **25**, 1–2.

Yonetani Y, Toritsuka Y, Yamada Y and Shino K (2005) Graft length changes in the bi-socket anterior cruciate ligament reconstruction: comparison between isometric and anatomic femoral tunnel placement. *Arthroscopy* **21**, 1317–22.

6

Meniscal lesions

Function

The role of the menisci of the knee is still debated, and it seems fruitless to list the different functions that have been suggested in any order of importance. The meniscus exerts a valuable and measurable effect on the capabilities and resilience of the knee joint, and its total removal hastens degenerative changes in the affected compartment. The menisci contribute to the following functions:

- Distribution of load – approximately 55 per cent through the lateral meniscus and 45 per cent through the medial meniscus when the knee is straight, when about half the body weight passes through the menisci (increasing to almost 90 per cent of body weight through the menisci when the knee is flexed more than 90° during squatting)
- Improvement of congruency
- Enhancement of stability
- Nutrition of articular cartilage
- Lubrication.

The first three actions are clearly interrelated, since the 'space-filler' effect of the menisci on the tibial condyles ensures an efficient transmission of stress through the joint, including their role as part of the guiding mechanism during rotatory movements.

Throughout flexion and extension the menisci move with the tibia, to which they are attached, but in rotation they are more influenced by the movement of the femoral condyles. Thus, during knee movements the tibia is able to pursue a winding or helicoid course across the distal end of the femur, rotating externally in extension (the converse of the internally directed 'screw home' action of the femur on the tibia), and internally on full flexion (Walker and Erkman 1975).

This precise tracking of the two bones upon each other is therefore determined collectively by the shape of the articulating condyles, the menisci, and the cruciate ligaments which act as guide-ropes. If this normal, accommodative rotation is prevented, the menisci may become trapped within the joint, resulting either in tears within the substance of the meniscus, or peripheral detachments. Both stretching and crushing forces are involved (Figure 6.1), although significant external force is not a characteristic in the majority of cases.

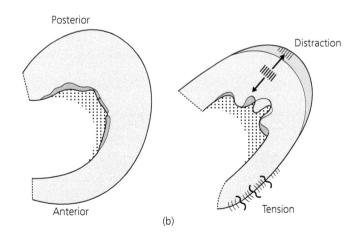

Figure 6.1 Minor distortion occurs under moderate load (a), while greater force causes anterior horn tension and distraction of the posterior half of the meniscus (b).

Structure

The anatomical and some of the functional differences of the two menisci are readily recognized. Although both structures are crescent-shaped when viewed from above, the lateral meniscus is more nearly a complete circle. The anterior horns are anchored to the non-articular region of the tibia, in front of the anterior cruciate ligament insertion on the intercondylar eminence. Both anterior horns are linked by the transverse ligament, which gives off bands of connective tissue that blend with the anterior cruciate ligament. The posterior horns are also attached to the intercondylar region of the tibia, but laterally there are additional anchorages since the lateral meniscus is moored to the medial femoral condyle in front of and behind the posterior cruciate ligament by the ligaments of Humphry and Wrisberg, respectively (the anterior and posterior meniscofemoral ligaments) (Figure 6.2a). A similar fibrous band may also link the medial meniscus to the posterior cruciate ligament.

In cross-section the menisci are triangular and, viewed from behind, the medial meniscus is narrower in front and broader posteriorly. The lateral meniscus is wider anteriorly than the medial meniscus and its width is more uniform, with a thicker outer margin. The peripheral attachments differ, since the medial meniscus is intimately blended with the capsule and the medial ligament, whereas the lateral meniscus is separated from the capsule posteriorly by the lateral ligament and the popliteus tendon. Hence the posterior half of the lateral meniscus is relatively free and can be drawn backwards by the popliteus muscle during internal rotation of the tibia on the femur (Figure 6.2b).

Histology

The menisci of the knee are formed of fibrocartilage, with some proteoglycan present. The collagen fibres are arranged in a predominantly circumferential orientation, which reflects the circumferential tension that develops in the meniscus during normal loading (Arnoczky and Warren 1983; Yasunaga *et al.* 2001). The extracellular matrix of the fibrocartilaginous menisci is composed of collagen and proteoglycan. Biochemical analysis has shown that collagen comprises over 75 per cent of the dry weight of meniscal fibrocartilage, whereas proteoglycan comprises only 2.5 per cent (Arnoczky and Warren 1982, 1983). Thus, fibrocartilage has a composition more like that of tendon than that of cartilaginous tissue (Yasunaga *et al.* 2001). Although the collagen in the meniscus is type I, similar to that found in bone and skin, the proteoglycans are in many ways similar to those found in hyaline cartilage (Yasunaga *et al.* 2001). The most obvious differences between the proteoglycan of meniscal fibrocartilage and hyaline cartilage are in their composition and concentration. Meniscal fibrocartilage contains only

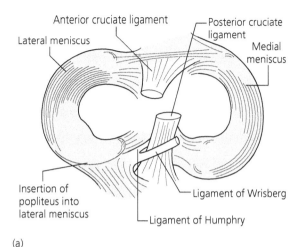

Figure 6.2 (a) Anatomy of the structures attached to the upper tibial surface, from in front: the anterior horn of the medial meniscus, the anterior cruciate ligament, the anterior and posterior horns of the lateral meniscus, the posterior horn of the medial meniscus, and the posterior cruciate ligament. (b) Anatomy of the popliteus muscle showing its partial insertion into the posterior horn of the lateral meniscus.

about one-eighth the proteoglycan concentration of hyaline cartilage. Also, glycosaminoglycan (GAG) composition differs, with dermatan sulphate making up 20 per cent of the GAG content of the meniscus. Keratin sulphate accounts for approximately a third of the GAG pool, with the rest being made up of chondroitin sulphate. In spite of these differences, the proteoglycan molecules of the menisci offer functional properties similar to those of articular cartilage proteoglycan (Arnoczky and Warren 1983; Yasunaga *et al.* 2001).

The fibres run circumferentially, resisting the bursting forces of weightbearing (Bullough *et al.* 1970), and are crossed, particularly in the central portion of the meniscus, by radial fibres (Figure 6.3). Nerves and blood vessels penetrate only the outer third and horns of the menisci, the remainder of the meniscus relying on synovial fluid and diffusion for nutrition. Some collagen fibres accompanying

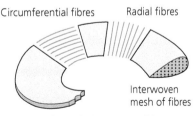

Figure 6.3 Histological structure of the meniscus showing the orientation of its collagen fibres.

123

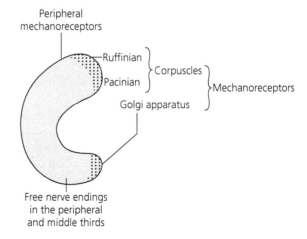

Figure 6.4 Innervation of the meniscus. Mechanoreceptors are congregated principally at both horns and along the peripheral margins.

the blood vessels in the periphery proceed radially through the circumferential fibres and form the inner edge of the meniscus. As these fibres are laminar rather than interwoven, they can be separated easily in the horizontal plane.

The innervation of the meniscus is shown in Figure 6.4. Mechanoreceptors are concentrated in the anterior and posterior horns, with a lesser distribution around the peripheral edge. Unmyelinated free nerve endings arborize as far as the middle third. Electron microscopy reveals that lymph channels extend throughout the full width of the meniscus and injection techniques define a network which may be absorptive, aiding in the nutrition of articular cartilage and meniscus. If the fluid percolating through the joint is considered to be a transudate from the articular surfaces of the femur and tibia, modulated by the synovium, then absorption is ensured by the menisci and other intra-articular soft tissues (Figure 6.5). The flow through the knee joint is therefore unidirectional, as with any other perfused organ in the body.

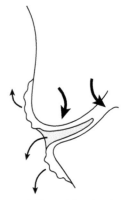

Figure 6.5 The unidirectional flow of fluid through the knee is depicted, forming as a modified transudate and being absorbed by the soft tissues, including the menisci.

Controversy exists within the orthopaedic literature regarding the ability of a meniscus or meniscus-like tissue to regenerate following total meniscectomy. This variance may have resulted from the extent of meniscectomy, partial versus total, or the fact that much of the data regarding meniscal regeneration have been limited to investigations in animals. Experiments in rabbits and dogs have demonstrated that, following total meniscectomy, there is regrowth of a structure similar in shape and texture to the removed meniscus. It is thought that, following removal of the meniscus, fibrocytes from the synovium and joint capsule migrate into the joint and are transformed into undifferentiated fibroblasts, which, in turn, form a loose, fibrous connective tissue (Arnoczky *et al.* 1988). In time, joint motion and the resultant hydrostatic pressure provide the proper environment for the transformation of these fibroblasts into fibrocartilage. Studies have shown that by 7 months, this tissue has the histological appearance of fibrocartilage and must be resected to expose the vascular synovial tissue or, in the case of subtotal meniscectomy, the excision must extend into the peripheral vasculature of the meniscus (Arnoczky and Warren 1982, 1983).

The importance of the peripheral synovial tissues for meniscal regeneration has been shown by experimental studies in rabbits. Animals in which total meniscectomy was accompanied by synovectomy showed no evidence of tissue regrowth at 12 weeks. However, total meniscectomy alone was followed by regrowth of a meniscus-like structure in 83 per cent of the knees. Evidence that the fibrous joint capsule may also be instrumental in the regeneration of fibrocartilaginous tissue within the joint space has been demonstrated by the presence of regenerated fibrocartilaginous rims in patients following total knee arthroplasty. Although these regenerated tissues do not grossly resemble normal menisci, histological examination reveals a fibrocartilaginous tissue consisting of chondrocytes in a dense connective tissue matrix (Albrecht-Olsen *et al.* 1999; Arnoczky and Warren 1983).

In 1936 King published his classic experiment on meniscal healing in dogs. He demonstrated that, for meniscal lesions to heal, they must communicate with the peripheral blood supply. Although this vascular supply appears to be an essential element in determining the potential for meniscal repair, of equal importance is the ability of this blood supply to support the inflammatory response characteristic of wound repair. Clinical and experimental observations have demonstrated that the peripheral meniscal blood supply is capable of producing a reparative response similar to that observed in other connective tissues (Albrecht-Olsen *et al.* 1999; Arnoczky and Warren 1982, 1983).

Following injury within the peripheral vascular zone, a fibrin clot forms that is rich in acute inflammatory cells (neutrophils and monocytes). Vessels from the perimeniscal capillary plexus spread within a fibrin scaffold, accompanied by the proliferation of undifferentiated mesenchymal cells. Eventually the lesion is filled with a cellular, fibrovascular scar tissue that glues the meniscal edges together and appears to be continuous with the adjacent normal meniscus fibrocartilage. Vessels from the perimeniscal capillary plexus, as well as a proliferative vascular pannus from the synovial fringe, penetrate the fibrous scar to provide a marked inflammatory (healing) response (Arnoczky and Warren 1982, 1983; Arnoczky *et al.* 1988).

Experimental studies have shown that radial lesions of the meniscus extending to the synovium are completely healed by fibrovascular scar tissue in 10 weeks. Modulation of this scar tissue into normal-appearing fibrocartilage, however, requires several months (Yasunaga *et al.* 2001). It should be stressed that the initial strength of this repair tissue, compared with normal meniscus, is minimal. Further study is required to delineate the biomechanical properties of this repair.

Classification of tears

Traumatic lesions of the meniscus generally occur vertically if they are produced acutely. The classic mechanism of injury comprises a rotational stress upon the semi-flexed and weightbearing knee. A valgus or varus component may also be recalled, particularly if the leg has been involved in a collision, or if ligament laxity is present. Males are more commonly affected and there are said to be racial differences. Horizontal cleavage lesions are produced more insidiously and are usually associated with chronic stresses acting on the meniscus in a knee that is already slightly osteoarthritic.

A variety of meniscal tears are encountered (Figure 6.6), although the different types frequently coexist at other sites. Trillat (1962) described the classic progression of a 'bucket handle' tear, commencing in the posterior third where arthroscopic access is most awkward. His anatomical classification was modified by Dandy (1990), but every surgeon with a large arthroscopic

Figure 6.6 Patterns of traumatic meniscal tears. (a) The upper six diagrams show how a vertical tear may progress; various forms of tear are shown, in most of which the peripheral half of the meniscus can be preserved. (b) A flap tear. (c) A fish mouth tear.

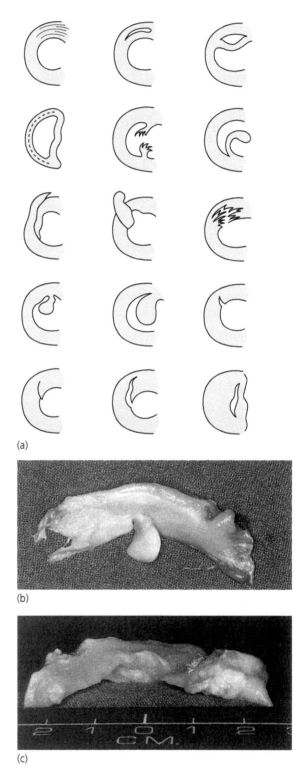

(a)

(b)

(c)

practice will have an individual impression of the pathological processes and their frequency. The components of the meniscal tears are:

- Vertical:
  - Longitudinal – incomplete/bucket handle/pedunculated tag
  - Radial
  - Combined (flap) (Figure 6.6b)
- Horizontal:
  - Posterior
  - Central
  - Anterior
  - Inner edge ('fish mouth' [Figure 6.6c] and 'parrot beak' tears)
- Complex:
  - Multiple vertical tears
  - Associated cystic changes (peripheral or central).

Cysts may also be encountered, affecting normal, congenitally abnormal and degenerative menisci. Figure 6.7 details the first author's audit of 1350 tears encountered over a 5-year period and gives an indication of the varying pathology that is encountered.

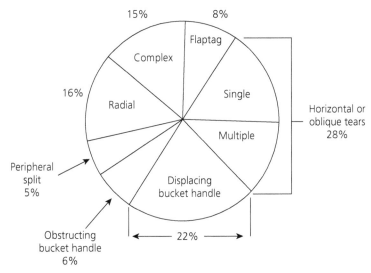

Figure 6.7 Incidence of meniscal tears (as a percentage of a consecutive total of 1350 lesions).

Symptoms

Meniscal tears will produce pain, loss of movement and instability of the joint. The interrelationship of these symptoms should be recognized. Pain arises from the stretching of the peripheral, sensory portions of the meniscus, and from the capsule and ligaments during the abnormal movement of the knee when an intra-articular obstruction is present. The body of the meniscus itself is insensitive.

Pain

Pain may be accompanied by clicking, or even a clunking sensation if the meniscus is displacing during flexion and extension. A limp may develop as the patient attempts to relieve the symptoms, and this protective gait may worsen towards the end of the day as the leg tires. 127

Pain over the medial joint line, with tenderness when the knees touch together, is frequently recalled if the patient is asked directly. This feature is noticed in bed at night, but is not, as is classically taught, solely caused by a horizontal cleavage lesion. Secondary patellar pain and crepitus develop as a result of the synovitis.

■ Effusion

An effusion may be painful if it is tense, but this is unusual following a tear of the meniscus. If the knee becomes very swollen, and rapidly so, then a haemarthrosis should be suspected. As the meniscus is relatively avascular, a tear of a ligament and possibly also of the associated capsule should be suspected. Meniscal tears produce a lesser degree of swelling, the effusion gradually forming over the 12-24 hours after the injury. Thereafter, the fluid tends to disappear, but recurs when the joint is twisted or stressed.

■ Abnormal function

Mechanical problems are manifest by a sense of restricted extension and flexion, a feeling of stiffness, and a tendency for the joint to give way. In early tears, where the surface of the meniscus is little altered, the loss of joint movement may be very subtle, or absent. Minimal losses of flexion and extension should be carefully elicited. Stiffness will tend to lessen as the knee is exercised, and hence is at its worst early in the morning or after rest. Instability, or buckling, results not only from the obstruction in the joint altering the normal pivot, but also from muscle weakness or quadriceps inhibition. The patient complains that the joint is weak, or does not feel 'true', and a catching sensation occurs when the patient kneels, squats, jumps or rotates the leg.

Signs

A torn meniscus produces joint line tenderness, often very localized, an effusion, which may be regional, or the more common total intrasynovial swelling, and locking. The last term describes not simply a loss of full extension, but also restriction of flexion and rotation. The loss of extension is rarely more than 10-20°, and a greater limitation suggests some other pathological lesion. In approximately 70 per cent of cases these are the three cardinal signs of a torn meniscus.

However, there may be quadriceps wasting in more chronic injuries, and a protrusion or localized area of oedema may be felt at the joint line. Ligaments may become tender and progressively lax owing to the abnormal mechanics of flexion, and patellofemoral pain and tenderness develop if the patient walks on a persistently flexed knee. Tenderness sometimes spreads over the femoral and tibial condyles so the clinical picture thereby becomes confusing.

The McMurray test describes the production of a clunk or snapping sensation when the tibia is rotated with the knee in full flexion (McMurray 1928) (see Chapter 2). The test may be positive if a vertical, longitudinal tear is present in the posterior segment of the meniscus, and the fingers of one hand should palpate the joint line in order to improve precision. A somewhat similar grinding test has been described by Apley, whereby axial pressure is directed along the tibia which is again rotated, this time with the patient prone and the knee flexed at a right angle.

These tests for meniscal pathology are open to misinterpretation but are sometimes confirmatory. Eliciting pain by these manoeuvres is not pathognomic of a meniscal tear, but

the production of a clunk or abnormal movement may cause the patient to remark that the symptoms of instability have been reproduced. It is always as well to check that a similar clunk cannot be elicited in the opposite knee and examination of the knee on different occasions is recommended, particularly if the assessments are separated by a few weeks. There is certainly nothing to suggest that such delay will adversely influence the eventual outcome.

With the advent of readily available magnetic resonance (MR) scanning (Figure 6.8) and arthroscopic examination (see Chapter 3), early diagnosis and treatment of meniscal tears is possible, but is limited in some parts of the world by healthcare restrictions and the availability of arthroscopically trained surgeons.

Figure 6.8 Magnetic resonance image of a bucket handle medial meniscal tear.

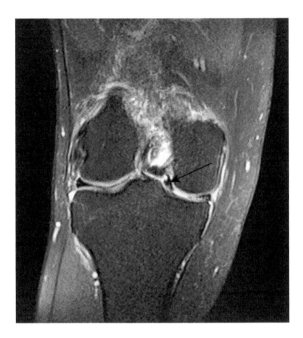

Meniscectomy

▨ Partial or total

Meniscal tears are the most common intra-articular knee injuries, comprising 75 per cent or more of all internal derangements of the knee (DeHaven 1999). Historically, symptomatic meniscal tears were dealt with by total meniscectomy through an open arthrotomy (Figure 6.9), regardless of the nature of the tear, its size and its location. This procedure, which was felt to be effective and purportedly allowed the formation of the 'neo-meniscus' discussed earlier, was subsequently shown to produce major long-term disability. Fairbank (1937) was the first to demonstrate clinically the deleterious effects of total meniscectomy. His classic description of radiographic joint space narrowing, flattening of the femoral condyle, and marginal osteophyte formation after meniscectomy, with subsequent progressive hyaline cartilage loss, remains a landmark in the treatment of meniscal tears.

The realization that the meniscus has a valuable function within the knee, even if only the peripheral portion is present, has led to a more conservative surgical policy when dealing with a tear (Noble and Erat, 1980). The principal argument for removing the whole meniscus at operation was centred upon the realistic concern that a further tear might otherwise be harboured within the remnant (Figure 6.10) and that regeneration of a pseudomeniscus was likely. Furthermore, an unstable residual rim of meniscus could, and indeed still can, be the

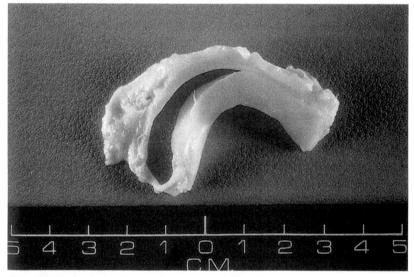

Figure 6.9 Total meniscectomy should not be carried out for a posterior 'bucket handle' tear if it is amenable to repair.

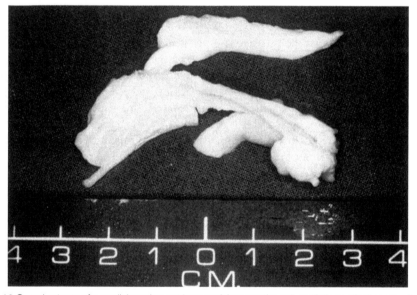

Figure 6.10 Complex tears of a medial meniscus where excision was the only realistic surgical approach.

source of continuing pain and instability. Equally, the peripheral remnant of meniscus is important as it not only constitutes part of the capsular and ligamentous complex, but is also capable of transmitting a significant proportion of load. Hence its preservation is preferable.

During the past decade, increasing understanding of the histological, biological and functional significance of the menisci has encouraged a more conservative philosophy. Today's selective approach includes non-operative treatment of meniscal tears, partial meniscectomy and meniscal repair as alternatives to routine meniscectomy. Since Thomas Annandale of Edinburgh reported the first meniscal repair in 1885, studies of the vascular anatomy of the meniscus have documented its healing potential (Arnoczky and Warren 1982; Henning *et al.* 1991). Annandale's patient was a Newcastle coal miner with a 10-month history. At arthrotomy a torn anterior horn of the medial meniscus was sutured to its peripheral attachment with restitution of knee function. Clinical reports of successful open and arthroscopic repairs eventually generated enthusiasm for these procedures. However, long-term follow-up of meniscal repair procedures is still essential to ascertain that repaired menisci will survive, function effectively and prevent the late degenerative changes seen after total meniscectomy (DeHaven *et al.* 1995; Hantes *et al.* 2006).

In the 1950s and 1960s, before knee arthroscopy, total meniscectomy was performed for almost any meniscal tear suggested by clinical examination. Sometimes the wrong side of the knee was opened initially, and a second posteromedial incision inflicted if the dissected meniscus tore, leaving a retained posterior third. In the last three decades, however, arthroscopy of the knee joint has provided us with a means of performing adequate meniscectomy following the technical rules laid down by several authors (Henning 1983; Cannon and Morgan 1994; DeHaven 1999).The period between 1970 and 1980 showed that, with a carefully executed arthroscopic partial meniscectomy confined to the tear region, restoration of satisfactory function was achieved in more than 90 per cent of cases. The short-term symptomatic results of these resections were comparable with those of open meniscectomy but postoperative recovery was enhanced. In the longer term, and in the event of total medial meniscectomy, factors such as varus malalignment and mechanical overload increased the risk of degeneration of the loadbearing cartilage in the medial compartment. Not only was the buffer function of the semilunar cartilage absent between the femoral condyle and medial tibial plateau, but stabilization from the meniscal rim was also lacking. As a result, there was an increased anteroposterior shift of the femoral condyle in relation to the tibial plateau. Any ligamentous laxity produced by the initial trauma increased the degenerative changes in the loadbearing area. Of even more importance, but medically often uncontrollable, is the magnitude of the mechanical load, depending on the weight of the patient and the intensity of occupational demand and sports-related activity.

The same principle applies to older age groups: the short-term results of accurate arthroscopic partial meniscectomy are superior to those of open total meniscectomy (DeHaven *et al.* 1995). Preservation of the meniscal rim is vital, while the quality of loadbearing articular cartilage will determine the functional outcome in this age group. In the long run, only 50 per cent of older patients will benefit from arthroscopic medial meniscectomy. These poor to fair results caution against an indiscriminate recommendation for arthroscopic 'meniscectomy'. Herrlin *et al.* (2007) recently confirmed that physiotherapy was equally effective as meniscal 'debridement' in a prospective randomized trial for patients with a degenerative medial meniscal tear.

Comparisons of the longer-term results following partial, instead of total, meniscectomy confirm the benefits of conservation surgery (McGinty *et al.* 1977; Dandy *et al.* 1983), confining the excision to unstable or severely distorted meniscal tissue. The details of arthroscopic technique can only be learnt by operative experience. Access and triangulation skills remain the pivotal factors in achieving successful surgical excision or repair, and the methodology is clearly described in surgical atlases (Johnson 1978; Dandy 1981). The displaced and displacing segments can be removed with punch forceps and other hand instruments including grasping forceps, or by the motorized shaver with high fluid flow and suction as required.

There is also some debate about whether a posterior horn remnant, not uncommonly left behind if access is difficult or if the meniscus ruptures in its central portion during attempted removal, should be dissected out *in toto* through the potentially injurious posteromedial approach. Such retained segments are probably better left initially, because a sizeable proportion of these cases will not become symptomatic after surgery. It is useful to request another MR scan or to re-arthroscope the knee before attempting a further excision as the

131

residual meniscus may be fairly smooth and non-obstructive. Even after removal of a retained portion of meniscus, post-meniscectomy symptoms may persist (Table 6.1).

■ Prognosis after meniscectomy

The prognosis after meniscectomy is adversely affected by the following factors:

• Presence of osteoarthritis
• Presence of significant ligament laxity or other injuries
• Other meniscus already removed
• Young patient (poor results common in the child)
• Female gender.

Complications following arthroscopic procedures are detailed in Table 3.4 (p. 49). The articular cartilage may be scuffed and lacerated by careless use of the instruments, and there is the risk that inadequate excision of abnormal tissue may occur in inexperienced hands. Nevertheless, convalescence after arthroscopic meniscectomy is certainly faster, characterized by efficient day case surgery and a speedier return to work and sport.

Osteoarthritic changes are hastened by meniscectomy, and are more obvious after total meniscectomy (Tapper and Hoover 1969; Parry *et al.* 1958). Indeed, it is now known that following a meniscectomy, approximately a third of patients will develop the clinical and radiographic signs of osteoarthritis, and a meniscectomy in childhood or adolescence introduces a 70 per cent risk of significant degenerative changes after 20 years (Suman *et al.* 1984; McNicholas *et al.* 2000). Degeneration of the articular cartilage not only occurs where it is exposed after surgery, but also appears below a regenerated neo-meniscus.

If a tear in the meniscus continues to block normal knee function, this too will bring about an arthritic process; yet there is little to suggest that the retention of an abnormal meniscus will lead to a greater deterioration in the knee than occurs after total meniscectomy, and the prevention of arthritis must never be promoted as a reason for meniscal excision. Rather, it should be the relief of pain and the improvement of function that act as indications for this form of surgery. Theoretically, ligament integrity is also preserved by the removal of an obstruction in the joint.

The radiographic features of osteoarthritis that follow meniscectomy, described first by Fairbank (1937) (Figure 6.11), also include femoral or tibial condylar ridging and coronal angular deformity. The signs are in no way specific so that the incidence of this complication is therefore difficult to gauge. The osteoarthritis is progressive, hence the incidence varies also with the length of follow-up.

Table 6.1 Grading of results following meniscectomy. Symptoms are more persistent if the knee is unstable or arthritic.

Grading of result	Criteria
Excellent	No symptoms, no loss of movement, no effusions
Good	Minor symptoms after vigorous activity, no loss of movement, occasional effusion
Fair	Symptoms prevent vigorous activity, slight loss of flexion, occasional effusion
Poor	Symptoms interfere with everyday activities, loss of flexion and extension, regular effusions

Adapted from Tapper and Hoover (1969).

Meniscal repair

The ability of meniscal lesions to heal has provided the rationale for the repair of a proportion of meniscal injuries, and several reports have demonstrated excellent results following primary repair of peripheral meniscal lesions (Clancy and Graf 1983; Cannon and Morgan 1994; DeHaven *et al.* 1995). Postoperative examination of these peripheral lesions reveals a repair process similar to that noted in animal models (Yasunaga *et al.* 2001). When damaged menisci are examined for potential repair, lesions are often classified by the location of the tear relative to the blood supply of the meniscus (Figure 6.12) and the vascular appearance of the peripheral and central surfaces of the tear (Arnoczky and Warren 1983). The red-red tear (peripheral capsular detachment) has a functional blood supply at both the capsular and meniscal sides of the lesion and thus has the best potential for healing. The red-white tear (meniscal rim tear through the perivascular zone) has an active peripheral blood supply, whereas the central (inner) surface of the lesion is devoid of functioning (perfused) vessels (Arnoczky and Warren 1983).

Theoretically, red-red and red-white lesions should have sufficient vascularity to heal by fibrovascular proliferation. White-white tears (meniscal lesion completely in the avascular zone) are without blood supply on either side of the lesion and are less likely to heal, other than in young patients (Noyes and Barber-Westin 2002). Although meniscal repair tends to be limited to the peripheral vascular area, a significant number of meniscal tears occur in the avascular portion of the meniscus (white-white tears), which is only nourished by synovial fluid imbibition through microscopic canaliculi. Experimental and clinical observations have suggested that these lesions are incapable of healing and thereby provided the rationale for partial meniscectomy. However, it is now appreciated that, if lesions in the avascular portion of the meniscus are connected to the peripheral vessels by vascular access channels or scarification of the synovial fringe, they are capable of healing through a process of fibrovascular scar proliferation, similar to that described in a vascular zone (Noyes and Barber-Westin 2002). Gallacher *et al.* (2010) found that two-thirds of such meniscal tears were capable of allowing acceptable function after repair with Mitek screws or fast T fix sutures

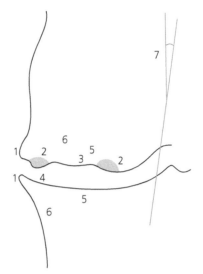

Figure 6.11 Post-meniscectomy radiographic changes. 1, osteophyte formation; 2, ridge formation; 3, generalized flattening of the marginal half of the femoral condyle; 4, narrowing of the joint space; 5, sclerosis of the subchondral plate on either side of the joint; 6, occasional cyst formation; 7, angulatory deformity of the knee.

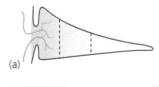

(a)

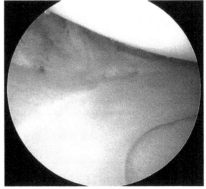

(b)

Figure 6.12 Vascularity of the meniscus.

(Smith and Nephew), provided that the tear was reducible without a rolled edge, degenerative changes were not evident, and the fixation was effective.

Although the vascular anatomy of the meniscus does not appear to change appreciably in adulthood, the ability of peripheral meniscus tears to heal in individuals over 40 years old is debatable (Roos *et al.* 1995). This contrasts with the fully vascularized meniscus in childhood and the receding front of central vascularity seen in adolescence. Although a meniscal blood supply is present in the older adult the structure of the meniscal tissue in these individuals may not be optimal for repair. Degenerative changes are even recognized in a high percentage of the contralateral, normally functioning medial menisci at this stage in life. Additional clinical evaluations are necessary before the limitation of age on meniscus repair can be determined (Yasunaga *et al.* 2001).

Research has shown that the meniscus is capable of repair within the scope of its vascularity, but little is known about the response of the meniscus to partial meniscectomy within the avascular zone (Rubman *et al.* 1998). As mentioned, previous clinical and experimental studies suggested that the meniscus is incapable of any reparative response within this zone, yet arthroscopic observations of menisci following partial meniscectomy have revealed remodelling of some of the transected surfaces (Rubman *et al.* 1998; Noyes and Barber-Westin 2002). Whether this remodelling process occurs in all cases and represents an intrinsic response of the meniscus, some type of extrameniscal accretion, or merely an attritional wearing away of the meniscus is unclear. However, experimental studies have shown that following partial meniscectomy (limited to the avascular zone), the meniscus may remodel through the organization and maturation of a fibrin clot that adheres to the cut edge of the meniscus. This clot presumably arises from the postoperative haemarthrosis, is populated with cells from the synovium and adjacent meniscus, and eventually differentiates into a fibrocartilage-like tissue. Thus, the remodelling represents an accretion of new tissue rather than an intrinsic regeneration. However, the mechanical (functional) character of this new tissue has not been determined (Bronstein *et al.* 1992).

If a haemarthrosis is not present or is insufficient to form a fibrin clot, the edge of the meniscus remains essentially unchanged. It is important to note that partial meniscectomy does not appear to predispose the remaining meniscus to further degeneration, although its effect on contiguous articular cartilage is variable (Yasunaga *et al.* 2001).

Based on observations of the ability of a fibrin clot to act as a scaffold and a stimulus for fibrocartilaginous tissue formation in the avascular portion of the meniscus, the use of a blood clot in the repair of avascular meniscal lesions has been proposed. In an experimental study, stable meniscal lesions in the avascular portion of canine medial menisci, filled with a fibrin clot, healed with the formation of dense connective tissue that modulated into fibrocartilaginous connective tissue by 6 months (Arnoczky and Warren 1983). Although this avascular repair tissue was morphologically different from normal meniscal tissue at 6 months, it was similar to the meniscal repair tissue seen following injury in the vascular portion of the meniscus.

Defects not filled with a fibrin clot showed no evidence of repair. In addition to providing a scaffold for the repair process, the clot contains chemotactic and mitogenic factors that stimulate the migration and proliferation of reparative cells. Although the exact origin of these cells is unclear, they are thought to arise from the adjacent meniscal tissue and synovium. Tissue culture studies have shown that meniscal cells are capable of proliferation and matrix synthesis when exposed to factors normally present in a fibrin clot. Long-term biochemical and biomechanical evaluation of this reparative tissue is needed before its true contribution to the avascular repair of meniscal tissue can be realized. Yet the results of experimental studies may warrant a rethinking of our traditional concepts of meniscal repair (Asik and Sener 2002; Borden *et al.* 2003).

Meniscal repair will now be considered more fully. The technique was popularized by Henning (1983) and DeHaven (1985), who published a 10-year experience. Cooper *et al.* (1991) provided detailed studies and refined the technique. Channels produced by the sutures allowed the ingrowth of cells, and it was recommended that the edges of the tear should be debrided. Successful healing is more likely in the stable knee (Hamberg *et al.* 1983; Steenbrugge *et al.* 2002, 2004a,b), when anatomical restoration can be anticipated in 90 per cent of the cases. Chondral congruity and compression is improved when the medial meniscus is under load. This also applies to the lateral compartment which contends with 55 per cent of transmitted weight, the convex lateral femoral condyle articulating with an almost convex lateral plateau. The contact area between both cartilaginous elements is flattened and widened because of the presence of the ring-shaped lateral meniscus so that its repair is vital (Glasgow *et al.* 1982; Ikeuchi 1982). Since a peripheral split of the medial or lateral meniscus is commonly encountered with anterior cruciate ligament tears, both the ligament and the meniscus should be dealt with concurrently. But grossly distorted and chronically displaced meniscal tears are unsuitable for suture. In summary, meniscal repair in a primarily stable knee results in 75 per cent good-to-excellent long-term results, whereas meniscal repair in a knee with a reconstructed (previously unstable) anterior cruciate ligament results in slightly fewer good-to-excellent results (Roos *et al.* 1995; Steenbrugge *et al.* 2005; Majewski *et al.* 2006; Meunier *et al.* 2007).

Techniques of repair include the use of a double-barrel curved cannula system, inserting long needles linked by a 2–0 PDS suture from inside-out (Figures 6.13–6.15) (Clancy and Graf 1983), an outside-in method where knotted PDS sutures are pulled peripherally (Warren 1985), and an inside-inside technique, suturing the meniscal portions together arthroscopically (Morgan *et al.* 1991). In the mid-1990s, the all-inside technique using meniscal darts was developed (Albrecht-Olsen *et al.* 1993). Other all-inside methods of stabilization soon followed and currently the third generation of devices for the all-inside technique include the Meniscal Cinch (Arthrex), Fast-Fix (Smith and Nephew) and Maxfire (Biomet). Their advantages are the stability they can immediately provide and the reduction in operating time. Chondral abrasion, implant failure or migration, synovitis and cyst formation have been reported as complications. The devices are also expensive (Turman and Diduch 2008).

The inside-out method can be further subdivided into double barrel cannula and single needle passage techniques. Since collagen bundles are oriented predominantly circumferentially at the periphery of the meniscus, it is advantageous to direct the individual insertions of the mattress suture in superior and inferior directions so that the suture is orientated vertically near the synovial attachment, thus securing more meniscal tissue for stronger fixation (Dervin *et al.* 1997; Asik and Sener 2002). A double-barrel system is more prone to suture pull-out and may not provide adequate meniscal coaptation unless it is used like a single-barrel system by rotating it between needle insertions to create vertically orientated sutures (DeHaven 1999). Common to all meniscal repair techniques is adequate preparation of the tear site and perimeniscal synovium, carried out using 2 mm and 3 mm rasps. A small, powered shaver may also be employed.

▨ Medial meniscal repair

A tourniquet is applied to the proximal thigh. A well-padded leg holder is placed distal to the tourniquet and, if meniscal repair is planned, the thigh should be flexed approximately 45° in 135

Figure 6.13a,b At arthroscopy a blunt hook confirms the presence of a displacing 'bucket handle' tear of the medial meniscus.

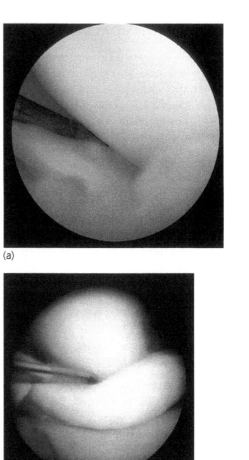

(a)

(b)

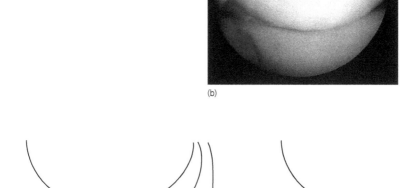

Figure 6.14 Sutures may be placed through the superior or inferior meniscal surface.

the leg holder to provide access to the posteromedial corner of the knee. It is important to pad the leg holder well and place it on the thigh distal to the tourniquet to prevent any pressure posteriorly on the sciatic nerve. Elevation of the thigh may not be necessary if the surgeon prefers to sit and flex the end of the table, but the thigh must extend far enough beyond the edge of the table break for access to the posterior corners of the knee. The leg may be kept in

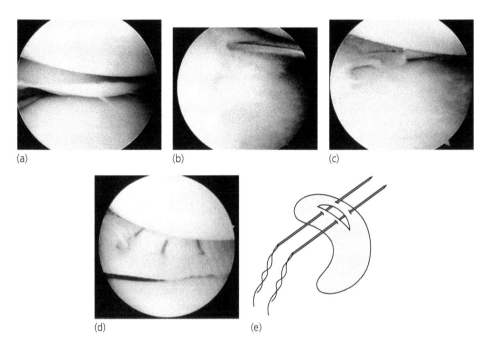

(a) (b) (c)

(d) (e)

Figure 6.15a–e Meniscal sutures retaining the reduced 'bucket handle' segment.

this position without redraping it if ACL reconstruction is to be carried out after meniscal repair (Henning 1983).

After diagnostic arthroscopy has established the need to repair the medial meniscus, a 6 cm longitudinal incision is made just behind the posterior border of the medial collateral ligament. The incision should be undertaken with the knee flexed so that the pes anserinus and the sartorial branch of the saphenous nerve will lie posterior to the joint line. Care must be taken throughout the procedure to avoid excessive retraction or entrapment of the nerve with sutures (Henning 1983; DeHaven 1999) so transillumination of the soft tissues at arthroscopy will aid in identifying it and the long saphenous vein (Kelly and Macnicol 2002).

Dissection is carried down to the posterior capsule, deep to the semimembranosus, and half-way across the medial head of the gastrocnemius. If the direct head of the semimembranosus is too tight, it may be necessary to release several millimetres of its attachment. When suturing of the mid-central portion of the meniscus is contemplated, subcutaneous tissue should be dissected off the medial collateral ligament anterior to the posteromedial incision. A popliteal retractor is then inserted behind the posterior capsule. From the anterolateral portal, the arthroscope is advanced medial to the posterior cruciate ligament to inspect the posteromedial compartment of the joint. Both sides of the tear should be freshened, especially if it is older than 8 weeks. The inferior surface of a posterior horn tear and the superior and inferior surfaces of a mid-central tear are best abraded with a burr or edge-cutting rasp introduced anteromedially. It is important to devote time to the careful abrasion of synovium under the inferior portion of the meniscus (DeHaven 1999).

Suturing is carried out using 2–0 non-absorbable Ethibond sutures with double-armed taper-ended needles. A 10–15° bend is made 4 cm from the needle tip, and a second 10–15° bend is made approximately 10 mm from the first bend in the same direction. The needle is then inserted into the needle holder. Suture placement for the posterior 137 horn of the medial meniscus is carried out from the anteromedial portal. A short cannula is placed through this portal, close to the medial edge of the patellar tendon. Suturing is commenced near the posterior horn origin of the tear, and the first suture should preferably be placed on the inferior surface of the meniscus. Once the needle has been inserted approximately 3–4 mm from the tear site and up to the second bend in the needle, a third bend should be created in the needle by pushing the cannula and needle holder into the intercondylar notch. The extra bend in the needle will allow easier needle retrieval from the posteromedial incision.

The first suture insertion should be directed from the inferior surface upward through the meniscus so as to include as much meniscal tissue in a vertical orientation as possible. The surgeon should then carefully palpate the posterior capsule to determine whether the exit site of the needle will allow it to be contained by the popliteal retractor. Once this has been established, the needle may be pushed through and grasped posteriorly with the needle holder. The needle should never be advanced while palpating posteriorly. After release of the needle anteriorly, it is pulled out through the posteromedial incision. The second throw of the first suture penetrates beyond the tear site near the meniscosynovial junction, thus creating a vertically oriented suture. In an alternative suturing technique, the second insertion of the suture is made approximately 3–4 mm from the first, thus creating a horizontal mattress suture. The needles should be passed in divergent directions so as to include as much meniscal tissue in a vertical orientation as possible.

Starting at the posterior horn origin, suture placement is alternated between the superior and inferior surfaces of the meniscus, spaced approximately 3 mm apart. If the tear extends into the middle third of the medial meniscus, the arthroscope should be switched to the anteromedial portal, and suturing should be carried out through the anterolateral portal. Sutures placed on the superior surface of the meniscus should have less of the suture loop exposed compared with those on the inferior surface. An attempt should be made to direct these sutures to the posteromedial incision site. The most anterior sutures may be directed out through a 1 cm incision placed between the posteromedial and the anteromedial incisions.

Sutures placed in this fashion will avoid shear forces that may result if they are directed obliquely out through the posteromedial incision (Asik and Sener 2002). If difficulty is encountered in adequately visualizing or placing sutures through the posterior horn fragment, a probe inserted through an accessory anteromedial portal may be used to bring the meniscal fragment anteriorly, or to tilt it so that suture placement can be optimized. Similarly, displaced bucket handle tears can be successfully repaired. If the anterior cruciate ligament is to be reconstructed, the sutures are not tied until the end of the reconstruction (DeHaven 1999). The sutures can be kept tight in the meantime by threading them through 7 cm pieces of intravenous extension tubing and cross-clamping the tubing.

Isolated meniscal repairs may be enhanced by fibrin clot introduced into the tear site before tying the sutures, although the postoperative haemarthrosis may itself provide a sufficiency of local blood clot. Approximately 50–75 mL of the patient's venous blood is placed in a plastic container and the blood stirred with one or two 10–20 mm glass syringe barrels for approximately 5–10 minutes until the clot adheres to the glass barrels. The clot is then removed and blotted with moistened gauze. An Ethibond suture (2–0) is placed and secured at each end of the clot. After introduction of a 6–7 mm cannula, the two free needles are bent in the same manner as for meniscal repair and loaded into the Henning needleholders. After passage through the cannula and under the inferior surface of the meniscus, through the meniscosynovial junction at the most posterior and anterior poles of the tear, they are

retrieved posteriorly.

When the clot has been tucked into the tear site, all sutures are tied. The single strands of the clot sutures are tied to adjacent meniscal repair sutures. Alternative methods of clot introduction include the use of a commercially available clot introducer, or the clot can be transferred through a 6 mm cannula with a blunt obturator or a glass syringe, using a blunt 13-gauge curved needle. The tear site is then pulled open with a probe and, with the joint evacuated of fluid so that the clot does not float away, the clot is placed under the inferior surface of the meniscus throughout the length of the tear. The sutures are pulled tight, trapping the fibrin clot, and then tied.

■ Lateral meniscus repair

The technique of lateral meniscal repair is similar to that for the medial meniscus. A 6 cm vertical incision is made at the posterolateral corner of the knee. A longitudinal incision is created in the deep fascia along the posterior margin of the iliotibial band and the biceps is retracted posteriorly with the knee flexed 90°. The lateral head of the gastrocnemius is dissected off the posterior capsule to a point where a nerve hook, passed from the anteromedial portal over the top of the posterior horn origin of the lateral meniscus, can be palpated through the posterolateral incision. With the knee flexed 90°, the peroneal nerve will lie posterior to the biceps except in the proximal portion of the incision, where it crosses over behind the biceps to lie closer to the posterior surface of the lateral head of the gastrocnemius. The nerve does not have to be dissected out and identified. Abrasion of both tear surfaces is carried out as described for the medial side. Suture placement is exclusively from the anteromedial portal. There should not be too much concern if a suture passes through the popliteus tendon, although, preferably, this should be avoided. Radial split tears of the posterior horn can be approximated by passing one suture through the posterior leaf close to the inner margin of the meniscus and the second suture through the anterior leaf of this tear. Since adequate healing of radial split tears is unlikely in the middle third of the lateral meniscus, they are probably best left alone (Ikeuchi 1982; Vandermeer and Cunningham 1989).

■ All-inside technique using the Biofix resorbable arrows (first generation all-inside technique)

The Biofix implant provides a horizontal fixation and has been designed to create optimal fixation of the meniscus (Albrecht-Olsen *et al.* 1993). A specially designed instrument set allows repair through standard arthroscopy portals, and consists of six cannulas with various curves, an obturator, a needle, perforator, pusher and hammer. After the rupture has been freshened and reduced, the chosen cannula with the blunt obturator inside is inserted via the portals. After withdrawal of the obturator the cannula is fixed 3–4 mm from the lesion, and the meniscus is kept reduced. With a special perforator, a hole for the arrow is made through the meniscus and into the joint capsule.

The irrigation is turned off, and the perforator is retracted. A tack is pushed into the cannula with the pusher and hammered into the meniscus. A special reciprocating instrument can be used for this procedure. Every 5–10 mm a new tack is inserted until the tear is stable. The implants have a diameter of 1.1 mm and are available in three lengths (10, 13 and 16 mm) for different meniscal tear sites. Third-generation devices are generally made of non-resorbable material. No cannulas are used and the device is usually pistol-shaped. The tags or arrows are fired and the prefabricated knot is then tied and cut. The tags can be adjusted in length. This further reduces operating time and the risk of device-related complications.

In the case of isolated meniscal repairs, partial weightbearing is initiated after 3 weeks. Full weightbearing is allowed from 3 to 6 weeks. More details about rehabilitation following meniscal repair are contained in Chapter 10.

◼ Meniscal transplantation

Garrett and Stevenson (1991) and Verdonk *et al.* (2007) proposed that transplantation of menisci will reduce the incidence of osteoarthritis after total meniscectomy and may also lessen instability in the anterior cruciate-deficient knee. Clinical experience with this technique is still limited to a few centres. As with meniscal repair, an associated anterior cruciate ligament rupture should be reconstructed since survival of the meniscus is otherwise endangered (Verdonk *et al.* 2007). Conversely, knee stability may be achieved by combining meniscal transplantation with anterior cruciate ligament surgery in cases where a total meniscectomy has been carried out. The provision of suitably sized and safe meniscal allografts may prove to be a limiting factor in the future. Furthermore, since the need for meniscal transplantation followed the era of total meniscectomy, partial meniscectomy has resulted in a reduction in the demand for allografts (Rodeo 2001; Noyes *et al.* 2004; Verdonk *et al.* 2007). The relative indications include:

- Patients over 50 years of age with a history of total meniscectomy, who have pain localized to the meniscus-deficient compartment. The knee joint should be stable, well aligned, and should not reveal articular cartilage lesions greater than grade III (International Cartilage Repair Society [ICRS] classification system). The cartilage defects should be focal and not generalized
- ACL-deficient patients who have undergone prior medial meniscectomy and who might benefit from the increased stability afforded by a functioning medial meniscus in conjunction with concomitant ACL reconstruction
- Young patients who have required complete meniscectomy may be considered as meniscal transplantation candidates before the onset of symptoms. That said, prophylactic meniscal transplantation is not routinely recommended.

The contraindications to meniscal allograft transplantation are:

- Advanced chondral degeneration, greater than grade III (ICRS classification). Radiographic evidence of significant osteophyte formation or femoral condyle flattening is associated with inferior postoperative results as these structural modifications alter the morphology of the femoral condyle
- Patients over 50 years of age may experience excessive cartilage breakdown and are suboptimal candidates
- Axial malalignment and flexion deformity (in cases of unicompartmental osteoarthritis, a unicompartmental prosthesis is now preferred to corrective osteotomy and meniscal transplantation)
- Miscellaneous conditions (obesity, skeletal immaturity, instability of the knee joint, synovial disease, inflammatory arthritis, previous joint infection).

Current research and experiments with collagen meniscal implants or scaffolds such as Menaflex (ReGen Medical, USA), Actifit and Ortec (Netherlands) offer a promising future. The indications are symptomatic, young adults following partial or subtotal meniscectomy. There should be a posterior horn remnant to allow implant attachment. The implant is 'off the shelf' and can be cut to shape as needed. The material is expensive and long-term follow-up has yet to prove its advantages in terms of restoration of normal knee function and the prevention of osteoarthritis (Rodkey *et al.* 2008).

■ The discoid lateral meniscus

The discoid meniscus probably forms as a result of its unusually mobile attachments, since the abnormality is not seen in other animals (Kaplan 1957). Classically the shapes have been divided into the complete (see Figure 4.39, p. 86), covering the lateral tibial condyle, the incomplete, and the highly mobile Wrisberg types (see Figure 4.38a, p. 85 and Figure 4.40, p. 86) (Watanabe *et al.* 1979). Fujikawa *et al.* (1978) proposed that a reduction in the lateral femoral condylar angle allowed the lateral meniscus to remain discoid (see Figure 4.38b, p. 85) and described an anterior 'megahorn' meniscus, which might develop if only the posterior half of the meniscus was resorbed normally.

The discoid anomaly appears to be more common in Chinese and Japanese patients, but in the West the frequency is approximately 2.5 per cent (Smillie 1948). Symptoms include snapping (Middleton 1936), pain, locking, limp, effusions and giving way (Glasgow *et al.* 1982). Aichroth *et al.* (1992) report that the classic clunk can be elicited in only 39 per cent of knees and in some cases movement within the lateral compartment is seen or felt without a snap. The joint line may feel full and is often tender (Papadopoulos *et al.* 2009).

Other causes of snapping knee are patellofemoral instability, a subluxing iliotibial band, subluxation of the tibiofemoral or proximal tibiofibular joints and other meniscal pathology, particularly cystic change. The diagnosis can be established by MR scanning and arthroscopy, which allow the morphology of the anomaly to be assessed, together with any tears involving the superior or inferior surfaces.

A conservative surgical approach is justifiable, so that medial edge tears should be saucerized and a partial, central meniscectomy carried out for more extensive lesions (Hayashi *et al.* 1988; Ikeuchi 1982). Excellent results have been reported in the short-term (Bellier *et al.* 1989), although other reviews are less optimistic (Vandermeer and Cunningham 1989). The troublesome Wrisberg type (see Figure 4.40, p. 86) merits complete excision, as do complete discoid menisci with major tears. In approximately 20 per cent of cases the anomaly is bilateral, yet symptoms rarely affect both knees (Ding *et al.* 2009).

Joint lubrication

The synovial membrane secretes a fluid which ensures that the coefficient of friction between the femur and the tibia, and the femur and the patella, is low. In articular joints the coefficient approaches 0.002, which compares very favourably with steel on ice (0.01). The coefficient of friction in artificial joints is in the region of 0.1.

Lubrication in the knee joint is of mixed type, with both fluid–film and boundary characteristics. In the fluid–film form, the apposing surfaces are separated by a thin film of fluid, many molecules thick. There are three forms of fluid–film lubrication:

* Hydrodynamic – which depends on the motion of one surface upon the other
* Elastohydrodynamic – which includes a component of elastic deformation of one or both surfaces as a result of contact pressures
* 'Squeeze' film – where loading of the joint surfaces wrings out fluid from the articular cartilage and thus ensures preservation of the fluid–film even with considerable loading.

The other form of lubrication is known as boundary lubrication, and here surface deformation occurs because a continuous fluid–film is not constantly present. It is also known that gel-like substances aggregate on the surface of articular cartilage, and this is proportional to the protein content of the synovial fluid (Caligaris *et al.* 2009).

In the knee joint, fluid–film and boundary lubrication exist together, although the fluid–film form is generally operant. When lubrication is insufficient, either as a result of injury or adverse metabolic processes, articular surfaces are subjected to greater stresses, both compressive and frictional. Repeated haemarthroses, or the presence of debris and loose bodies, will also exert an adverse effect on the properties of synovial fluid, and the increased wear within the joint will lead to osteoarthritis. It is apposite to conclude this chapter with the reminder that the menisci combine with the synovium and its secreted fluid to ensure that the articular cartilage of the knee joint is effectively lubricated and nourished (Katta *et al.* 2009).

References

Aichroth PM, Patel DV and Marx CL (1992) Congenital discoid lateral meniscus: a long-term follow-up study. In: Aichroth PM and Cannon WD (eds) *Knee Surgery: Current Practice.* London: Martin Dunitz, pp. 540-5.

Albrecht-Olsen P, Kristensen G and Törmälä P (1993) Meniscus bucket-handle fixation with an absorbable Biofix tack: development of a new technique. *Knee Surg Sports Traumatol Arthrosc* **1**, 104-6.

Albrecht-Olsen P, Kristensen G, Burgaard P, *et al.* (1999) The arrow versus horizontal suture in arthroscopic meniscus repair. A prospective randomized study, with arthroscopic evaluation. *Knee Surg Sports Traumatol Arthrosc* **7**, 268-73.

Annandale T (1885) An operation for displaced semilunar cartilage. *Br Med J* **i**, 779-81.

Apley AG (1959) *A system of orthopaedics and fractures.* London: Butterwort.

Arnoczky SP and Warren RF (1982) Microvasculature of the human meniscus. *Am J Sports Med* **10**, 90-5.

Arnoczky SP and Warren RF (1983) The microvasculature of the meniscus and its response to injury: An experimental study in the dog. *Am J Sports Med* **11**, 131-41.

Arnoczky SP, Warren RF and Spivak JM (1988) Meniscal repair using an exogenous fibrin clot – an experimental study in dogs. *J Bone Joint Surg Am* **70**, 1209-20.

Asik M and Sener N (2002) Failure strength of repair devices versus meniscus suturing techniques. *Knee Surg Sports Traumatol Arthrosc* **10**, 25-9.

Bellier G, Dupont JY, Larrain M, *et al.* (1989) Lateral discoid menisci in children. *Arthroscopy* **5**, 52-6.

Borden P, Nyland J, Caborn DN, *et al.* (2003) Biomechanical comparison of the FasT-Fix Meniscal repair suture system with vertical mattress sutures and meniscus arrows. *Am J Sports Med* **31**, 374-8.

Bronstein R, Kirk P and Hurley J (1992) The usefulness of MRI in evaluating menisci after repair. *Orthopedics* **15**, 149-52.

Bullough P, Munera L, Murphy J and Weinstein AM (1970) The strength of the menisci as it relates to their fine structure. *J Bone Joint Surg Br* **52**, 64-70.

Caligaris M, Canal CE, Ahmad CS, *et al.* (2009) Investigation of the frictional response of osteoarthritic human tibiofemoral joints and the potential beneficial tribological effect of healthy synovial fluid. *Osteoarthritis Cartilage* **17**, 1327-32.

Cannon WD and Morgan CD (1994) Meniscal repair. *J Bone Joint Surg Am* **76**, 294-311.

Clancy WG and Graf BK (1983) Arthroscopic meniscal repair. *Orthopaedics* **6**, 1125-8.

Cooper DE, Arnoczky SP and Warren RF (1991) Meniscal repair. *Clin Sports Med* **10**, 529-48.

Dandy DJ (1981) *Arthroscopic Surgery of the Knee.* Edinburgh: Churchill Livingstone.

Dandy DJ (1990) Arthroscopic anatomy of symptomatic meniscal lesions. *J Bone Joint Surg Br* **72**, 628-31.

Dandy DJ, Northmore-Ball MD and Jackson RW (1983) Arthroscopic, open partial and total meniscectomy: a comparative study. *J Bone Joint Surg Br* **65**, 400-4.

DeHaven KE (1985) Meniscus repair in the athlete. *Clin Orthop* **198**, 31–5.

DeHaven KE (1999) Meniscus repair: current concepts. *Am J Sports Med* **27**, 242–50.

DeHaven KE, Lohrer WA and Lovelock JE (1995) Long-term results of open meniscus repair. *Am J Sports Med* **23**, 524–30.

Dervin GF, Downing BE, Kenee CR and McBride DG (1997) Failure strengths of suture versus biodegradable arrow for meniscus repair: an in vitro study. *Arthroscopy* **13**, 296–330.

Ding J, Zhao J, He Y, *et al.* (2009) Risk factors for articular cartilage lesions in symptomatic discoid lateral meniscus. *Arthroscopy* **25**, 1423–6.

Fairbank HAT (1937) Internal derangement of the knee in children and adolescents. *Proc R Soc Med* **30**, 427–32.

Fujikawa K, Tomatsu T and Malso K (1978) Morphological analysis of meniscus and articular cartilage in the knee joint by means of arthrogram. *J Jpn Orthop Assoc* **52**, 203–15.

Gallacher PD, Gilbert RE, Kanes G, *et al.* (2010) White on white meniscal tears: to fix or not to fix? *Knee* **17**, 270–3.

Garrett JC and Stevenson RN (1991) Meniscal transplantation in the human knee: a preliminary report. *Arthroscopy* **7**, 52–62.

Glasgow MMS, Aichroth PM and Baird PRE (1982) The discoid lateral meniscus: a clinical review. *J Bone Joint Surg Br* **64**, 245–50.

Hamberg P, Gillquist J and Lysholm J (1983) Suture of new and old peripheral meniscus tears. *J Bone Joint Surg Am* **65**, 193–7.

Hantes ME, Zachos VC, Varitimidis SE *et al.* (2006) Arthroscopic meniscal repair: a comparative study between three different surgical techniques. *Knee Surg Sports Traumatol Arthrosc* **14**, 1232–7.

Hayashi LK, Yamaga H, Ida K, *et al.* (1988) Arthroscopic meniscectomy for discoid lateral meniscus in children. *J Bone Joint Surg Am* **70**, 1495–500.

Henning CE (1983) Arthroscopic repair of meniscus tears. *Orthopedics* **6**, 1130–2.

Henning CE, Yearout M, Vequist SW, *et al.* (1991) Use of the fascia sheath coverage and exogenous fibrin clot in the treatment of complex meniscal tears. *Am J Sports Med* **19**, 626–31.

Herrlin S, Hallander M, Wange P, *et al.* (2007) Arthroscopic or surgical treatment of degenerative medial meniscal tears: a prospective randomized trial. *Knee Surg Sports Traumatol Arthritis* **15**, 393–401.

Ikeuchi H (1982) Arthroscopic treatment of the discoid lateral meniscus: technique and long-term results. *Clin Orthop* **167**, 19–28.

Johnson LL (1978) *Diagnostic and Surgical Arthroscopy*, 3rd edn. St Louis: Mosby.

Kaplan EB (1957) Discoid lateral meniscus of the knee joint. Nature, mechanism and operative treatment. *J Bone Joint Surg Am* **39**, 77–87.

Katta J, Jin Z, Ingham E, *et al.* (2009) Effect of nominal stress on the long term friction, deformation and wear of native and glycosaminoglycan deficient articular cartilage. *Osteoarthritis Cartilage* **17**, 662–8.

Kelly M and Macnicol M F (2002) Identification of the saphenous nerve at arthroscopy. *Arthroscopy* **14**, L312–14.

King D (1936) The healing of semilunar cartilages. *J Bone Joint Surg Br* **18**, 333–42.

Majewski M, Stoll R, Widmer H, *et al.* (2006) Midterm and long-term results after arthroscopic suture repair of isolated, longitudinal, vertical meniscal tears in stable knees. *Am J Sports Med* **34**, 1072–6.

McGinty JB, Geuss LE and Marvin RA (1977) Partial or total meniscectomy. A comparative analysis. *J Bone Joint Surg Am* **59**, 763–6.

McMurray TP (1928) The diagnosis of internal derangements of the knee. In: *Robert Jones Birthday Volume*. Oxford: Oxford Medical Publications, pp. 301–5.

McNicholas MJ, Rowley DI, McGurty D *et al.* (2000) Total meniscectomy in adolescence. *J Bone Joint Surg Br* **82**, 217–21.

Meunier A, Odensten M and Good L (2007) Long-term results after primary repair or non-surgical treatment of anterior cruciate ligament rupture: a randomized study with a 15-year follow-up. *Scand J Med Sci Sports* **17**, 320–7.

Middleton DS (1936) Congenital disc-shaped lateral meniscus with snapping knee. *Br J Surg* **24**, 246–55.

Morgan CD, Wojtys EM, Casscells CD, *et al.* (1991) Arthroscopic meniscal repair evaluated by second-look arthroscopy. *Am J Sports Med* **19**, 632–8.

Noble J and Erat K (1980) In defence of the meniscus; a prospective study of two hundred meniscectomy patients. *J Bone Joint Surg Br* **62**, 6–11.

Noyes FR and Barber-Westin SD (2002) Arthroscopic repair of meniscal tears extending into the avascular zone in patients younger than twenty years of age. *Am J Sports Med* **30**, 589–600.

Noyes FR, Barber-Westin SD and Rankin M (2004) Meniscal transplantation in symptomatic patients less then fifty years old. *J Bone Joint Surg Am* **86**, 1392–404.

Papadopoulos A, Kirkos JM, Kapetanos GA(2009) Histomorphologic study of discoid meniscus. *Arthroscopy* **25**, 262–8.

Parry CBW, Nichols PJR and Lewis NR (1958) Meniscectomy: a review of 1,723 cases. *Ann Phys Med* **4**, 201–9.

Rodeo SA (2001) Meniscal allografts: where do we stand? *Am J Sports Med* **29**, 246–61.

Rodkey WG, DeHaven KE, Montgomery WH 3rd, *et al.* (2008) Comparison of the collagen meniscus implant with partial meniscectomy. A prospective randomized trial. *J Bone Joint Surg Am* **90**, 1413–26.

Roos H, Adalbrecht T, Dahlberg L and Lohmander LS (1995) Osteoarthritis of the knee after injury to the anterior cruciate ligament or meniscus: the influence of time and age. *Osteoarthritis Cartilage* **3**, 261–7.

Rubman MR, Noyes FR, Barber-Westin SD (1998) Arthroscopic repair of meniscal tears that extend into the avascular zone: a review of 198 single and complex tears. *Am J Sports Med* **26**, 87–95.

Smillie IS (1948) The congenital discoid meniscus. *J Bone Joint Surg Br* **30**, 671–82.

Steenbrugge F, Verdonk R and Verstraete K (2002) Allograft reconstructions for chronic ruptures of the anterior cruciate ligament: augmentation versus non-augmentation. *Eur J Orthop Surg Traumatol* **12**, 8–11.

Steenbrugge F, Verdonk R, Hürel C and Verstraete K (2004a) Arthroscopic meniscus repair: inside-out vs. Biofix meniscus arrow. *Knee Surg Sports Traumatol Arthrosc* **12**, 43–9.

Steenbrugge F, Verdonk R and Verstraete K (2004b) Magnetic resonance imaging of the surgically repaired meniscus: a 13-year follow-up study. *Acta Orthop Scand* **75**, 323–7.

Steenbrugge F, Van Nieuwenhuyse W, Verdonk R and Verstraete K (2005) Arthroscopic meniscus repair in the ACL-deficient knee. *Int Orthop* **29**, 109–12.

Suman RK, Stother IG and Illingworth G (1984) Diagnostic arthroscopy of the knee in children. *J Bone Joint Surg Br* **66**, 535–7.

Tapper E and Hoover N (1969) Late results after meniscectomy. *J Bone Joint Surg Am* **51**, 517–26.

Trillat A (1962) Lésions traumatique du ménisque interne du genu. Classement anatomique et diagnostic clinique. *Rev Chir Orthop* **48**, 551–63.

Turman KA and Diduch DR (2008) Meniscal repair: indications and techniques. *J Knee Surg* **21**, 154–62.

Vandermeer RD and Cunningham FK (1989) Arthroscopic treatment of the discoid lateral meniscus: results of long-term follow-up. *Arthroscopy* **5**, 101–9.

Verdonk R, Almqvist KF, Huysse W and Verdonk PC (2007) Meniscal allografts: indications and outcomes. *Sports Med Arthrosc Rev* **15**, 121–5.

Walker PS and Erkman MH (1975) The role of the menisci in force transmission across the knee. *Clin Orthop* **104**, 184–93.

Warren RF (1985) Arthroscopic meniscus repair. *Arthroscopy* **1**, 170–2.

Watanabe M, Takeda S and Ikeuchi H (1979) *Atlas of Arthroscopy*. Tokyo: Igaku Shoin.

Yasunaga T, Kimura M and Kikuchi S (2001) Histologic change of the meniscus and cartilage tissue after meniscal suture. *Clin Orthop* **387**, 232–40.

7

Patellofemoral problems

Introduction

The injury that provokes patellar symptoms may be recalled clearly as a single event by the patient or may be cumulative. In many instances, no trauma can be recalled, the patellofemoral joint aching during periods of rapid growth in early adolescence or after repetitive use of the knee during certain occupations or in athletics. Although it is important to differentiate between the group of patients whose patellae are dislocating or subluxing and those whose patellar tracking appears to be normal, the two groups are not easy to separate and there are undoubtedly patients with subclinical (undetectable) subluxation of the patellofemoral joint. In certain instances the patella may tilt rather than sublux, and the term 'patellar instability' is to be preferred in these cases.

Yates and Grana (1990) use the term 'patellofemoral dysplasia' to describe a continuum of anatomical variations which predispose the child to patellar symptoms. Many of these reside at sites distant from the patellofemoral joint (Figures 7.1, 7.2), combining torsional abnormalities with deficient connective tissue strength and morphological oddities of the joint itself. One important factor in most cases of dislocation during earlier childhood is relative shortening of the quadriceps mechanism. This is invariably present in the congenital forms of knee dislocation and subluxation (see Chapter 4 and Figure 4.6), where recurvatum and restricted flexion are the norm.

Patellar dislocation is conveniently graded as:

- Congenital – in association with other gross anomalies noted at birth
- Habitual – coming to light in the first half of childhood:
  - During flexion
  - During extension
  - Persistent, where the patella remains permanently out of the femoral groove
- Recurrent – often after relatively trivial injury:
  - Acute onset with subsequent repeated episodes
  - Chronic, with gradual onset of instability.

Although dislocation is usually lateral (Figure 7.3), inferior, superior (vertical) and medial displacement may also occur. Patella alta (Figures 7.4, p. 150) and variations in the congruency angle of the patellofemoral joint have been defined radiographically (Merchant *et al.* 1974) (Figure 7.5, p. 150) and by computed tomography (CT) (Fulkerson *et al.* 1987). These measurements are applicable clinically but do not fully reflect the complexity of patellar biomechanics. Additionally, magnetic resonance (MR) scanning has revealed that the articular cartilage contours often concord poorly with the calcified bone evident on skyline radiographs.

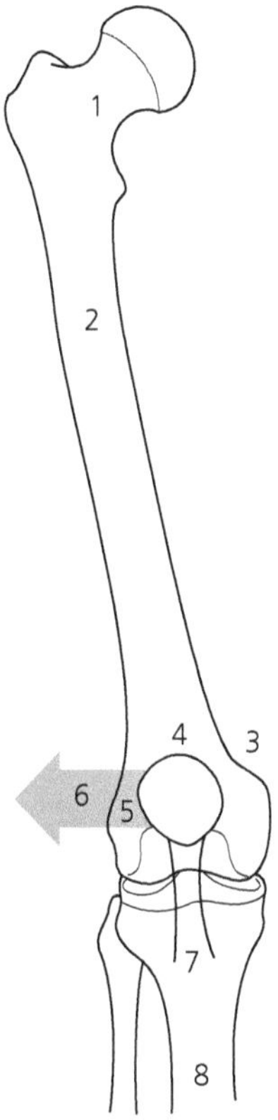

Congenital dislocation

Congenital dislocation (see also Chapter 4 for the neonatal presentation) is often associated with a skeletal dysplasia or motor retardation. The child is slow to walk or may be unable to weightbear effectively on the leg. Previous surgery may have been attempted. In addition to the quadriceps contracture the femoral condylar groove is shallow with poor development of the lateral femoral condyle. The patella is usually oval and dysplastic, and its distal attachment may be laterally placed. Torsional deformities of the femur and tibia, soft tissue laxity or contracture, and foot abnormalities are common.

Since stretching and splintage of the knee in flexion usually fails when there is fixed deformity, treatment of the condition involves a lengthening of the rectus femoris and vastus lateralis, release of vastus intermedius and double breasting of the medial parapatellar structures, including vastus medialis (Goa *et al.* 1990). Distal realignment of the patellar tendon should be achieved by rerouting its lateral half medially by means of the Roux–Goldthwait technique. Significant external tibial rotation is sometimes encountered and a concomitant pesplasty is then advisable. However, extensive realignment of musculotendinous units around the knee should not be undertaken lightly and it is often better to stage procedures, correcting the short quadriceps mechanism and lateral tethers first, and the torsional abnormalities in later childhood if patellar stability is not secured.

Following this extensive surgical release the knee is splinted in 20–30° of flexion for 6 weeks. The child is readmitted to hospital when the plaster is bivalved and physiotherapy

Figure 7.1 Sites where morphological abnormalities may predispose towards lateral patellar dislocation or subluxation: 1, increased femoral neck anteversion; 2, internal (medial) femoral torsion; 3, weak vastus medialis muscle; 4, high or abnormally shaped patella; 5, deficient lateral femoral condyle; 6, tight lateral retinacular bands; 7, laterally placed tibial tuberosity; 8, external tibial torsion.

is arranged as an inpatient. Full flexion is rarely restored, but a flexion arc of over 90° can usually be obtained. If the fascia lata remains tight the Ober test (Ober 1936) will be positive, demonstrated by the presence of an abductor contracture of the hip when the knee is extended.

Habitual dislocation

In children where the quadriceps mechanism is relatively short, marked genu recurvatum will not be present but the patella rests high in the sulcus (femoral trochlea) or above it. Coupled with this are other features of knee dysplasia, including a shallow sulcus, axial and angulatory malalignment and ligament laxity. These are constitutional abnormalities, differentiating the problem from acquired quadriceps fibrosis following injections into the thigh during infancy

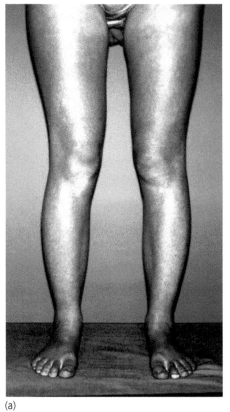 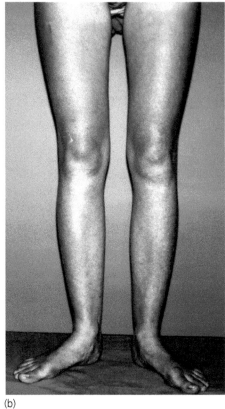

(a)   (b)

Figure 7.2 Persistent femoral anteversion producing inward squinting patellae (a) and compensatory external tibial torsion (b).

(Gunn 1964). Williams (1968) described patellar dislocation secondary to injections later in childhood, in contrast to the restricted knee flexion (without patellar dislocation) encountered in the infantile form of this iatrogenic condition.

Habitual dislocation may be familial and is seen in ligament laxity syndromes (Carter 1960) and the hypermobility associated with the Ehlers–Danlos, Marfan's, Down's and Ellis–van Creveld syndromes, or other skeletal dysplasias such as onycho-osteodysplasia (nail-patella syndrome) and osteogenesis imperfecta. The onset of symptoms is gradual with no convincing trauma as a precipitant. Patella alta is usually obvious and the patella either shifts laterally under load during the last 20° of extension (inverted 'J tracking') or subluxes as the knee is flexed (Figure 7.6). In the latter variety an abnormal attachment of the iliotibial band into the lateral border of the patella may be palpable. In some children the patella tracks in a sinusoidal manner, moving out of the femoral sulcus in both extension and mid-flexion.

When these abnormalities of tracking become painful the child ceases to cope with sports; even walking and sitting become troublesome. Physiotherapy may help in a proportion of cases, but persistence of the symptoms is common and disabling. Lateral release alone is ineffectual unless the dislocation occurs in flexion and a lateral tether can be demonstrated. If the quadriceps mechanism is short, a V–Y or Z-lengthening is indicated, combined with a Roux–Goldthwait medialization of the patellar tendon. The leg is splinted in a cast postoperatively,

Figure 7.3 Lateral patellar dislocation viewed on (a) 'skyline' and (b) oblique radiographs.

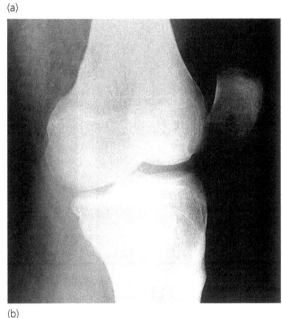

(a)

(b)

and after 6 weeks a period of intensive physiotherapy is required. Once again, the child may require inpatient supervision and recovery of knee function is slow. Scarring is often widened and long-term patellar stability is not assured.

Recurrent subluxation and dislocation

This disorder manifests towards the end of childhood and during adolescence. Girls are twice as commonly affected until the mid-teenage years when boys present more often. The characteristics of patellar tracking are usually demonstrably abnormal, although the changes may be subtle and best shown by dynamic CT (Fulkerson *et al.* 1987). The classification of recurrent dislocation has been discussed by Jackson (1992), who divides the condition in the second and third decades of life into:

- Lateral subluxation of the patella in extension ('J tracking')
- Lateral subluxation in flexion
- Dislocation with no evidence of maltracking.

149

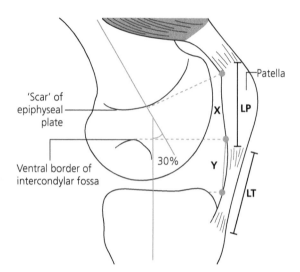

Figure 7.4 Suggested measurements to describe patella alta. (1) Blumensaat (1932) considered that the patella normally lies between the dotted lines, which are extensions of the epiphyseal line and the intercondylar fossa with the knee in 30° of flexion. (2) Insall and Salvati (1971) stated that LT: LP should not exceed 1.2; the distal end of the patellar tendon, and hence the length of LT, is difficult to define radiographically. (3) Blackburne and Peel (1977) used the ratio Y: X because this uses the upper end of the tibia as a point of reference; normal values are less than 1.0.

A family history of patellofemoral problems is often present and internal torsion of the femur, with or without external torsion of the tibia, predisposes to instability by producing a large Q-angle (Figure 7.7). The femoral sulcus may be shallow and a variety of patterns of patellofemoral incongruency have been described (Laurin *et al.* 1979; Merchant *et al.* 1974; Merchant 1992). Genu valgum is no more common than in asymptomatic children.

The diagnosis is often missed by the inexperienced since episodes of giving way and medial discomfort are wrongly ascribed to meniscal pathology. The patella rarely presents in its dislocated position and an effusion is only seen acutely. The apprehension sign is positive, patellar manipulation is painful and the opposite knee may also be symptomatic. The patella may be laterally displaced or tilted on the skyline radiographic projection but variations in the osseous patellar shape do not appear to be of much consequence. The patellofemoral relationship in the first 30° of flexion is of significance, and avulsion and osteochondral fragments may be present.

Direct trauma can, however, produce a dislocation in a normal knee, and this may be accompanied by a shearing, osteochondral fracture of the patella or the contiguous lateral femoral condyle (Figure 7.8). The patella usually dislocates laterally but may also jam inferiorly, superiorly or medially.

Indirect violence, for example when the patient twists on the weightbearing leg, may be sufficient to cause an inherently weak patellofemoral articulation to dislocate spontaneously. Nevertheless, it is often difficult to state

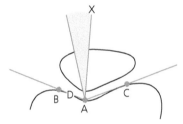

Figure 7.5 The sulcus (condylar groove or trochlear) angle BAC is constructed by the highest points of the medial (B) and lateral (C) condyles and the deepest part of the sulcus (A). The congruence angle XAD is the angle between the line bisecting the sulcus angle (AX) and the line linking the apex of the patella (D) and A. A congruence angle of over 5° suggests patellar subluxation (after Merchant *et al.* 1974).

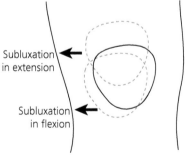

Figure 7.6 Subluxation may occur in extension, in flexion or in both positions, particularly if the patient is asked to exercise under load.

with certainty whether factors such as patella alta, a shallow femoral groove, torsional abnormalities of the legs, ligament laxity or quadriceps weakness are directly responsible for the resultant instability of the patellofemoral joint.

After an acute lateral patellar dislocation a haemarthrosis develops, unless an extensive synovial tear has occurred, in which case the blood escapes to form a boggy and ill-defined haematoma or ecchymosis. MR scanning should be combined with skyline radiographic views of the patella (see Chapter 3) in order to define the presence of an intra-articular fracture and loose body formation which may interfere with later function of the patellofemoral joint. The medial retinacular fibres of the patella and medial patellofemoral ligament are invariably partially or completely ruptured, and the stretched vastus medialis muscle will be incompetent for several weeks. Arthroscopy may be indicated if the intra-articular pathology is significant. Repair or reconstruction of the medial patellofemoral ligament (see Figure 4.3 p. 60) is advocated by some but is usually reserved for the recurrent problem.

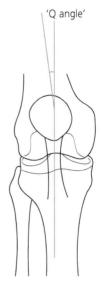

Figure 7.7 The Q-angle is formed by a line drawn from the anterior superior iliac spine to the centre of the patella, and a second line from that point to the tibial tuberosity. An increased angle may predispose the patella to lateral subluxation, and therefore a medial vector of force, shown by the arrow, has to be provided by the vastus medialis muscle and patellar retinacular fibres.

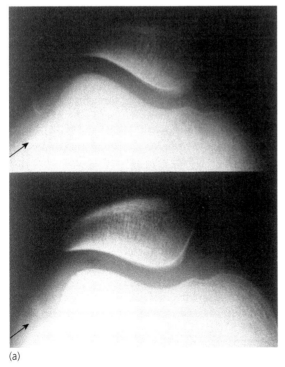

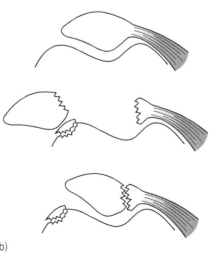

(a)   (b)

Figure 7.8 A lateral femoral condylar shear fracture (a) with a loose body that became fixed and enlarged with time (below). Medial avulsion (marginal) fracture of the patella may coexist (b).

151

Treatment of adolescent patellar instability

■ Acute dislocation

Acute, traumatic dislocation is classically treated conservatively by a splint or brace; aspiration of the haemarthrosis will lessen pain. The aims of treatment are:

- To ensure the patella is reduced with gentle knee extension (it may have relocated already, possibly inflicting further damage to the lateral condylar edge of the sulcus)
- To assess the knee for osteochondral loose bodies
- To prevent recurrent dislocations. Radiographs should therefore be scrutinized for the presence of osteochondral injury and a fat–blood interface, although the films are often of poor quality since the patient is distressed. A later MR scan may refine the diagnosis.

Splintage for 4 weeks allows the torn medial retinaculum to heal with the minimum of lengthening. Surgical repair is unnecessary but the interior of the knee is examined arthroscopically later if an osteochondral fragment is present. Nikku *et al.* (2005) found that recurrence was just as likely after operative repair of the soft tissues than after conservative management, instability episodes occurring in 40–45 per cent of both groups of patients after 7 years. Recurrent dislocation usually occurred within 2 years of the first episode, and was more likely in immature girls with bilateral patellar symptoms and an osteochondral fracture. Since the medial capsule is breached, arthroscopic review, if indicated, should be delayed for 2 weeks. Some articular cartilage lesions may merit replacement and fixation, but usually the fragments are small and can be removed. Fibrin glue does not offer sufficient bonding of the displaced osteochondral lesion and therefore temporary fixation of larger fragments with K-wires is appropriate. Rehabilitation is usually slow, with gradual resumption of the knee flexion and physiotherapy, as described in Chapter 10. Strengthening the vastus medialis (Figure 7.9) should stabilize patellar tracking in the majority of cases.

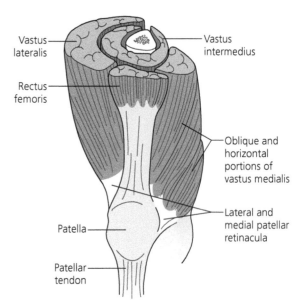

Figure 7.9 The control of patellar tracking depends upon the quadriceps muscle groups and the retinacular fibres.

Vastus lateralis

Vastus intermedius

Rectus femoris

Oblique and horizontal portions of vastus medialis

Lateral and medial patellar retinacula

Patella

Patellar tendon

■ Chronic dislocation

If conservative measures fail to control patellar instability the patient will continue to experience regular episodes of locking and giving way, and less frequent complete patellar dislocation. A variety of proximal and distal realignment procedures have been described so that it is important to define the nature of the patellar dislocation before deciding upon surgical correction. If the instability and lateral shift occur when the knee is extended, lateral release will only worsen the tracking unless it is combined with distal realignment of the patella. Recurrence of patellar instability is fairly common after surgery. Arnbjörnsson *et al.* (1992) reported the results of unilateral operation for bilateral patellar dislocation. At an average of 14 years after surgery they found that the surgically treated knee generally functioned worse than the conservatively managed joint, even though the preoperative problem was approximately the same on both sides. The rate of redislocation was reduced to around 5–10 per cent, but at the expense of the later onset of osteoarthritis. Concerns about the induction of arthritic change were also expressed by Hampson and Hill (1975) and Barbari *et al.* (1990), where the danger of distal transfer of the tibial tuberosity was described, and by Crosby and Insall (1976) who advised against more than soft tissue realignment. The frequency of patellar dislocation lessens with age (Larsen and Lauridsen 1982), but is itself associated with the onset of mild patellofemoral degenerative change.

When repeated and disabling episodes of patellar dislocation are accompanied by effusions, and the child or adolescent is severely restricted by the disability, a conservative policy of management should on rare occasions be abandoned. A simple lateral release for patellar dislocation in flexion may prove sufficient, although this procedure alone affects patellar tracking very little since the reciprocal shapes of the patellar and femoral articular surfaces dictate in large measure the position of the patella during various stages of knee flexion.

Both proximal and distal surgical realignment of the patellar mechanism have been advocated, and sometimes a combination of these procedures is necessary (Figure 7.10). However, the variation in patellar morphology and uncertainty about the source of the symptoms that are produced by the patellofemoral joint make the outcome of surgery very unpredictable. In the

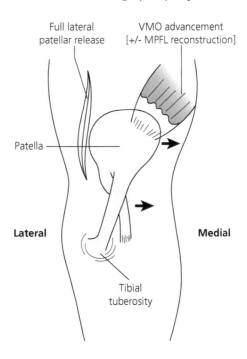

Figure 7.10 Distal patellar realignment is achieved by moving a lamina of the patellar tendon medially or by transposing the whole of the tuberosity medially after the end of skeletal growth. Proximal realignment employs some form of reefing, using vastus medialis or some other dynamic structure. An extensive lateral patellar release should accompany these procedures.

Full lateral patellar release

VMO advancement [+/- MPFL reconstruction]

Patella

Lateral

Medial

Tibial tuberosity

absence of clearly identified patellar subluxation, surgery to the quadriceps muscle or patellar tendon should be avoided, as changes in the distribution and degree of loading on the knee cap will not necessarily prove beneficial.

The variety of proximal and distal realignment procedures that have been described in association with a lateral release prevent a dogmatic approach, so most surgeons keep their interventions as simple as possible. Proximally, the vastus medialis can be plicated, and thus tightened; however, paradoxically, this may impair the function of that muscle and the surgeon must be at pains to avoid weakening the medial vector of force which controls patellar tracking. Various connective tissue structures, including the tendon of the semitendinosus muscle, can be used to medialize the position of the quadriceps mechanism.

Reconstruction of the medial patellofemoral ligament is now in vogue. The anatomy of this structure has been defined (see Figure 4.3, p. 60), and the fact that it tightens in knee extension (thus mooring the patella) and relaxes during flexion. The gracilis or semitendinosus may be used to augment the stretched ligament although, with time, any transferred connective tissue will tend to elongate and there may be no substantial improvement in patellar tracking (Mountney *et al.* 2005). Artificial ligament augmentation is also being trialled. Once again, it should be recalled that muscle tone may be reduced by these procedures. However, the results of this reinforcement are encouraging, provided the reconstruction is correctly attached to the adductor tubercle and the proximal, medial border of the patella (Steensen *et al.* 2004; Thaunat and Erasmus 2007).

The tibial tubercle–patellar sulcus 'offset' can be defined by CT scanning (Mulford 2007). This measurement is a predisposing factor towards patellar lateral instability if it is greater than 15 mm but any skeletal, rotational correction should be delayed until late adolescence. Surgery to correct a shallow sulcus or flattened lateral femoral condyle (Dejour and Saggin 2010) is not recommended. The results are unpredictable and the procedure may worsen pain and stiffness. In the longer term, osteoarthritis is likely to be hastened.

Distal realignment is a somewhat simpler technique, but the danger here lies in producing an excessive degree of medial and distal positioning of the patellar tendon. The Roux-Goldthwait procedure employs only the lateral half of the patellar tendon, which is transposed beneath the medial half of the tendon and inserted medial to the tibial tuberosity using periosteal sutures (Figure 7.10, p. 153). Additionally, a small block of bone can be transferred to ensure good healing. The use of a compression screw and washer anchors the new attachment effectively but the presence of a screw at this rather sensitive site over the upper shin is often a source of symptoms. Furthermore, scarring over the tibial tuberosity is usually tender for a prolonged period. Fortunately, soft tissue suturing between the tendon and the tibial periosteum is usually sufficient for the paediatric distal realignment.

Procedures that move the whole insertion of the patellar tendon, including a block of bone, are now usually avoided. An excessive degree of distal as well as medial realignment produces osteoarthritis of the knee, and damage to the growth plate in the younger patient may result in a hyperextension deformity of the proximal tibia (see Figure 4.7, p. 63). The bone block procedure is therefore contraindicated in the adolescent. Both proximal and distal soft tissue procedures are usually indicated when gross patellar instability is present, but there is always the risk that patellar tracking will remain abnormal and pain actually increase.

Retropatellar pain syndrome

There is no one term that adequately and specifically defines this troublesome condition which affects so many young people and has already been briefly discussed in Chapter 4. The term 'chondromalacia patellae' suggests that the articular surfaces of the patella and the associated femoral condyles are breaking down, leading to fibrillation (Outerbridge 1961; Abernethy *et al.* 1978). This is very rarely the case in younger patients, and an absence of any characteristic cartilaginous lesion apart from slight softening (Mori *et al.* 1991) has only highlighted the general dissatisfaction experienced by patient and doctor alike, when dealing with this perplexing condition. The term 'anterior knee pain' is so bland and non-specific that it is perhaps preferable. Common sites where pain and tenderness are experienced (see Figure 1.10, p. 8) do not necessarily relate to structures directly at those localities and discomfort may be experienced at several places.

Patellar pain is produced by a large number of subtle abnormalities (Fulkerson and Shea 1990), some of which are related to the patella and others which are distant to it (Table 7.1). It is therefore helpful to distinguish between pain and tenderness:

- Directly localized to the patella
- Principally in parapatellar structures
- More generalized, but principally in the front of the knee.

Patellar pain is frequently seen in the child actively involved with sport. There is no convincing evidence that the symptoms worsen during a 'growth spurt', although stress through the patellofemoral joint may increase from both overuse and rapid elongation of the lower limb. Straight-leg raising is often restricted due to 'tight' hamstrings. Milgrom *et al.* (1991) studied male army recruits prospectively and found that 15 per cent developed anterior knee pain. The only predictive factors were isometric quadriceps strength (which rather confounds the basis of physiotherapy for this condition) and mild varus alignment.

Royle *et al.* (1991), in a prospective study of knee arthroscopy cases, found that 40 per cent of patients without patellar pain presented with chondral fibrillation (Figure 7.11), whereas 40 per cent with anterior symptoms had no patellar cartilage changes. The lack of correlation between the clinical symptoms and definable pathology has been appreciated for some time (Abernethy *et al.* 1978) and therefore a large array of aetiological factors has to be considered (Table 7.1). Obvious osteochondral lesions are uncommon. The management of osteochondritis dissecans patellae (Figure 7.12) (Edwards and Bentley 1977) follows the same principles of management as osteochondritis dissecans at other sites in the knee (see Chapters 4 and 9).

The problems associated with malalignment syndromes and variations in patellar shape, tracking and loading usually prove complex to understand, let alone to modify by operation, and the presence of ligament laxity adversely affects the surgical intentions of realignment (Insall 1982).

Arnoldi (1991) has implicated an elevation of intraosseous venous pressure in patellar pain syndromes, similar to the disturbance in venous drainage seen in osteoarthritis. However, intraosseous phlebography is open to considerable errors in measurement and the significance of the alteration in patellar vascularity remains uncertain but intriguing. Similarly, the patterns of chondropathy (Mori *et al.* 1991) do not correlate convincingly with observed symptoms.

Abnormalities in ossification, particularly of the superolateral secondary ossification centre of the patella (Chapter 4), may also result in tenderness and pain in the region of the patella (Figure 7.13). At the end of skeletal growth the bipartite patella may become asymptomatic or may continue to cause disability (Weaver 1977). Excision of one or more ununited fragments or lateral patellar release (Osborne and Fulford 1982) will usually alleviate the pain. Acute, marginal fracture is easily distinguishable from bipartite patella but may confuse the unwary. Osteolytic lesions may occur as a result of neoplastic change (Linscheid and Dahlin 1966), including chondroblastoma, giant cell tumour, aneurysmal bone cysts, plasmacytoma

Table 7.1 Different pathological conditions producing anterior knee pain

Site	Pathology
Patellar	Trauma (osteochondral, avulsion or stress fracture)
	Abnormal pressure or shear stress:
	– Increased or decreased
	– With or without patellofemoral instability
	– With or without patellar tilting
	– From chronic knee flexion (neurological, 'long leg dysplasia')
	Abnormal ossification centres (bipartite, tripartite or more)
	Neoplasia
	Sinding–Larsen–Johansson syndrome
	Patellofemoral arthropathy
	'True' chondromalacia patellae
	Patella baja, including after anterior cruciate ligament reconstruction
	Osteoarthritis
Peripatellar	Synovial fringe lesion
	Medial fat pad syndrome
	Synovitis
	Loose body
	Plica syndrome
Quadriceps mechanism	Chronic quadriceps weakness
	Quadriceps tendon partial rupture
	'Jumper's knee' (patellar tendonitis with partial tear)
	Ligament laxity
Superficial	Prepatellar, infrapatellar or suprapatellar bursitis
	Neuroma (especially of the infrapatellar branch of the saphenous nerve) and complex regional pain syndrome following cutaneous nerve injury
	Scarring
	Dermatological conditions
Other	Intra-articular (meniscal tear, ligament rupture, osteochondritis dissecans, bone bruising with synovial reaction, villonodular synovitis, haemangioma)
	Referred from spine or hip joint
	Psychosomatic
	Idiopathic

(McLeod and Macnicol 1990) and metastases. Infection is rare but should not be forgotten (Figure 7.14).

Other local abnormalities to be considered include the presence of a plica, generally over the medial femoral condyle. The plica represents a hypertrophied synovial fold, and may be post-traumatic. Figure 2.9 (p. 19) shows the sites of the plicae which have been described, but these are generally only symptomatic when they enlarge to the extent that they rub against the femoral condyle or any other prominent bony margin of the knee. A contiguous lesion

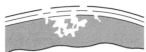

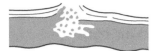

Normal

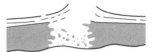

Stage I fasciculation

Stage II fasciculation
(fibrillation)

Erosions (ulceration)

Figure 7.11 The stages in articular cartilage breakdown.

Figure 7.12 Osteochondritis
dissecans patellae.

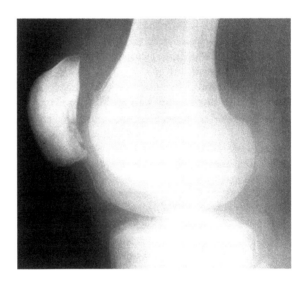

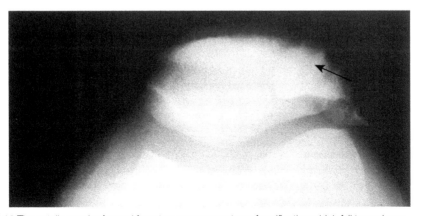

Figure 7.13 The patella may be formed from two or more centres of ossification which fail to coalesce.

157

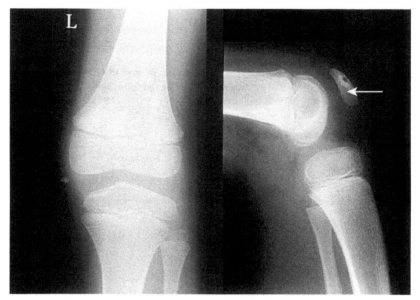

Figure 7.14 A subacute osteomyelitic focus in the patella.

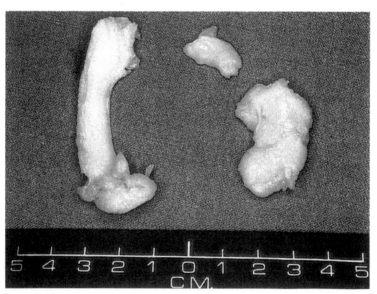

Figure 7.15 An excised plica which resembles a meniscus owing to its hypertrophy in response to chronic friction against the medial femoral condyle.

should therefore be identified over an articular surface, along with the thickened band (Figure 7.15). Whether the plica is truly causing friction against the medial femoral condyle is difficult to confirm arthroscopically as the knee joint cavity is distended. Fat pad lesions (Hoffa 1904) are rare and inferior pole tenderness is usually secondary to bursitis, chronic patellar tendon avulsion (Figure 7.16) (Sinding-Larsen 1921) and other stress lesions of the patellar attachment.

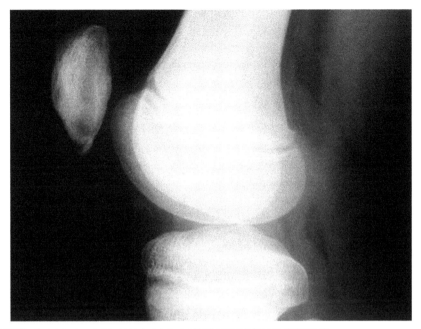

Figure 7.16 Sinding-Larsen–Johansson syndrome affecting the inferior patellar pole.

A non-specific discomfort in the patellofemoral joint will occur after a patient has walked on a flexed knee, whatever the reason, for more than a few days. Children with cerebral palsy may also experience patellar pain and stress fractures if they develop knee flexion contractures from hamstring dominance. In the years of skeletal maturation, pain in and around the knee is quite common and may be due to 'growing pains' brought on by relatively tight hamstrings. These can be exacerbated by sport, where the patellofemoral mechanism, for example, is further stressed by strenuous activities. Generally, at the end of growth, any increase in the musculotendinous tension secondary to bone elongation will lessen and the pain should settle after 1–2 years.

However, other abnormalities must be ruled out, and this requires a careful history and examination of the symptomatic lower limb. It must never be forgotten that the cause of pain over the medial aspect of the knee may reside in the hip and, in any examination of the knee, the hip, spine and lower leg and foot should be carefully assessed. Referred pain in this manner, which radiates down a branch of the obturator nerve from the hip joint, occurs in cases of slipped epiphysis, Perthes' disease and osteonecrosis, septic and inflammatory arthritis, and in any other condition where the hip joint capsule is distended by an effusion. Thus, another common cause of knee pain occurs in the child with a transient synovitis of the hip, where symptoms may be felt over the medial aspect of the knee rather than proximally.

In many cases, retropatellar pain is apparently idiopathic. It is important to try to establish the cause if possible, and in this respect the age and sex of the patient, and also any abnormality of body build, should be noted. Dynamic testing includes a review of gait as the patient may walk with knee caps squinting inwards owing to persistent femoral anteversion. Obvious knock-knee or other angulatory or torsional abnormalities will be also be identified (Figure 7.2, p. 148). Next, the patient sits with the legs dangling over the edge of the examination couch: patellar tracking is readily observed under load as each knee in turn is straightened against gravity.

Investigations should include radiographs to rule out skeletal lesions and MR scanning to define chondral and soft tissue pathology (Figueroa *et al.* 2007). In cases where the pain gives cause for concern imaging can be augmented by isotope bone scanning and CT. However, in most cases of patellar pain a careful physical examination is all that is required (Ficat and Hungerford 1977; Bentley and Dowd 1984). Arthroscopy will fail to detect changes deep to the articular cartilage (Imai and Tomatsu 1991) and the expense of MR scanning is such that it should be used only in the chronic and unresponsive case.

■ Treatment of patellar pain

Symptoms in adolescence tend to remit with time, although Karlstrom (1940) found that after 20 years many patients were still symptomatic. Sandow and Goodfellow (1985) reported that counselling and physiotherapy alleviated the symptoms in half of a group of adolescent girls, but symptoms persisted in the rest. In a prospective study of 30 adolescents, O'Neill *et al.* (1992) found that symptomatic relief was achieved in 85 per cent of cases by isometric quadriceps strengthening coupled with hamstring and iliotibial band stretching. McConnell (1986) also popularized the conservative approach to anterior knee pain (see Chapter 10) and it is assumed that these alterations in loading at the patellofemoral joint reduce the shear and compressive forces to which the patella is subjected. The effects of physiotherapy may be short-lived, particularly if the exercise programme is abandoned. Yet the conservative approach at least succeeds in demonstrating that the symptoms can be controlled by conscious effort in the majority of patients.

Lateral patellar release is recommended less frequently for patellar pain than used to be the case (Osborne and Fulford 1982). The indiscriminate use of this release was based upon the mistaken belief that the procedure was a safe and benign intervention, particularly if carried out arthroscopically. Hughston and Deese (1989) described the risk of producing medial patellar subluxation postoperatively if the vastus lateralis is wasted; and haemarthrosis, reflex sympathetic dystrophy and painful clicking at the lateral patellar edge may complicate the operation. Demonstrable tightness of the lateral parapatellar tissues and an absence of patellar hypermobility were considered to be important preconditions of successful lateral patellar release by Gecha and Torg (1990). Fulkerson and Shea (1990) also stressed the importance of identifying the lateral retinaculum as pathologically tight before interfering with a structure which balances the patella during tracking.

Lateral release also offers an analgesic effect but the results are unpredictable, so that after 2–3 years there is a return of symptoms in a substantial portion of patients. Denervation of the lateral capsule has been shown to occur anatomically (Abraham *et al.* 1989) and reinnervation may account for the resumption of symptoms.

When severe patellar pain persists after lateral patellar release, and in the absence of any intra-articular knee pathology, overt patella maltracking or alternative disease process, the Maquet (1976) procedure and patellar osteotomy (Morscher and Dick 1980; Macnicol 1985, 1994) have been proposed as alternatives to patellectomy. If there seems to be an 'excess' of retropatellar pressure, such as when sitting or climbing stairs, then there may be a place for raising the patella anteriorly away from the femoral groove. Maquet suggested an operation where the distal tibial attachment is elevated, in the belief that a 1 cm shift of the tuberosity anteriorly reduces patellar pressure by 20–40 per cent. However, this concept is based on cadaveric studies, and the dynamics of the patellofemoral joint following this procedure in the living are unknown. There is also the risk that moving the patella anteriorly will increase its likelihood of either subluxing or tilting laterally, while the prominence of the tibial tuberosity postoperatively may adversely affect wound healing and leave the proximal shin significantly tender (Radin 1986; Radin and Pan 1993).

An alternative approach has been to recommend a patellectomy for cases of intractable anterior knee pain. This does not guarantee success, and extension of the knee is weakened by at least 15 per cent. Paradoxically the anterior knee pain regularly persists in the absence of the patella. In order to preserve the patella, a patellar osteotomy can be of value in these very difficult cases and it is of interest to note that the cancellous bone of the patella often appears very dry and avascular during this procedure, suggesting that

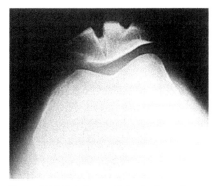

Figure 7.17 Patellar sagittal osteotomy for intractable anterior knee pain.

an 'osteodystrophy' is responsible for the anterior knee pain in a proportion of cases. However, the osteotomy may hasten osteoarthritic changes in the patellofemoral joint, if it breaches the subchondral plate, and only a sagittal cut should be utilized so that proximal patellar blood supply is not impaired (Scapinelli 1967) (Figure 7.17).

Whichever surgical procedure is recommended, the surgeon must be aware of the complications that may ensue and the fact that many patients will respond poorly to an operation which addresses a syndrome where the cause of the symptoms is still so little understood. If surgery is advised it should only be after a prolonged period of physiotherapy, possibly with some form of supportive strapping or bracing for the knee cap, and a modification of activities.

It is also important to stress to the patient, and the parents, that anterior knee pain, from whatever cause, may have to be accepted, and that there may be a modest, but never complete, reduction in symptoms with time. The use of anti-inflammatory analgesics over a prolonged period is inadvisable, although there was a vogue for salicylate therapy used for short periods. If the anxiety of the patient (and parents) can be reduced, and an acceptable level of sporting activity prescribed, many individuals seem quite ready to live within the limits set by their patellofemoral symptoms. As a general rule, surgery should be conservative and restricted to soft tissue only in the growing child.

Thereafter any procedure which is directed towards the articular cartilage must be justified carefully, and it is probably better to confine surgery to a distal realignment procedure where patellar maltracking is obvious, or to, at most, an arthroscopic irrigation and full intra-articular inspection in those with no obvious abnormality of patellar movement. Patellectomy should be avoided if at all possible, particularly as osteoarthritis of the knee will be hastened. Yet there is a small group of patients who seem to benefit from patellectomy and the difficulty lies in defining this group. Resurfacing operations for the patellofemoral joint are gaining in popularity but have no place as yet in the management of the younger patient.

Bipartite patella

This condition has already been discussed in this chapter. It should be appreciated that the patella ossifies from a number of centres beginning at the age of 3 years onwards. Traction from the quadriceps mechanism may result in an apophysitis, most commonly at the supero-lateral corner of the (bipartite) patella (Figure 7.13, p. 157) or between the main patella and two separate centres (tripartite). Pain is induced by exertion or squatting. If the force is sufficient the ossification centre may avulse. It should then be reattached with a compression screw. Removal of a symptomatic ossicle should be avoided unless it is small. Physiotherapy, including muscle stretching and the use of a local anti-inflammatory gel, should tide the patient over the period until the skeleton matures.

Sleeve fracture of the patella

This fracture accounts for just over half the patellar fractures in childhood. It is comparable to avulsion fracture of the intercondylar eminence, the tibial tuberosity or the femoral epicondyle. The incidence peaks at the age of 12–13 years. The separation occurs through the zone of chondro-osseous transformation such that the 'sleeve' consists of both articular and pre-osseous cartilage, and periosteum (Figure 7.18). Collagen fibrils of the patellar tendon blend directly with the lower pole for there are no Sharpey–Schafer fibres at this site.

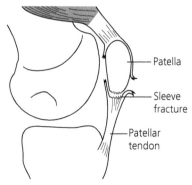

Figure 7.18 The line of pathological separation in the patella sleeve fracture.

The clinical signs are important to elicit (Houghton and Ackroyd 1979) since this fracture is often missed initially. Patella alta is obvious when both knees are compared in extension and a gap is palpable at the lower patellar pole. The patient is unable to weight-bear on the affected leg and straight leg raising is only partially possible (with an 'extensor lag'), by using the intact patellar retinacular fibres. A boggy swelling or spreading ecchymosis develops at the site of avulsion, and the patellar tendon feels lax.

Radiographs reveal the proximal position of the patella and a thin shell of cancellous bone which thickens with time if the diagnosis is delayed (Figure 7.19). An

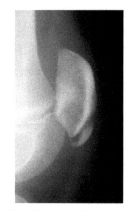

Figure 7.19 A lateral radiograph showing the extent of the lesion, following a delay in diagnosis.

ultrasound scan defines the tissues well and is therefore diagnostic. Careful open reduction is possible anatomically in the acute case, with fixation using a wire loop or tension band wire. Repair of the retinacular fibres is also advised. After a 3-week period of extension splintage and crutches to reduce loading through the leg, flexion and increasing weight bearing are permitted progressively over 3-months. Very rarely, the superior patellar pole may be avulsed, singly or in combination with the lower pole.

◼ Sinding-Larsen–Johansson syndrome

Pain over the lower pole of the patella may be associated with a small avulsion of bone (Sinding-Larsen 1921). In rare cases an ossicle forms and the symptoms persist (Figure 7.16, p. 159). The combination of rapid growth and repetitive sport triggers this overuse syndrome which is seen most commonly between the ages of 9 and 14 years. Rest is all that is required in the majority of cases, and it is preferable to avoid the use of a plaster cylinder. Local ultrasound and the application of a non-steroidal anti-inflammatory gel may lessen the discomfort. The child and parents should be reassured that the condition will heal slowly. In rare instances the attachment to the inferior patellar pole merits drilling and a mobile ossicle should be excised if it is painful when manipulated. The acute sleeve fracture should be suspected when sudden pain occurs at the lower pole; ultrasound scanning and radiographs are diagnostic, although X-rays rarely show the true size of the separated osteochondral fragment.

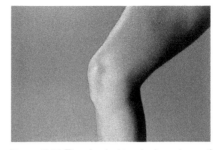

Figure 7.20 The classical tender, bony lump of Osgood–Schlatter's condition.

Osgood–Schlatter condition

This common complaint was described separately by Osgood (1903) and Schlatter (1903). Ogden and Southwick (1976) reviewed the developmental changes in the tuberosity with growth, and the pattern of ossification. Under the stress of skeletal growth and active sport the pre-osseous cartilage is partially avulsed and the trauma leads to hypertrophy (Figure 7.20). Boys are affected three times more commonly than girls and the contralateral tuberosity may become symptomatic 6–18 months later in approximately a quarter of cases. Once again it is most common in late childhood and usually resolves during adolescence, leaving variable enlargement of the tendon insertion. It affects athletic youngsters (Kujala *et al.* 1985) and hypertrophy of both it and Gerdy's tubercle are seen in many sprinters, soccer players and gymnasts.

A reduction in sport and counselling about the temporary nature of the condition is usually all that is required, although symptoms persist for several years in most patients. Kneeling and squatting are avoided by the patient quite naturally, and local treatment may be helpful but only gives short-term relief. Splintage should be used sparingly as there is a risk that the introspective child will develop more morbid symptoms.

If an ossicle develops in adolescence its excision may relieve the symptoms although this is by no means assured. Drilling of the tuberosity, and partial reduction of its size, are more speculative procedures, occasionally advocated if disabling symptoms persist. As with any anterior knee pain syndrome, surgical intervention should never be considered before a period of conservative treatment.

Patellar tendonitis

Tenderness in relation to the patellar tendon is usually localized to one or other end of the tendon attachment in childhood. This differs from the adult where symptoms occur from a microtear of the proximal tendon itself, often in association with a prepatellar or infrapatellar bursitis, or a similar inflammatory process between the tendon and the upper tibia. Blazina *et al.* (1973) coined the phrase 'jumper's knee' for a variety of conditions that affect the patellar tendon and its attachments. Overuse, particularly repetitive eccentric loading, triggers symptoms which may be present bilaterally in approximately 20 per cent of patients. Inflammatory change results from microtrauma either in the tendon or at its interface with bone. Cystic changes may develop, revealed by ultrasound examination (Fritschy and De Gautard 1988), and the tendon later feels thickened as fibrosis develops. The pathological changes can also be detected by MR scanning (Figure 7.21).

Rest and anti-inflammatory agents are usually prescribed, but enforced inactivity is rarely acceptable to the elite athlete. Stretching exercises and local friction massage may prove beneficial symptomatically. Changes in training technique and orthotic adjustment of the shoes may help those involved with basketball, volleyball, tennis and athletics, but the symptoms persist in a proportion. Sometimes a leg-length discrepancy is evident and should be corrected by a contralateral shoe insert.

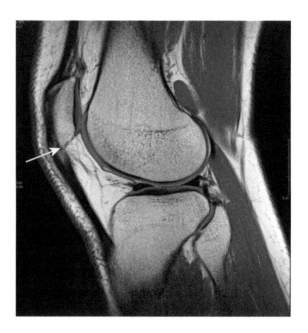

Figure 7.21 Magnetic resonance scan of patellar tendonitis shows a bright signal depicting the chronic interstitial tear.

Peers *et al.* (2003) have reported success with the use of extracorporeal shock wave therapy. This method has the advantage of being non-invasive and is more effective than pulsed ultrasound. Steroid injection is not advisable because of the risks of worsening the lesion, so that surgical exploration and paratenon release may be the only effective recourse in the chronic and unresponsive case (Colosimo and Bassett 1990). This helps to relieve any fibrotic constriction and rekindles the healing process within the chronic tear. Excision and detachment of portions of the tendon is illogical and risky, but removal of a chronic prepatellar or infrapatellar bursitic lesion may be justifiable.

References

Abernethy PJ, Townsend PR, Rose RM and Radin EL (1978) Is chondromalacia patellae a separate clinical entity? *J Bone Joint Surg Br* **60**, 205–10.

Abraham E, Washington E and Huang T-L (1989) Insall proximal realignment for disorders of the patella. *Clin Orthop* **248**, 61–5.

Arnbjörnsson A, Egund N, Rydling O, *et al.* (1992) The natural history of recurrent dislocation of the patella. *J Bone Joint Surg Br* **74**, 140–2.

Arnoldi CC (1991) The patellar pain syndrome. *Acta Orthop Scand* **62**(Suppl), 1–29.

Barbari S, Raugstad TS, Lichtenberg N and Refrem D (1990) The Hauser operation for patellar dislocation. *Acta Orthop Scand* **61**, 32–5.

Bentley G and Dowd G (1984) Current concepts in the etiology and treatment of chondromalacia patellae. *Clin Orthop* **189**, 209–28.

Blackburne JS and Peel TE (1977) A new method of measuring patellar height. *J Bone Joint Surg Br* **59**, 241–2.

Blazina ME, Kerlan RK, Jobe FW, *et al.* (1973) Jumper's knee. *Orthop Clin North Am* **4**, 665–78.

Blumensaat C (1932) Die Lageabweichungen und verrenkungen der kniescheibe. *Ergebn Chir Orthop* **31**, 149–223.

Carter CO (1960) Recurrent dislocation of the patella and of the shoulder. *J Bone Joint Surg Br* **42**, 721–7.

Colosimo AJ and Bassett FH (1990) Jumper's knee: diagnosis and treatment. *Orthop Rev* **19**, 139–49.

Crosby EB and Insall J (1976) Recurrent dislocation of the patella: relation of treatment to osteoarthritis. *J Bone Joint Surg Am* **58**, 9–13.

Dejour D and Saggin P (2010) The sulcus deepening trochleoplasty: the Lyon procedure. *Int Orthop* **34**, 311–16.

Edwards DH and Bentley G (1977) Osteochondritis dissecans patellae. *J Bone Joint Surg Br* **59**, 58–61.

Ficat RP and Hungerford DS (1977) *Disorders of the Patellofemoral Joint*. Baltimore, MD: Lippincott Williams & Wilkins.

Figueroa D, Calvo R, Valsman A, *et al.* (2007) Knee chondral lesions: incidence and correlation between arthroscopic and magnetic resonance findings. *Arthroscopy* **23**, 312–15.

Fritschy D and De Gautard R (1988) Jumper's knee and ultrasonography. *Am J Sports Med* **16**, 637–40.

Fulkerson JP and Shea KP (1990) Current concepts review: disorders of patellofemoral alignment. *J Bone joint Surg Am* **72**, 1424–9.

Fulkerson JP, Schutzer SF, Ramsby GR and Bernstein RA (1987) Computerised tomography of the patellofemoral joint before and after lateral release or realignment. *Arthroscopy* **3**, 19–24.

Gecha SR and Torg JS (1990) Clinical prognosticators for the efficacy of retinacular release surgery to treat patellofemoral pain. *Clin Orthop* **253**, 203–8.

Goa GX, Lee EH and Bose K (1990) Surgical management of congenital and habitual dislocation of the patellae. *J Pediatr Orthop* **10**, 255–60.

Gunn DR (1964) Contracture of the quadriceps muscle. *J Bone Joint Surg Br* **46**, 492–7.

Hampson WGJ and Hill P (1975) Late results of transfer of the tibial tubercle for recurrent dislocation of the patella. *J Bone Joint Surg Br* **57**, 209–13.

Hoffa A (1904) The influence of the adipose tissue with regard to the pathology of the knee joint. *J Am Med Assoc* **43**, 795–6.

Houghton GR and Ackroyd CE (1979) Sleeve fractures of the patellar in children. *J Bone Joint Surg Br* **61**, 165.

Hughston JC and Deese M (1989) Medial subluxation of the patella as a complication of lateral retinacular release. *Adv Orthop Surg* **12**, 170–1.

Imai N and Tomatsu T (1991) Cartilage lesions in the knee of adolescents and young adults: arthroscopic analysis. *Arthroscopy* **7**, 198–203.

Insall J (1982) Current concepts review: patellar pain. *J Bone Joint Surg Am* **64**, 147–52.

Insall J and Salvati E (1971) Patella position in the normal knee joint. *Radiology* **101**, 101–4.

Jackson AM (1992) Recurrent dislocation of the patella. *J Bone Joint Surg Br* **74**, 2–4.

Karlstrom S (1940) Chondromalacia patellae. *Acta Chir Scand* **64**, 347–81.

Kujala V, Kuist M and Heinonen O (1985) Osgood-Schlatter's disease in adolescent athletes. *Am J Sports Med* **13**, 236–41.

Larsen E and Lauridsen E (1982) Conservative treatment of patella dislocations. *Clin Orthop* **171**, 131–6.

Laurin CA, Dussault R and Levesque HP (1979) The tangential x-ray investigation of the patellofemoral joint. *Clin Orthop* **144**, 16–26.

Linscheid RL and Dahlin DC (1966) Unusual lesions of the patella. *J Bone Joint Surg Am* **48**, 1359–66.

Macnicol MF (1985) Patellar osteotomy for intractable anterior knee pain. *J Bone Joint Surg Br* **67**, 156.

Macnicol MF (1994) Patellar osteotomy for intractable patellar pain. *Knee* **1**, 41–5.

Maquet P (1976) Advancement of the tibial tuberosity. *Clin Orthop* **115**, 225–60.

McConnell J (1986) The management of chondromalacia patellae: a long-term solution. *Aust J Physiotherapy* **32**, 215–20.

McLeod GC and Macnicol MF (1990) Plasmacytoma of the patella. *J R Coll Surg Edinb* **35**, 195–6.

Merchant AC (1992) Radiologic evaluation of the patellofemoral joint. In: Aichroth PM and Cannon WD (eds) *Knee Surgery*. London: Martin Dunitz, pp. 380–8.

Merchant AC, Mercer RL, Jacobsen RH and Cool CR (1974) Roentgenographic analysis of paellofemoral congruence. *J Bone Joint Surg Am* **56**, 1391–6.

Milgrom C, Finestone A, Eldad A and Shlamkovitch N (1991) Patellofemoral pain caused by overactivity: a prospective study of risk factors in infantry recruits. *J Bone Joint Surg Am* **73**, 1041–3.

Mori Y, Kuroki Y, Yamamoto R, *et al.* (1991) Clinical and histological study of patellar chondropathy in adolescents. *Arthroscopy* **7**, 182–97.

Morscher E and Dick W (1980) Sagittal patellar osteotomy in chondromalacia patellae. *Orthop Prax* **16**, 692–5.

Mountney J, Senavongse W, Amis AA, *et al.* (2005) Tensile strength of the medial patellofemoral ligament before and after repair or reconstruction. *J Bone Joint Surg Br* **87**, 36–40.

Mulford JS (2007) Assessment and management of chronic patellofemoral instability. *J Bone Joint Surg Br* **89**, 709–16.

Nikku R, Nietosvaara Y, Aalto K, *et al.* (2005) Operative treatment of primary patellar dislocation does not improve medium-term outcome. A 7-year follow-up report and risk analysis of 127 randomized patients. *Acta Orthop Scand* **76**, 699–70.

Ober FR (1936) The role of the iliotibial band and fascias: a factor in the causation of low back disabilities and sciatica. *J Bone Joint Surg Am* **18**, 105–11.

Ogden JA and Southwick WO (1976) Osgood-Schlatter's disease and tibial tuberosity development. *Clin Orthop* **116**, 180–6.

O'Neill DB, Micheli LJ and Warner JP (1992) Patellofemoral stress: a prospective analysis of exercise treatment in adolescents and adults. *Am J Sports Med* **20**, 151–6.

Osborne AH and Fulford PC (1982) Lateral release for chondromalacia patellae. *J Bone Joint Surg Br* **64**, 202–5.

Osgood R (1903) Lesions of the tibial tubercle occurring during adolescence. *Boston Med Surg J* **148**, 114–18.

Outerbridge RE (1961) The aetiology of chondromalacia patellae. *J Bone Joint Surg Br* **43**, 313–21.

Peers KH, Lysens RJ, Brys P and Bellemans J (2003) Cross-sectional outcome analysis of athletes with chronic patellar tendinopathy treated surgically and by extracorporeal shock wave therapy. *Clin J Sports Med* **13**, 79–83.

Radin EL (1986) The Maquet procedure – anterior displacement of the tibial tubercle. Indications, contraindications, and precautions. *Clin Orthop Rel Res* **213**, 241–8.

Radin EL and Pan HQ (1993) Long-term follow-up study on the Maquet procedure with special reference to the causes of failure. *Clin Orthop Rel Res* **290**, 253–8.

Royle SG, Noble J, Davies DRA and Kay PR (1991) The significance of chondromalacic changes on the patella. *Arthroscopy* **7**, 158–60.

Sandow MJ and Goodfellow JW (1985) The natural history of anterior knee pain in adolescents. *J Bone Joint Surg Br* **67**, 36–9.

Scapinelli R (1967) Blood supply of the human patella. *J Bone Joint Surg Br* **44**, 563–71.

Schlatter C (1903) Verletzungen des schnabelformigen Forsatzes der oberen Tibiaepiphyse. *Beitr Klin Chir* **38**, 874–7.

Sinding-Larsen MF (1921) A hitherto unknown affection of the patella in children. *Acta Radiol* **1**, 171–5.

Steensen RN, Dopirak RM and McDonald WG (2004) The anatomy and isometry of the medial patellofemoral ligament. *Am J Sports Med* **32**, 1509–13.

Thaunat M and Erasmus PJ (2007) Favourable anisometry: an original concept for MPFL reconstruction. *Knee* **14**, 424–8.

Weaver JK (1977) Bipartite patellae as the cause of disability in the athlete. *Am J Sports Med* **5**, 137–43.

Williams PF (1968) Quadriceps contracture. *J Bone Joint Surg Br* **50**, 278–84.

Yates CK and Grana WK (1990) Patellofemoral pain in children. *Clin Orthop* **255**, 36–43.

8

Fractures around the knee

Introduction

Fractures involving the knee are relatively common, and often involve the articular surface of the joint. In childhood and old age the bone may yield before any major ligament tear occurs, whereas in the adult a ligament disruption commonly precedes and accompanies the fracture.

Initial treatment

When a significant and unstable fracture has been sustained, the early management should include emergency splintage of the limb, appropriate surgical care of any wound, and attention to other injuries. If a fracture involving the knee is associated with multiple injuries, the patient will require resuscitation with a blood transfusion and electrolyte solutions and the primary aim should be to ensure that there is no life-threatening condition. Unfortunately, serious injuries to the knee may be overlooked, or their treatment delayed, when a patient is admitted with multiple or head injuries. In addition, if displaced fractures of the femur or tibia have been sustained, the assessment of any ligamentous or bony damage around the knee may prove difficult initially.

Principles of fracture care

The four Rs of fracture care are:

- *Respect* the soft tissues, remembering that the blood supply to bone is reliant upon their integrity, as is wound healing
- *Reduce* the fracture, and maintain this reduction by external splintage, traction, internal fixation or external fixation
- *Restore* function by ensuring that fixation of the fracture is adequate and that joint movement can be regained as rapidly as possible
- *Remember* that one is dealing with the whole patient. The emotional, social and economic concerns of the patient must be dealt with as effectively as possible, and every effort should be made to motivate the patient towards a successful recovery.

Tibial fractures

Undisplaced fractures are best treated conservatively by fixed splintage and then cast bracing (Hohl and Luck 1956), although the displacement of fragments may be underestimated

Table 8.1 Fractures involving the knee

Patellar	
Osteochondral	Medial avulsion
	Lateral shear
	Central shear
Transverse	Undisplaced
	Displaced
Polar	Upper
	Lower (including cartilaginous 'sleeve' fracture in child)
Vertical	
Comminuted	
Tibial	
Plateau	Undisplaced
	- Medial – anterior, posterior or total
	- Lateral – anterior, posterior or total
	- Comminuted medial and lateral
	Displaced
	- Split (single fragment) – sagittal or coronal; vertical or oblique
	- Compression (more than articular 3 mm depression of the surface)*
	- Split-compression
	- Comminuted
Intercondylar eminence (including tibial spines)	Tilted up anteriorly
	- Minor displacement
	- Major displacement
	Complete separation
	- No rotation
	- Rotated
Tuberosity	Undisplaced
	- Displaced
	- Comminuted
Femoral	
Supracondylar	Undisplaced
	- Transverse
	- T or Y configuration Impacted
	Displaced
	- Transverse
	- T or Y configuration comminuted
Condylar	Undisplaced
	- Medial
	- Lateral
	- Both condyles
	Displaced
	- Medial
	- Lateral
	- Both condyles
	- Coronal

*Anterior, posterior, marginal, central or total – use tomography with the film directed 15° distally and centred over the knee joint since the slope of the plateaux to the tibial shaft is 105° (otherwise the amount of depression is falsely-magnified if there is a posterior depression, and underestimated for a central or anterior depression). Magnetic resonance and computed tomography (CT) scanning is of value, including three-dimensional CT. Open reduction if more than 20° coronal tilting with the knee flexed approximately 20°, or depression of the joint surface of 5 mm or more.

radiographically. Percutaneous fixation is an effective solution if reduction is unnecessary. Table 8.1 details the classic descriptive terminology for tibial plateau fractures. The AO group (Müller *et al.* 1988) has produced its universal grouping as follows:

A – extra-articular
B_1 – pure split
B_2 – pure depression
B_3 – split and depression
C_1 – simple articular and simple metaphyseal
C_2 – simple articular and multifragmentary metaphyseal
C_3 – multifragmentary or comminuted.

Roughly three-quarters of all fractures are in the B category (Figure 8.1) and much debate centres on the acceptable level of displacement. Porter (1970) showed that fibrocartilage will fill in moderate splits and depressions, and early movement (Apley 1956) has long been recommended to preserve range of motion and the joint surfaces. Fixation after reduction should be attempted with greater than 4 mm depression (Rasmussen and Sörensen 1973) and depends upon the experience and skills of the surgeon (Burri *et al.* 1979; Schatzker *et al.* 1979). Arthroscopic review of the joint surfaces will help to monitor reduction of splitting or depressed plateau fractures (O'Dwyer and Bobic 1992) and meniscal interposition. Associated meniscal tears are reported in varying degree (17–85 per cent) and peripheral separations should certainly be repaired.

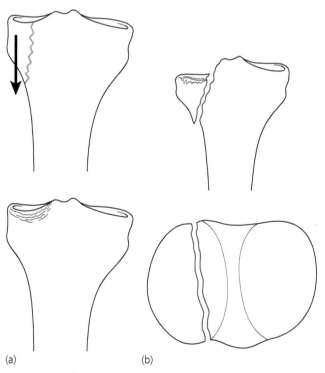

(a)   (b)

Figure 8.1 Minimally displaced type B tibial condylar fractures (pure split above and partial depression below) (a) and displaced split and depression fractures (b).

The C group of fractures involve the tibial condyles and were previously described by Schatzker *et al.* (1979) as medial condylar (type IV), lateral condylar with valgus tilting (type V) and bicondylar (type VI). Honkonen and Jarvinen (1992) subdivided the bicondylar group into those tilted medially and those tilted laterally, believing that fixation and prognosis were different.

Proximal tibial fractures are difficult lesions to treat because of the involvement of the articular surface, the frequent comminution, and the precarious condition of the soft tissues, especially following high-energy trauma. The POLYAX Locked Plating System (Depuy, Warsaw, USA) allows screws to be inserted and locked into the plate at any desired angle within a 30° cone of angulation. The system is designed to give surgeons maximum flexibility with the use of fixed-angle locking, variable-angle locking, and non-locking screw options, as well as percutaneous instrumentation (Mallina *et al.* 2010).

Ligament injuries are unusual, and difficult to treat in association with major joint surface displacement (Porter 1970). Laxity is usually the result of split/depression fractures and proves very disabling. Osteoarthritis correlates with malalignment, pathological laxity and extensive articular involvement, especially if there has been significant loss of meniscal substance. Knee replacement may be appropriate in elderly patients with severe fracture patterns but the long-term outcome is unpredictable.

Femoral fractures

Fracture patterns of the distal femur are described in Table 8.1. The AO classification (Müller *et al.* 1988) prefers the use of a coding system which can be applied universally as follows:

A_1 – extra-articular – simple
A_2 – extra-articular – metaphyseal wedge
A_3 – extra-articular – metaphyseal complex
B_1 – partially articular – lateral condylar sagittal
B_2 – partially articular – medial condylar sagittal
B_3 – partially articular – condylar in the frontal plane
C_1 – completely articular–articular simple, metaphyseal simple
C_2 – completely articular–articular simple, metaphyseal multifragmentary
C_3 – multifragmentary.

Although fractures of the femoral condyles can be treated with traction (Rockwood and Green 1991) it is impossible to ensure precise reduction. Internal fixation is advised if facilities permit especially when displacement is major, (Figure 8.2), when the fracture is irreducible (often due to soft tissue interposition and the effect of dynamic forces) and when a significant neurovascular deficit is present. Olerud (1972) presented one of the first major series of operative fixation, although the infection rate was almost 5 per cent. Non-union can be avoided completely by anatomical reduction (Giles *et al.* 1982), confirmed by Siliski *et al.* (1989), who stressed the importance of avoiding residual varus and internal deformities of the distal segment (Figure 8.3).

A lateral incision and 95° AO blade plate (Müller *et al.* 1970) or Richards device permit good fixation in the majority of cases, augmented with further intercondylar compression screws as necessary. Sanders *et al.* (1991) recommended the use of double plating, adding a medial buttress plate for comminuted, unstable fractures. Stability should then allow early movement, although the soft tissue dissection may result in stiffening from adhesions. An interlocking 171

Figure 8.2 Condylar fractures of the distal femur may occur in different planes (a). AO screws, blade plates and buttress plates offer an excellent means of fixation (b).

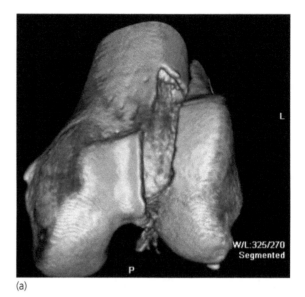

(a)

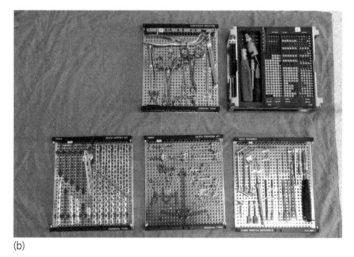

(b)

intramedullary nail has a role in some supracondylar and extensive intercondylar fractures (Leung *et al.* 1992). Bone grafting and the impaction of metaphyseal bone in the elderly should ensure that non-union is minimized.

The 'less invasive stabilization system' (LISS) is an extramedullary, internal fixation method (Figure 8.4). It incorporates technical innovations such as: closed, indirect reduction techniques; implants with minimal bone contact; modified internal fixators; and further advances in extramedullary force carriers. Its main features are an atraumatic insertion technique, minimal bone contact and a locked, fixed-angle construct (Liu *et al.* 2009).

Femoral shaft fractures are also accompanied by a significant incidence of knee injuries, Vangsness *et al.* (1993) finding at arthroscopy that complex and radial tears of the medial and lateral menisci were present in over 25 per cent of patients. Almost half their cases demonstrated ligament laxity, although not necessarily in association with meniscal damage. A large portion of these lesions heal or become asymptomatic, but knee injury should always

Figure 8.3 Residual varus after poor fixation of a left distal femoral fracture.

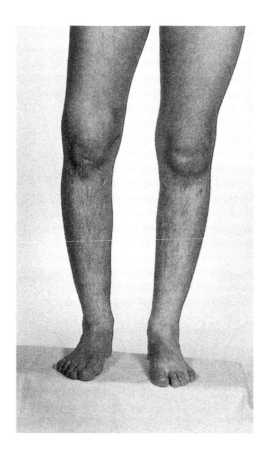

be assessed in patients with femoral fractures and with high-velocity tibial or hindfoot injuries. MR scanning ensures a clear depiction of associated soft tissue trauma.

Rehabilitation

Active and passive movement of the knee is encouraged immediately postoperatively, and continuous passive motion is beneficial. Progressive weightbearing is encouraged and union is usually complete by the fourth month after injury.

With both tibial and femoral fractures, serious vascular or neurological injuries may coexist at the level of the knee. It is then advisable to fix the fracture internally acutely so that any vessel repair can be protected. After neurological injury, either to the leg itself or in the wider context of a patient with a major head injury, rehabilitation will be more rapid if the fracture is operated on and stabilized, although the risks of infection must always be balanced against the advantages of early and anatomical restoration of the fractured bone.

Low-intensity pulsed ultrasound (LIPUS) is a relatively new technique for the acceleration of fracture healing in fresh fractures and non-unions. It has a frequency of 1.5 MHz, a signal burst width of 200 μm, a signal repetition frequency of 1 kHz, and an intensity of 30 mW/cm^2. In 1994 and 1997, two milestone double-blind randomized controlled trials revealed the benefits of LIPUS for the acceleration of fracture healing in the tibia and radius (Heckman et al. 1994; Kristiansen et al. 1997). The studies showed that LIPUS accelerated the fracture healing rate from 24 per cent to 42 per cent for fresh fractures although other reports have described no positive effects. The beneficial effect of acceleration of fracture healing by LIPUS

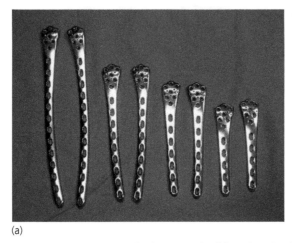

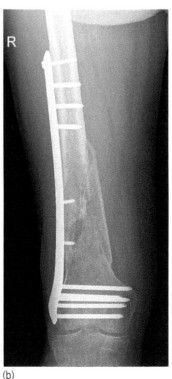

(a)   (b)

Figure 8.4a,b 'Less invasive stabilization system' (LISS) plating of a distal femoral fracture.

is considered to be larger in the group of patients or fractures with potentially negative factors for fracture healing. The incidence of delayed union and non-union is 5–10 per cent for all fractures. In delayed union and non-union cases, the overall success rate of LIPUS therapy is approximately 67 per cent (humerus), 90 per cent (radius/radius-ulna), 82 per cent (femur), and 87 per cent (tibia/tibia-fibula). Although LIPUS appears to enhance the maturation of callus in distraction osteogenesis, thus reducing the time to union, its therapeutic value in fracture healing remains unproven because of the heterogeneity of results in clinical trials involving fresh fractures, and the lack of controlled trials for delayed union and non-union (Watanabe *et al.* 2010).

The efficacy of recombinant human bone morphogenetic protein-2 (rhBMP-2), as an adjunct to the standard of care, has been investigated in the BMP-2 Evaluation in Surgery for Tibial Trauma (BESTT) study. A review of the Cochrane Database shows that there is limited evidence to suggest that BMP is more effective than controls for acute tibial fracture healing and that the use of BMP for treating a non-union remains unclear. The limited evidence currently available indicates that BMP treatment may only be economically justified when used in patients with the most severe fractures (Garrison *et al.* 2010).

Patellar fractures

Fractures patterns of the patella are described in Table 8.1 (p. 169). Sometimes a secondary ossification centre is confused with an acute fracture, although the outline of the former is always smooth and rounded and does not resemble the appearances after acute injury. Avulsion fractures of the patella (Dowd 1982) may occur after a lateral patellar dislocation (Figure 8.5)

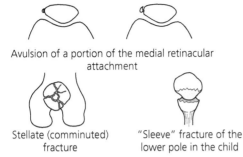
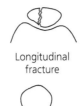
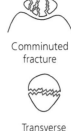

Avulsion of a portion of the medial retinacular attachment

Longitudinal fracture

Comminuted fracture

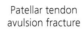

Stellate (comminuted) fracture

"Sleeve" fracture of the lower pole in the child

Patellar tendon avulsion fracture

Transverse fracture

Figure 8.5 The different types of patellar fracture.

and there may be associated shearing fractures of the osteochondral surfaces of the lateral edge of the sulcus or posteromedial patella (Figure 8.6).

A sudden contraction of the quadriceps muscle, in the absence of any direct injury to the front of the knee, may produce a transverse fracture of the patella which may be either undisplaced or displaced. In the child, such an avulsion fracture, involving the lower pole of the patella, pulls off a 'sleeve' of cartilage (see Chapters 4 and 7). This fragment may look innocuous radiographically, but constitutes a reason for internal fixation of what then turns out to be a fairly major fragment.

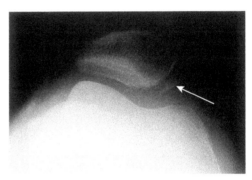

Figure 8.6 An osteochondral shear fracture of the patella seen on a 'skyline' radiograph.

Where the patellar fracture is relatively simple, with either a major transverse or vertical component to it, internal fixation with circumferential wires and a tension band wiring system is recommended. This allows early movement of the knee and should restore the posterior articular surface of the patella. Injury to the articular surface of the femoral groove may coexist and will obviously have an adverse effect upon subsequent patellofemoral function.

The comminuted patellar fracture is best treated by early excision of the fragments. An attempt can be made to reduce the fragments and produce a reasonably smooth articular surface, but this must be reviewed at the time of surgery and if incongruencies exist, a patellectomy is more likely to relieve the patient of symptoms than a united but abnormal patella. Patellectomy results in an appreciable loss of knee extensor power, but if the medial and lateral retinacular fibres are carefully repaired and the capsule of the patella sutured to form a ligamentous structure, the end results of patellectomy are acceptable.

Osteochondral fractures

Osteochondral and chondral fractures occur frequently in relation to the patellofemoral joint, as a result of lateral patellar dislocations. The details of this injury have been discussed in Chapter 4 and 7. Very rarely, the tibial plateau may also be the site of such a fracture.

175

If these separation fragments are small, they can be removed arthroscopically (Hubbard 1987). Larger fragments may be worth preserving, particularly if there is a bleeding base of cancellous bone (Figure 8.7, and see Figure 4.42, p. 87). When fragments do not heal back adequately, they will separate and produce a loose body in the joint (Dandy 1992).

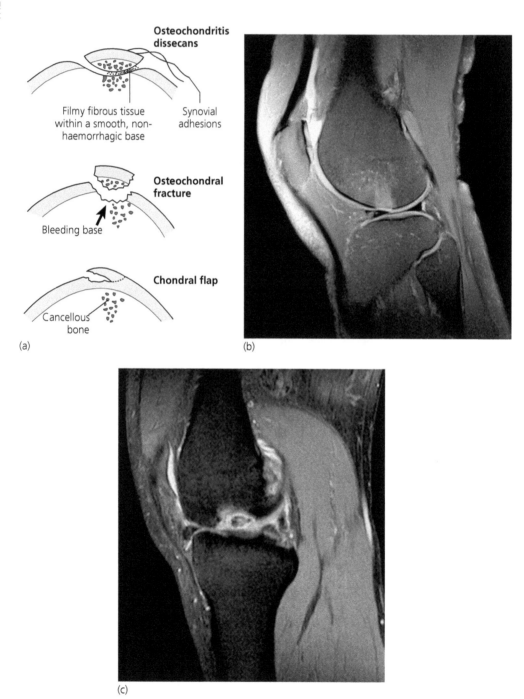

Figure 8.7 (a) The differentiation between osteochondritis dissecans, osteochondral fracture and a chondral flap. (b) Magnetic resonance (MR) image of an osteochondral fracture. (c) MR image of osteochondritis dissecans.

Alternative forms of fixation of larger osteochondral fractures include the use of pins, small fragment compression screws, absorbable implants or retrograde Kirschner wires. It must be remembered that whenever an osteochondral fracture has occurred, a significant ligament or retinacular tear may coexist and prove to be a significant cause of subsequent morbidity (O'Donoghue 1966).

Stem cells are now being produced as a means of healing significant articular (hyaline) cartilage defects. Ideally, they should be easy to harvest, producing a reasonable population density with the potential to differentiate. Sources for the younger patient include the synovial fat pad, the periosteum and bone marrow. The mesenchymal cell is encouraged biologically to form chondrocytes rather than osteocytes, fibrocytes or adipocytes. Scaffolds of collagen gel, fibrin or alginate are combined with growth factors and gene therapy to produce a favourable milieu for tissue growth, differentiation and adherence to the articular surface (Khan *et al.* 2010).

Epiphyseal fractures

In children, fractures may involve the growth plate, although metaphyseal and diaphyseal fractures are more common and variations in frequency depend on age (Figure 8.8). The distal femoral or proximal tibial epiphyses may be displaced to varying degree from the shafts of the respective bones (Beaty and Kasser 2009). Figure 8.9 details the various types

Figure 8.8 Patterns of knee injury at the different stages of childhood. (From Skak *et al.* 1987.)

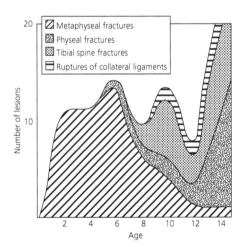

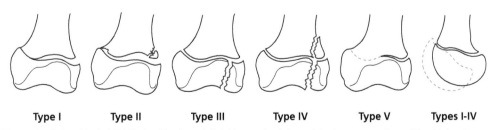

Type I   **Type II**   **Type III**   **Type IV**   **Type V**   **Types I-IV**

Figure 8.9 Salter-Harris (1963) classification of distal femoral epiphyseal fracture-separations. Direct injury to the perichondrial ring from an open, abrading wound may cause a partial growth arrest, which also complicates types II–V fractures in ascending order of frequency.

of epiphyseal/growth plate fracture (Salter and Harris 1963). Damage to the germinal layer of the growth plate, with resultant growth arrest, is most likely with the type V, crushing fracture. However, types II–IV may also be associated with a partial growth plate arrest and children with these injuries should be reviewed over a minimum of 2 years and preferably until maturity. Malunion occurs readily following the type IV fracture, and internal fixation of both types III and IV fracture is usually necessary (Macnicol and Murray 2010). In children the tibial tuberosity may also be avulsed, with or without articular involvement (Figures 8.10). The tuberosity should be reduced and secured with one or more screws if there is displacement.

Epiphyseal separations are four or five times more common at the distal tibia or fibula than at the knee, where the distal femur is displaced twice as often as the proximal tibia (Figure 8.11). Proximal femoral and fibular separations are rare. The distal femoral epiphysis fracture, despite being a type I or II in most cases, may lead on to partial growth arrest because of the extreme, shearing force that produces the separation and abrasion damage

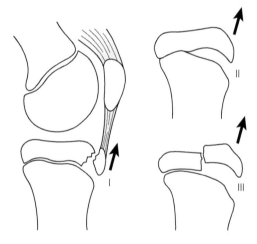

Figure 8.10 Variations of proximal tibial epiphyseal fractures produced by the pull of the patellar tendon (separation of the whole epiphysis is rare owing to the tethering effect of the collateral ligaments and tendons). In the adult, rupture of the patellar tendon is the corresponding injury.

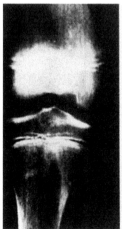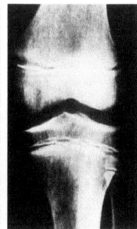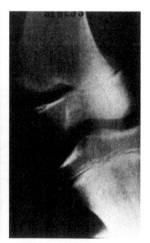

Figure 8.11 A stress view radiograph reveals major displacement of the distal femoral epiphysis.

to the germinal layer of the physis. Gross displacement also accounts for the frequency of neurovascular injury, the metaphysis shifting backwards against the popliteal vessels after the knee has been subjected to major hyperextension or coronal forces. The distal femoral epiphysis comes to lie anterior to the shaft of the femur and is pathologically rotated (Figure 8.12, p. 180). Stress radiographs, angiography if indicated, and careful closed or open reduction should protect the vitality of the limb. Tissue interposition may persist after closed reduction, an indication for surgical exploration. Crossed, smooth K-wires (Figure 8.13, p. 179), or one or two compression screws in the Thurston–Holland fragment (Figure 8.14, p. 180) ensure effective stabilization when combined with a plaster cast for 4–6 weeks. Later MR or CT scanning improves the precision of follow-up, disclosing late complications, including growth plate arrest. Leg-length discrepancy occurs in almost one-third of cases, followed in frequency by angular deformity, knee stiffness, peroneal nerve injury and acute popliteal artery damage.

Proximal tibial epiphyseal fractures are intrinsically more stable because the collateral ligamentous attachments cross the growth plate (Figures 8.15, p. 180). In order of frequency, the Salter–Harris grading

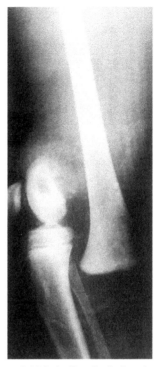

Figure 8.12 A significantly displaced type II fracture of the distal femoral epiphysis. Injury to the popliteal vessels and nerves is of principal concern.

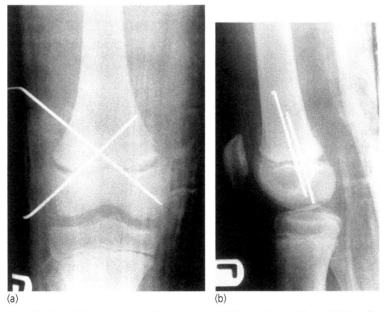

(a)　　　　　　　　　　(b)

Figure 8.13 Internal fixation with percutaneous Kirschner wires (of the fracture in Figure 8.12) is effective in the younger child after closed reduction, provided that there is no soft tissue interposition and the limb is supported in a plaster cast.

is II > IV > III > I > V. Half of type I fractures are undisplaced compared with a third of type II fractures. The type III fracture occurs close to skeletal maturity and represents a shearing or avulsion injury. Angular deformity and total growth plate arrest (Figures 4.7, p. 63, and Figure 4.32, p. 80), respectively, may complicate type IV and V fractures. Other complications are neurovascular damage, compartment syndrome, meniscal tears and infection (if open), in the early stages, and later residual ligament laxity, stiffness and chronic pain.

Combined and transitional fractures, akin to biplanar and triplanar fracture of the distal tibia, are rare but may require careful CT scan analysis and discussion about possible reduction and fixation if displacement warrants this (Beaty and Kumar 1994). Loss of joint movement is less likely in children than in adults, but the principles of management remain the same, in that early movement of the knee is recommended. Cast bracing and partial weightbearing using crutches are both valuable techniques in the older child and adult.

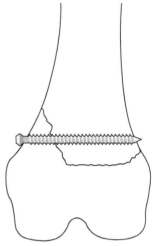

Figure 8.14 If the metaphyseal fragment is large enough fixation with an interfragmentary compression screw should be augmented with plaster cast support.

Stress fractures

Repetitive stresses to the leg may produce hairline stress fractures, particularly in the tibial shaft (Figure 8.16, p. 181), but also in the fibula and rarely in the femur. These should be suspected in children or athletes who perform repetitive activities, whether at work, during leisure (Devas 1963) or when resuming sports, particularly road-running. The diagnosis can often be made by suspecting the injury and undertaking an ultrasound or magnetic resonance (MR) scan acutely.

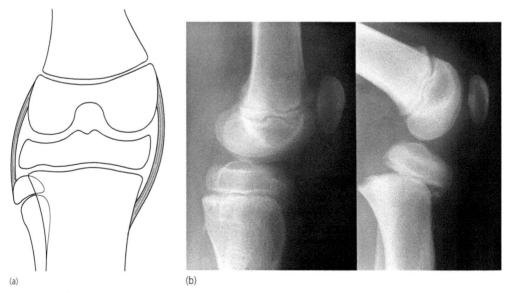

(a) (b)

Figure 8.15 The collateral ligaments of the knee offer more support to the proximal tibial epiphysis because they are attached to the metaphysis (a) and thus proximal tibial displacement is usually minimal (b).

Figure 8.16 A stress fracture of the proximal tibial shaft.

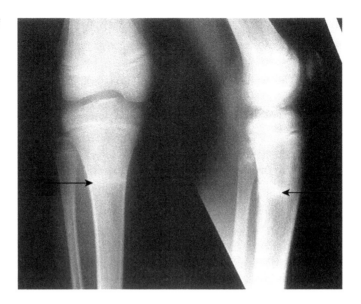

A standard radiograph, 2–3 weeks after the onset of symptoms, will usually reveal periosteal and osseous changes. A bone scan is rarely necessary but demonstrates increased blood flow at the site of the established stress fracture. Occasionally these changes may be difficult to differentiate from the early stages of a bone tumour, and a careful history and follow-up is essential (Mattila *et al.* 2007).

During growth a form of stress fracture occurs in relation to the attachment of tendons to bone. These 'osteochondroses' are numerous throughout the skeleton, and in the region of the knee involve the tibial tuberosity (Osgood–Schlatter disease) and the lower pole of the patella (Sinding-Larsen–Johansson syndrome) (Figure 8.17, p. 182, see also Chapter 7). Treatment is conservative, including an initial period of rest and advice, and reassurance for both the child and the parents. Most of these 'growing pains' will settle at the end of skeletal growth.

Occasionally the symptoms from Osgood–Schlatter disease may become chronic and this is said to be more common if an ossicle forms in relation to the patellar tendon distally (Figure 8.18, p. 182). Excision of this ossicle in late adolescence or early adult life may relieve symptoms, but in other respects these developmental injuries are best managed conservatively.

Complications of fractures

Early complications include:

- Haemarthrosis of the knee, which may merit an aspiration for the purpose of diagnosis and the relief of symptoms
- Major nerve or vessel damage, which is not uncommon when a compound fracture involves the knee
- Compartment syndrome, which should be relieved within 8 hours of its occurrence if permanent disability is to be avoided. This syndrome is discussed further in Chapter 9.
- Infection of a compound fracture or following surgical intervention.

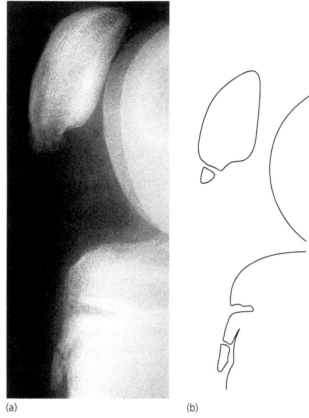

(a)   (b)

Figure 8.17 Chronic stress changes are evident at both ends of the patellar tendon.

Figure 8.18 An ossicle has formed within the distal patellar tendon secondary to Osgood–Schlatter's disease.

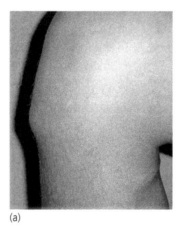 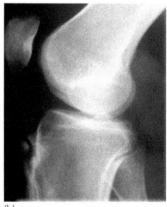

(a)   (b)

Later complications include:

- Chronic infection
- Malunion
- Degenerative changes and eventual osteoarthritis
- Complex regional pain syndrome type 1
- Stiffness.

Stiffness of the knee was a major problem after conservatively managed femoral fractures, particularly if the fracture had been significantly displaced and if movement of the knee was not encouraged at an early stage (Charnley 1947). Stiffness is the result of both extra-articular adhesions, binding the quadriceps mechanism to the femoral shaft (Judet 1954), and intra-articular adhesions when the joint is involved. The additional factors of muscle weakness and residual deformity will also worsen any restriction.

Distal femoral fractures complicated by infection are far more likely to develop significant stiffness. Inappropriate internal fixation will also reduce knee movement by implant impingement. Usually, periosteal scar and callus reabsorb and remodel so that recovery of knee movement occurs slowly over the ensuing 18 months after injury. This progress must not be inadvisedly hastened by forcible manipulation of the knee since passive stretching and muscle tearing may promote myositis ossificans and inhibit subsequent muscle function.

If stiffness of the knee cannot be avoided by physiotherapy throughout the period of convalescence, a distal quadricepsplasty may be required (Nicoll 1963). Adhesions between the muscles and the bone must be released and the knee moved as soon as possible thereafter. The use of a commercial knee 'mobilizer' may be of great value in maintaining movement of the knee during the early postoperative period, and regular, passive movement of the knee at this stage is not particularly painful. Although distal quadricepsplasty may address the problems at the site of the fracture, there is the danger that an extension lag may persist. A proximal quadricepsplasty combined with a release of all adhesions may therefore be preferred.

More general complications which may follow any fracture of the lower limb include deep venous thrombosis (Chapter 9), pulmonary embolism, chest infection, malnutrition and osteoporosis. These complications are beyond the scope of this book but will obviously influence the recovery following fractures of the knee.

References

Apley AG (1956) Fracture of the lateral tibial condyle treated by skeletal traction and early mobilisation. *J Bone Joint Surg Br* **38**, 699–708.

Beaty JH and Kumar A (1994) Fractures about the knee in children. Current concepts review. *J Bone Joint Surg Am* **76**, 1870–80.

Beaty JH and Kasser JR (eds) (2009) *Rockwood and Wilkins' Fractures in Children*, 7th edn. Philadelphia, PA: Waters Kluwert/Lippincott, William and Wilkins.

Burri C, Bartzke G, Coldewey J and Muggier E (1979) Fractures of the tibial plateau. *Clin. Orthop* **138**, 84–93.

Charnley J (1947) Knee movement following fractures of the femoral shaft. *J Bone Joint Surg Am* **29**, 679–86.

Dandy DJ (1992) Chondral and osteochondral lesions of the femoral condyles. In: Aichroth PM and Cannon WD (eds) *Knee Surgery: Current Practice*. London: Martin Dunitz, pp. 443–9.

Devas MB (1963) Stress fractures in children. *J Bone Joint Surg Br* **45**, 528–41.

Dowd GE (1982) Marginal fractures of the patella. *Injury* **14**, 287–91.

Garrison KR, Shemilt I, Donell ST, *et al.* (2010) Bone morphogenetic protein (BMP) for fracture healing in adults. *Cochrane Database Syst Rev* **16**, CD006950.

Giles JB, DeLee JC, Heckman JD, *et al.* (1982) Supracondylar–intercondylar fractures of the femur treated with a supracondylar plate and lag screw. *J Bone Joint Surg Am* **64**, 864–70.

Heckman JD, Ryaby JP, McCabe J, *et al.* (1994) Acceleration of tibial fracture-healing by non-invasive, low-intensity pulsed ultrasound. *J Bone Joint Surg Am* **76**, 26–34.

Hohl M and Luck JV (1956) Fractures of the tibial condyle. A clinical and experimental study. *J Bone Joint Surg Am* **38**, 1001–18.

Honkonen SE and Jarvinen MJ (1992) Classification of fractures of the tibial condyles. *J Bone Joint Surg Br* **74**, 840–7.

Hubbard MJS (1987) Arthroscopic surgery for chondral flaps in the knee. *J Bone Joint Surg Br* **69**, 794–6.

Judet R (1954) Mobilisation of the stiff knee. *J Bone Joint Surg Br* **41**, 856–7.

Khan WS, Johnson DS and Hardingham TE (2010) The potential of stem cells in the treatment of knee cartilage defects. *Knee* **17**, 369–74.

Kristiansen TK, Ryaby JP, McCabe J, *et al.* (1997) Accelerated healing of distal radial fractures with the use of specific, low-intensity ultrasound. A multicenter, prospective, randomized, double-blind, placebo-controlled study. *J Bone Joint Surg Am* **79**, 961–73.

Leung KS, Shen WY, So WS, *et al.* (1992) Interlocking intrameduallary nailing for supracondylar and intercondylar fractures of the distal part of the femur. *J Bone Joint Surg Am* **73**, 332–40.

Liu F, Tao R, Cao Y, *et al.* (2009) The role of LISS (less invasive stabilisation system) in the treatment of peri-knee fractures. *Injury* **40**, 1187–94.

Macnicol MF and Murray AW (2010) Principles of fracture care. In: Benson MKD, Fixsen JA, Macnicol MF and Parsch K (eds) *Children's Orthopaedics and Fractures*, 3rd edn. London: Springer-Verlag, pp. 651–64.

Mallina R, Kanakaris NK and Giannoudis PV (2010) Peri-articular fractures of the knee: an update on current issues. *Knee* **17**, 181–6.

Mattila VM, Niva M, Kiuru M, *et al.* (2007) Risk factors for bone stress injuries: a follow-up study of 102,515 person-years. *Med Sci Sports Exerc* **39**, 1061–6.

Müller ME, Allgower M and Willenegger H (1970) *Manual of Internal Fixation. Technique Recommended by the AO Group*. Berlin: Springer-Verlag.

Müller ME, Nayeria S and Koch P (1988) *The AO Classification of Fractures*. Berlin: Springer-Verlag.

Nicoll EA (1963) Quadricepsplasty. *J Bone Joint Surg Br* **45**, 483–90.

O'Donoghue DH (1966) Chondral and osteochondral fractures. *J Trauma* **6**, 469–81.

O'Dwyer KJ and Bobic VR (1992) Arthroscopic management of tibial plateau fractures. *Injury* **23**, 261–4.

Olerud S (1972) Operative treatment of supracondylar–intercondylar fractures of the femur. *J Bone Joint Surg Am* **54**, 1015–32.

Porter BB (1970) Crush fractures of the lateral tibial table. *J Bone Joint Surg Br* **52**, 676–87.

Rasmussen PS and Sörensen SE (1973) Tibial condylar fractures. *Injury* **4**, 265–8.

Rockwood CA and Green RP (eds) (1991) *Fractures*, 3rd edn. Philadelphia: JB Lippincott.

Salter RB and Harris WR (1963) Injuries involving the epiphyseal plate. *J Bone Joint Surg Am* **45**, 587–92.

Sanders R, Swiontkowski M, Rosen H and Helfet D (1991) Double-plating of comminuted, unstable fractures of the distal part of the femur. *J Bone Joint Surg Am* **73**, 341–6.

Schatzker J, McBroom R and Bruce D (1979) The tibial plateau fracture. *Clin Orthop* **138**, 94–104.

Skak SV, Jensen TT, Poulsen TD, *et al.* (1987) Epidemiology of knee injuries in children. *Acta Orthop Scand* **58**, 78–81.

Siliski JM, Mahsing M and Hofer HP (1989) Supracondylar–intercondylar fractures of the femur. *J Bone Joint Surg Am* **71**, 95–104.

Vangsness C Jr, DeCampos J, Merritt PO and Wiss DA (1993) Meniscal injury associated with femoral shaft fractures. *J Bone Joint Surg Br* **75**, 207–9.

Watanabe Y, Matsushita T, Bhandari M, *et al.* (2010) Ultrasound for fracture healing: current evidence. *J Orthop Trauma* **24**, S56–61.

9

Non-traumatic conditions

Introduction

A number of 'intrinsic problems' may affect the knee and confuse the clinical assessment of the joint that is painful after presumed trauma. An underlying disease process or congenital abnormality will predispose the knee to symptoms which are then precipitated by an injury, often of fairly minor degree. When considering congenital abnormalities, the following variations from normal should be remembered:

* Ligament laxity, which may be familial or in association with muscular dystrophy, Marfan's syndrome, osteogenesis imperfecta, spinal muscular atrophy, Down's syndrome and certain skeletal dysplasias
* Anomalies of the meniscus, particularly:
  – The discoid lateral meniscus
  – Cysts at the periphery of, or within, either the lateral or medial meniscus
* Absence of one or both cruciate ligaments (sometimes in association with major skeletal abnormalities)
* Haemophilia and other bleeding disorders
* Malalignment syndromes, such as persistent femoral anteversion and torsional deformities of the tibia.

A number of developmental conditions may also afflict the knee in the child or young adult and these include osteochondritis dissecans, synovitis and arthropathies, metabolic diseases, tumours and infections. Many of these problems have been discussed in other sections of the book; this chapter will deal with inflammatory arthritis, including infection, synovial pathology, haemophilia, osteonecrosis and osteochondritis dissecans, Blount's disease and tumours. Compartment syndrome, deep venous thrombosis and pressure sores will also be described briefly insofar as they influence the function of the knee.

Inflammatory arthritis

In younger patients the knee is most commonly involved if a monarticular synovitis develops, acting as a signal for the beginning of a systemic disease. It is therefore important to obtain a detailed medical history which should include questions about:

- Symptoms from inflammatory conditions of the eye, including iritis, scleritis and conjunctivitis
- Mucosal ulceration
- Respiratory and abdominal symptoms
- Urethritis
- Skin rashes
- Non-specific symptoms such as malaise, loss of weight or fevers
- A family history, with specific questioning about iritis, inflammatory bowel disease, psoriasis, gout and stiff and painful joints.

■ Synovitis

When a synovitis develops, a minor degree of trauma may be advanced by the patient as the cause of the symptoms. A systemic condition should be suspected when the synovitic features remain or if the history is not convincingly that of trauma. A synovitis will cause the knee to feel rather doughy and warm, and may be associated with an effusion. If the skin appears reddened, infection or a crystal synovitis should be suspected and in these instances a synovial fluid assay is diagnostic.

■ Synovial fluid

Synovial fluid and tissue, if available, should be examined microscopically for the presence of pus cells and crystals (Table 9.1). The Gram stain is an early discriminant for infection but bacteriological culture should also be requested to define an organism's antibiotic sensitivity. An anti-staphylococcal antibiotic is started until the causative organism is known. The culture should include media for anaerobic and tuberculous organisms in addition to standard plating. Thermography and scanning with radioisotopes may be indicated but have been largely superseded by the availability of MR scanning. Undoubtedly the most direct assessment is provided by arthroscopy which permits both an evaluation of the intra-articular fluid and a synovial biopsy (Figure 9.1).

Certain blood tests are of value, but may not necessarily provide more than a clue to the diagnosis. The erythrocyte sedimentation rate (ESR) is often raised, but is a non-specific test.

Table 9.1 Synovial fluid analysis as an aid to diagnosis

Blood	Fracture, ligament rupture, synovial tear (haemophilia, haemangioma)
Fat	Osteochondral fracture, fat pad lesion
Debris	Articular cartilage damage including chondromalacia, meniscal tear
Cells	Monocyte predominance in osteoarthritis
	Polymorphonuclear cell predominance in inflammatory synovitis including rheumatoid arthritis and septic arthritis
Crystals	Gout (urate) – feathery crystals
	Pseudogout (monophosphate) – rectangular crystals
Lactate, acidity and lysosomal enzymes	Increased in inflammatory conditions
Lysosomal enzymes	Increased in painful synovitis
Complement	Increased in Reiter's syndrome and gout
	Increased in osteoarthritis
	Decreased in rheumatoid arthritis

The white blood cell count and C-reactive protein are elevated. The rheumatoid factor, representing the production of a macro-immunoglobulin against IgG, may be negative in the majority of cases with juvenile chronic arthritis in childhood and in 30 per cent of adults with rheumatoid arthritis. Tests for the serum uric acid and titres against staphylococcus and streptococcus may be helpful, and an anti-streptococcal titre consistently below 200 units makes rheumatic fever unlikely. The HLA-B27 antigen is positive in 5–10 per cent of the normal population, but may be a useful pointer in a patient with ankylosing spondylitis, Reiter's syndrome or an arthritis that is associated with inflammatory bowel disease.

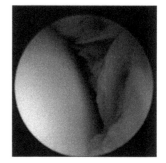

Figure 9.1 Arthroscopic appearance of synovitis.

Synovial biopsy

Arthroscopic examination will not only allow an accurate sampling of the inflamed synovium, but will also help to rule out the following mechanical lesions that may cause a synovitis:

- Meniscus tear
- Loose body
- Articular cartilage abnormality
- Plica/impingement
- Fracture.

Synovial biopsy, although a very direct test, can again only indicate the presence of an inflammatory condition; the following histological changes may be observed:

- Hypertrophy of the synovial fronds
- Proliferation of the superficial synovial cells
- A chronic inflammatory cell infiltrate, occasionally with the development of lymphoid follicles
- Cell necrosis in patches of the synovial tissue
- Deposition of fibrin both within and on the surface of the synovium.

The synovial biopsy will aid in diagnosing gout and pseudogout (crystal synovitis), pigmented villonodular synovitis, sarcoidosis, synovial chondromatosis (Figure 9.2), malignant synovioma and specific infections, including tuberculosis.

Treatment

If an inflammatory arthritis is considered to be present, a number of relatively conservative measures can be used to lessen symptoms and preserve function in the joint. Splintage in extension may be of value in the early stages, when the inflammation is poorly controlled, but prolonged immobilization will lead to disuse atrophy of muscle and stiffness. Hence, a balanced approach must be ensured, with preservation of muscle bulk by means of isometric exercises, and the subsequent maintenance of a functional arc of movement by controlled and carefully directed physiotherapy.

Ice packs may lessen pain from muscle spasm, and mild heat in the form of hydrotherapy or wax baths may permit a greater degree of function in the joint. Unfortunately, the benefits from these techniques are short lived, and some other means of reducing the synovitis is usually necessary. In this context, radiant heat, including short-wave diathermy, may markedly worsen symptoms, as will over-vigorous physiotherapy.

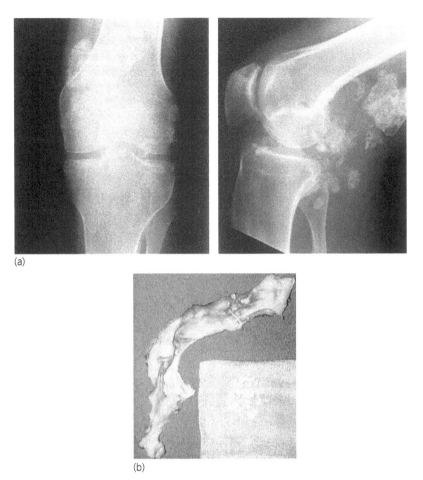

(a)

(b)

Figure 9.2 (a) Synovial chondromatosis. (b) Synovial chondromatosis with a segment of hypertrophic synovium.

Anti-inflammatory analgesia is usually beneficial, although no one drug will remain effective indefinitely, and various patients will react in different ways to the different preparations. A policy of monitoring symptoms and alternating the drug treatments is therefore advisable.

Table 9.2 lists the various anti-inflammatory analgesic agents that can be used. These drugs are unsafe if combined with oral anti-coagulants, hypoglycaemic agents and other highly protein-bound compounds. Gastrointestinal bleeding may also be produced. Various enteric-coated drugs are therefore available, and analgesics may also be given in suppository form.

■ Synovectomy

If the synovitis fails to respond to these measures, a synovectomy may be necessary and still finds a place in the treatment of the patient with rheumatoid arthritis and the younger patient with haemophilia. Subtotal synovectomy is quite possible surgically, but must be offered in good time, before the articular cartilage has been extensively affected. There is always a risk that the range of movement will lessen owing to the postoperative scarring, and the principal indication for synovectomy is unremitting pain, particularly if the range of movement is lessening rapidly.

Subtotal synovectomy is effective arthroscopically using a motorized shaver. Rehabilitation is usually more rapid than after open synovectomy, but great care must be taken with the

Table 9.2 Anti-inflammatory analgesic drugs

Simple analgesics	Low doses of acetyl salicylic acid
	Paracetamol
	Codeine phosphate
Non-steroidal anti-inflammatory agents	*Weaker preparations:*
	Ibuprofen
	Naproxen
	Fenoprofen
	Sulindac
	Piroxicam
	Azapropazone
	Diclofenac sodium
	Mefenamic acid
	Celecoxib (cyclo-oxygenase-2 inhibitor)
	Stronger preparations:
	Full doses of acetyl salicylic acid
	Indocid (indometacin)
Local corticosteroid injections	Methylprednisolone acetate
	Hydrocortisone acetate
	Triamcinolone acetonide

placement of portals and protection of the articular surfaces. Medical synovectomy using radioactive gold or yttrium-90 may be more appropriate in older patients or for those with recurrent symptoms.

■ Septic arthritis

The knee is the most common site of sepsis in later childhood and adult life, although classic, long-bone metaphyseal osteomyelitis is on the wane, with atypical and deeper skeletal infection (for example in the pelvis) causing diagnostic difficulties (Macnicol 2001). In the pre-school child, and especially during infancy, the hip is the prime target joint, partly because the femoral metaphysis is intra-articular so that infection readily spreads from a proximal femoral osteomyelitis. Subacute osteomyelitic foci may result *de novo*, or as a result of inadequate antibiotic therapy, but do not endanger the knee joint as the infection is rarely metaphyseal. However, the patella may harbour the subacute form (see Figure 7.14, p. 158) which may lead to a secondary knee septic arthritis. Multifocal septic arthritis should always be suspected in the septicaemic patient, particularly if the host is known to be immunocompromised.

Magnetic resonance (MR) and ultrasound scans have revolutionized the management of bone and joint infection. Arthroscopy allows ready access to the knee joint without the uncertainties of joint aspiration. Irrigation of the joint is of value, and the combination of parenteral antibiotic treatment and arthroscopic lavage prevents collagen destruction more effectively than antibiotics and aspiration alone (Daniel *et al.* 1976). Nevertheless, the biochemical effects of the irrigant may also be deleterious, and therefore Ringer's lactate is preferred to other solutions and should neither be chilled nor used in excessive volume.

The differential diagnosis includes the various arthropathies of childhood, whether
seronegative or seropositive, synovitis in association with rheumatic fever and the exanthemata,

and neoplastic conditions of the synovium and skeleton. Delay in diagnosis and inadequate decompression remain the critical factors (Goldenberg *et al.* 1975) and a series of papers has confirmed the value of the arthroscope (Ivey and Clark 1985; Skyhar and Mubarak 1987; Stanitski *et al.* 1989; Ohl *et al.* 1991). This form of treatment is superior to aspiration where approximately one in three cases will be left with residual necrotic and fibrinous debris and adhesion formation. The smaller diameter (3.8 mm rather than 5 mm) arthroscope may be indicated in pre-school children, but the larger sheath is more effective and will allow a cannula to be inserted into the joint for intermittent lavage. Every 8 hours for 2–3 days 10 mL of isotonic Ringer's lactate can be instilled, combined with bupivacaine (Marcain) and morphine if pain is severe. Antibiotic should be given intravenously since the potentially harmful effects of concentrated antibiotic upon articular cartilage mean that concentrated drug solutions should not be inserted in the joint.

General anaesthesia is recommended rather than local anaesthesia when arthroscopy is being considered for the child, although Jarrett *et al.* (1981) found that regional or local block was satisfactory in adults. The essence of arthroscopic treatment is that it should ensure complete decompression of the joint, with the breakdown of adhesions and loculations using a blunt trocar, and that all recesses of the cavity should be thoroughly irrigated with a non-irritant fluid. Even if a cannula is left *in situ* to allow intermittent lavage, the use of continuous passive motion and early active movement should be encouraged. Reaccumulation of pus and the return of pain should be dealt with by further irrigation and by repeat arthroscopy if necessary. In the early case this approach will ensure a satisfactory functional recovery with minimal postoperative morbidity. In the chronic or recurrent case the outcome is less certain (Baker and Macnicol 2007) and residual stiffness and articular cartilage damage are likely to persist.

The range of organisms cultured from the infected knee does not differ from that seen in other large joints, particularly the hip. Staphylococcal organisms (including meticillin-resistant strains, [MRSA]) are the most likely, but streptococcal, Gram-negative and anaerobic organisms must also be suspected, sometimes in combination:

- *Staphylococcus aureus*
- *Staph. epidermidis*
- *Streptococcus pyogenes*
- *Haemophilus influenza*
- *Strep. pneumoniae*
- *Pseudomonas aeruginosa*
- *Strep. faecalis*
- *Escherichia coli*
- *Proteus* spp., *Klebsiella* spp., *Salmonella* spp.
- *Clostridium difficile*
- Anaerobic organisms (rare).

Immunodeficiency is less common after the neonatal period (Macnicol 1986), but may play a part in the indolent septic arthritis encountered in older, arthritic patients and in those with polyarthropathy. Drug abuse and acquired immune deficiency syndrome (AIDS) (human immunodeficiency virus [HIV] positivity) also exert a devastating effect on the immune system. The antibiotic of choice will depend on sensitivity patterns, and should commence with the intravenous administration of a 'best guess' agent, such as flucloxacillin and co-amoxiclav (Augmentin), followed by alternative drugs as indicated. The antibiotic therapy which follows is dependent on hospital policy and subsequent cultures: flucloxacillin, gentamicin, clindamycin, fusidic acid, cefuroxime, cefotaxime, co-trimoxazole, ampicillin and other bactericidal agents in combination.

Ohl *et al.* (1991) reported a 10-month follow-up of 16 septic knees in children, with good initial results following early weightbearing after arthroscopic debridement. However, the long-term results following infection are poorly recorded and permanent articular cartilage loss is inevitable after late treatment. Extensive surgery may be required to correct late deformity if the growth plate has been involved (Figure 9.3).

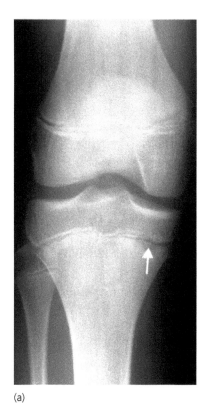

(a)

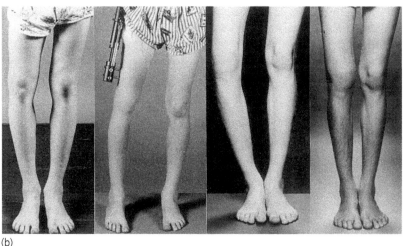

(b)

Figure 9.3 (a) Subacute osteomyelitis of the proximal tibial growth plate (arrow) resulted in a varus knee deformity at maturity. (b) Infantile septic arthritis of the right knee produced distal femoral growth arrest (shortening and varus), corrected by leg lengthening and distal femoral valgus osteotomy.

Synovial conditions

Haemangioma of the fat pad (see Figure 4.30b, p. 79) and other synovial lesions may impinge between the surfaces of the knee and cause episodes of haemarthrosis and locking (Figure 4.30a, p. 79). Eventually this leads to loss of movement if the bleeds go unchecked (Paley and Jackson 1986; Juhl and Krebs 1989). Stimulus of the growth plate may result in slight overgrowth of the limb whereas a flexion deformity will cause shortening. Arthroscopic treatment is effective in dealing with these lesions, as it may also be in haemophilia, provided the appropriate factor cover is given intravenously immediately before, during and after surgery (Klein *et al.* 1987; Limbird and Dennis 1987).

Synovial chondromatosis (Carey 1983; Coolican and Dandy 1989; Kistler 1991) is a rare but recognized acquired condition in childhood (Figure 9.2, p. 189). Pain, swelling, catching and locking are again the features, which may also characterize torsion of a synovial polyp, pigmented villonodular synovitis (Giron *et al.* 1991) and synovioma. A generalized synovitis is pathognomonic of juvenile chronic arthritis but may also be seen in mild haemophilia, in Lyme disease (Schoen *et al.* 1991) and after viral illnesses. Skin conditions such as eczema and psoriasis also seem to predispose the younger patient to knee effusions.

The plica syndrome generated much interest a decade ago and is now accepted as one of a number of causes of anterior knee pain. When a thickened band can be palpated as it rolls or clicks over the medial femoral condyle, the diagnosis can be sustained, particularly when abrasion is present over the articular edge of the condyle. Excision of the thickened band or shelf of synovium (Figure 7.15, p. 158) is sometimes effective (Koshino and Okamoto 1985; Patel 1986) but the interior of the knee must be thoroughly inspected for other pathology at the time of arthroscopy and extra-articular lesions should always be considered by appropriate preoperative examination and investigations (Joyce and Mankin 1983).

A popliteal cyst commonly presents in mid-childhood (Figure 9.4) without the knowledge of the patient but to parents' alarm. The swelling is usually a semimembranosus bursa which communicates with the knee joint but is not a pathological process. Histology of the wall of the cyst reveals a non-specific inflammatory reaction, with a fibrotic response proportional to the

Figure 9.4 The popliteal cyst in childhood usually resolves.

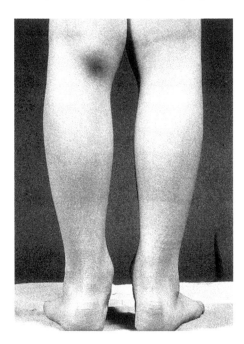

chronicity of the lesion. Radiography is advisable to rule out skeletal changes, but ultrasound, arthrographic and MR assessment are rarely indicated.

In childhood the cyst usually disappears and its excision is quite unnecessary. Aspiration is appropriate if the knee appears synovitic, but this will only aid in diagnosis and is not therapeutic. In older patients a popliteal cyst develops as a manifestation of repeated effusions in the knee. When associated with osteoarthritis the term 'Baker's cyst' is often used and the swelling may communicate with a degenerative lesion of the medial meniscus. Excision of a large cyst may be indicated if the symptoms are severe, but recurrence is likely if the primary inflammatory process is not addressed or the meniscal chronic tear is not excised arthroscopically. The injection of local steroid preparations after aspiration of the cyst is therefore preferable, at least initially, and may be enough to reassure the patient.

Rupture of a Baker's cyst may produce symptoms that mimic a deep venous thrombosis in the calf. Arthrographic ultrasound or MR imaging is diagnostic and the condition is treated symptomatically with supportive stockings, physiotherapy to maintain power and knee motion, and short-term anti-inflammatory analgesia.

Haemophilia

Haemophilia is a genetically determined coagulation disorder which occurs predominantly in males (types A and B) with an incidence of approximately 1 in 8000. Haemophilia C (von Willebrand's disease) affects both men and women, the female being an asymptomatic carrier of the sex-linked recessive gene. Haemophilia A is caused by a deficiency of factor VIII (anti-haemophilic factor: AHF) and constitutes 80 per cent of all cases. Haemophilia B (Christmas disease) results from a deficiency of factor IX (Christmas factor or plasma thromboplastin component).

The general clinical manifestations of haemophilia include a tendency to bleed readily from lacerations and mucosal surfaces. Haemarthroses are common, causing pain, distension and warmth of the joint (Figure 9.5). Typically, a haemophiliac patient will feel that there is a bleed within a joint before the clinical signs become evident (Skeith *et al.* 2010). Haematomas and haemophilic cysts may develop in the thigh, buttock, abdomen, calf and hand. The cysts are either simple, contained within muscle fascia, or deeper, in which case they may be either juxtacortical, between muscle attachment and bone, or subperiosteal, which is the most common site.

Pathology

After a haemarthrosis has developed in the knee, there is a subsequent release of haemosiderin as blood corpuscles break down. This irritant material in relatively large dosage produces a

Figure 9.5 Chronic synovitis produces increased heat emission on thermography.

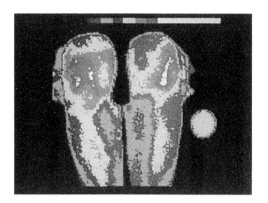

synovial haemosiderosis. An initial low-grade synovitis eventually becomes fulminating, and as severe as any rheumatoid arthritis. Worse still, the synovial haemosiderosis predisposes the joint to further bleeds.

In time the synovitis progresses to a fibrotic stage, producing contracture of the capsule. The articular cartilage becomes eroded by lysosomal enzymes, released from the inflamed synovium which grows across the joint as a pannus. The chondrocytes perish from an excess of iron pigment, and an associated pressure necrosis.

The knee joint is involved in at least 50 per cent of all patients with haemophilic arthropathy and the presentation clinically may be acute, subacute or chronic. Occasionally, the patient is unaware of having a particular bleeding tendency, but recurrent haemarthroses in a joint such as the knee should alert the clinician to this possibility. Spontaneous bleeding may also occur from localized haemangiomas within the knee, but are rarely as troublesome as the recurrent haemarthroses in severe, untreated haemophilia.

Radiography

The radiographic features of a knee affected by haemophilic arthropathy include soft tissue swelling, epiphyseal overgrowth (Figure 9.6), osteoporosis and thickening of the haemosiderotic synovium. Cysts and subchondral sclerosis develop around the margins of the knee joint in the more chronic cases and eventually the standard osteoarthritic changes of narrowing of the joint space, increasing sclerosis and deformity occur. Petterson *et al.* (1980) developed a grading system, scoring from 0 to 13, based on these radiographic changes. The progression of the arthropathy can therefore be described and applied to reviews of therapy.

A characteristic squaring of the patella is seen, and in association with this the intercondylar femoral notch becomes deepened and widened (Figure 9.7). The femoral condyles may become indented by impaction of the anterior tibial articular surface, and this is hastened by the fact that the tibia gradually subluxes posteriorly and externally (Figure 9.8). A flexion deformity therefore becomes irreversible, not only because of the fibrotic component, but as a result of impingement between the tibia and femur.

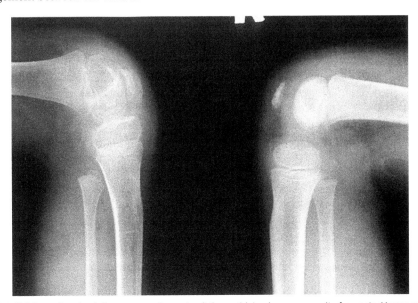

Figure 9.6 Epiphyseal and patellar overgrowth, and soft tissue thickening, as a result of repeated haemarthroses. Note the Harris growth arrest lines.

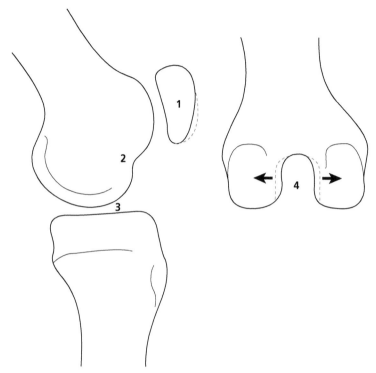

Figure 9.7 The changes which characterize haemophilic arthropathy of the knee (1, 'squaring' of the patella; 2, notching of the femoral condyle; 3, narrowing and sclerosis of the joint; 4, widening of the femoral intercondylar notch).

Figure 9.8 Gross radiographic changes of haemophilic arthropathy include posterior subluxation of the tibia and an irreversible flexion deformity.

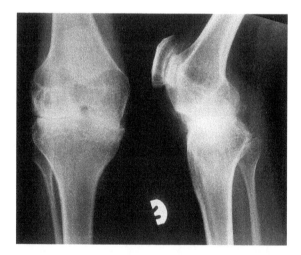

■ Treatment

Treatment should embrace two principles:

- Prevention of haemorrhages by prompt treatment with factor VIII or IX prophylaxis
- Preservation of a useful arc of knee movement and patellar mobility.

Factor VIII or IX is given by intravenous infusion to produce normal concentrations in the circulation. The knee should be immobilized in a backshell, which can be readily fashioned with polypropylene, and compression is applied by circumferential elasticated bandaging. Aspiration of the joint should be avoided; instead, static quadriceps exercises are instructed in order to increase intra-articular pressure. By this means the swelling should decrease progressively over 1–2 weeks. Extension should be preserved as fully as possible by ensuring quadriceps muscle tone, and thereafter flexion is regained by hamstring drill. The team approach is essential, combining the skills of the physician, orthopaedic surgeon, physiotherapist, general practitioner, specialist nurse and social worker.

In cases where a chronic synovitis has developed but the joint surfaces are still relatively well preserved, a case can be made for surgical synovectomy. This is necessarily subtotal, but will reduce the incidence of subsequent haemorrhage, although possibly at the expense of movement since fibrosis is produced by the surgery. Therefore patellofemoral mobility and knee extension must be ensured. Limbird and Dennis (1987) recommended the use of continuous passive motion after synovectomy, combined with full factor VIII or IX cover. Arthroscopic intervention early in the course of the disease may help to control haemorrhage from localized sites in the knee and the morbidity is thereby much reduced (Weidel 1990; Verma *et al.* 2007). Effective prophylaxis with heat-treated or recombinant factor VIII, preferably by educating the patients to the benefits of home therapy, has also reduced the severe disability that used to result from a progressive haemophilic arthropathy. Ultrasound and MR scanning, reveal early articular and synovial changes before they become apparent radiographically, and will also define subchondral and soft tissue cysts.

In association with appropriate physiotherapy, to improve all components of the quadriceps group, the use of posterior splints and wedging casts is of value, and there may be a place for 'reverse dynamic slings', which distract and gradually extend the flexed joint (Flower 2007). However, in cases where tibiofemoral impingement is occurring anteriorly, such measures are doomed to fail and may promote further haemorrhage within the joint. In these cases, particularly if pain is troublesome and haemarthroses recurrent, a total joint replacement or arthrodesis (Figure 9.9) may have to be considered. Surgery may also be required if a painful muscle haematoma or cyst develops.

Osteonecrosis

Osteonecrosis affects the older patient but may occasionally be seen in younger individuals with Gaucher's disease, systemic lupus erythematosus and rheumatoid-related conditions (Zywiel *et al.* 2009). Sickle cell disease and other haemoglobinopathies may also precipitate a

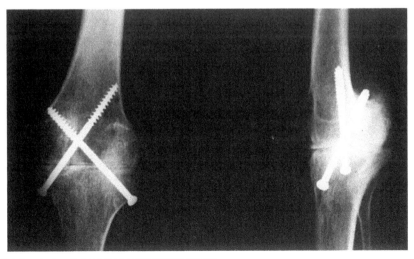

Figure 9.9 Arthrodesis using crossed compression screws.

problem, as may irradiation. Corticosteroid therapy for autoimmune disease or following renal transplantation, and in conditions such as severe asthma or the lymphomas, accounts for most of the drug-related cases. The association with alcoholism and with Caisson disease is well-established. The position and size of the lesion is prognostically significant, as are the alignment of the limb and the speed of enlargement of the infarction. Involvement of more than half the medial femoral condyle in the varus knee inevitably leads to osteoarthritis and disabling pain.

Ahlbäck *et al.* (1968) are credited with the first recognition of the idiopathic form which progresses from the stage of normal radiographs to slight flattening of the weightbearing segment, as in Perthes' disease. At this stage radioisotope bone scanning and MR imaging will define the extent of the lesion accurately. A radiolucent area gradually becomes apparent, surrounded by a sclerotic halo (Motohashi *et al.* 1991). As the subchondral plate collapses and deforms, the affected femorotibial compartment becomes increasingly irregular and arthritic.

Treatment of the early lesion includes protected weightbearing, thigh exercises and anti-inflammatory agents. Surgical intervention is based upon the merits of each case, aided by the use of arthroscopy. Core decompression (Jacobs *et al.* 1989), tibial realignment osteotomy (Koshino 1982), allografts and knee replacement all have a place in treatment (Kraenzlin *et al.* 2010).

Osteochondritis dissecans

This condition has already been discussed in Chapter 4, as it affects children as well as young adults. Paré first described loose bodies of the knee in 1558, and Paget (1870) considered that they resulted from avascular separation, the so-called 'quiet necrosis'. The osteochondritic change in childhood is relatively benign, the juvenile form sometimes representing an alteration in distal femoral ossification rather than a progressive lesion. Males are twice as commonly affected and trauma is often implicated.

An ischaemic necrosis of the bone seems unlikely since there are no end-arteries in the distal femur, which is the usual site of osteochondritis dissecans (Figures 4.21 [p. 72], 9.10). Histological examination rarely shows cellular necrosis. In this sense, osteochondritis dissecans should be distinguished from the other forms of osteochondritis (the osteochondroses) where there is a definite loss of blood supply. Although a positive family history may be recorded, the hereditary evidence is conflicting and usually the condition appears sporadically.

It seems most likely that in the teenager and adult trauma plays a significant part in the development of the lesion, possibly in as many as 50 per cent of the cases reported. Perhaps the injury produces a stress fracture but it is not known whether this trauma is exogenous, in which case very major forces have to be applied to the knee, or is endogenous, as a result of regular impaction against the femoral condyle by a prominent tibial spine, a discoid lateral

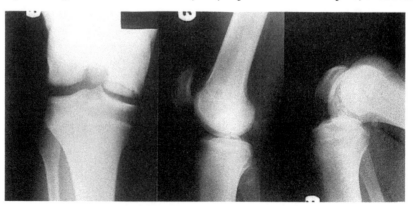

Figure 9.10 A large medial inferior–central osteochondritic separation.

meniscus or a subluxing patella. The healing capacity of the osteochondritic fragment is very variable, but is poor if the true 'dissecans' or separating form is present.

Both the juvenile and adult lesions should be distinguished from a true, acute osteochondral fracture, which separates from a bed of bleeding cancellous bone. The osteochondritic fragment, in contrast, is covered with fibrous tissue or hyperplastic cartilage, and is associated with an effusion, but not with a haemarthrosis, since the defect is relatively avascular.

Sites where osteochondritis dissecans may be encountered radiographically have already been shown in Chapter 4. The condition may be bilateral in up to a quarter of cases. A loose body is found in between a third and a half of all knees, and males are affected twice as commonly as females. There may be a correlation with genu recurvatum, valgus or varus deformity of the knee and patellar subluxation, and an association with anomalies such as discoid lateral meniscus and epiphyseal dysplasia has been described. The classic site is at the lateral aspect of the medial femoral condyle, and it is now believed that the prognosis is better in these cases (Garrett 1991; Twyman *et al.* 1991). The lateral femoral condyle is affected in some 20 per cent of cases (Aichroth 1971), and rarely the process affects the femoral sulcus (Smith 1990) or the patella (Figure 7.12, p. 157) (Edwards and Bentley 1977).

Constitutional factors are of importance, with a positive family history in some patients and the association with discoid lateral meniscus in others. Symptoms are relatively non-specific: aching pain, locking or clicking, recurrent effusions and limp. Wilson's sign is based on the fact that the tibial spines may impinge against the femoral condyle when the tibia is internally rotated with the knee extended (Wilson 1967), and tapping over the femoral condyle elicits tenderness compared with the rest of the knee.

■ Management

Evaluation requires four radiographic views of the knee augmented by tomography, and MR scans as necessary. Monitoring is best achieved with the MR scan, whereas arthroscopic review may improve the accuracy of staging the lesion. If the area is demarcated by softened hyaline cartilage but there is no breach in its surface, a conservative approach is indicated, particularly in patients before skeletal maturity. Athletic activities should be restricted, but there is no benefit from immobilization or non-weightbearing.

Arthroscopic drilling of the lesion may relieve the symptoms and is considered to hasten healing (Bradley and Dandy 1989), although there are no controlled trials to confirm this. Drilling attempts to traumatize the base of the fragment without undue articular cartilage injury. Both retrograde and reversed drilling have been promoted, each technique purporting to bring in fresh blood supply and possibly cells to the line of cleavage. Removal of a hinging fragment, curettage of the base, and re-fixation will be effective if the lesion is large (more than 1 cm in diameter) and reasonably congruent. Excision and removal should only be considered with small or fragmented lesions, particularly away from the weightbearing surface of the condyle, or if the fragment cannot be reduced anatomically. The depth of the bone base can be increased to accommodate the lesion which should never be left proud of the joint surface.

Smillie (1957) used pins or screws to stabilize the lesion, and Hughston *et al.* (1984) felt that fixation with K-wires produced better results than excision. Herbert screw fixation for smaller fragments (Thomson 1987) and countersunk small fragment AO compression screws are now established as effective implants. In arthroscopy, a small cannula should be used to prevent the guide wire from breaking, and a cannulated screw system should be used. The implant must be accurately positioned, using at least two mini-screws for larger fragments, and the knee monitored for 6 months postoperatively, checking the position of the screws radiographically as well as the appearances of the lesion.

Bone pins (Lindholm and Pylkkänen 1974) and absorbable pins have yet to prove themselves as safe and effective options (Stewart *et al.* 2008). Osteochondral allografting (Garrett 1991) may be appropriate when facilities permit but, when possible, the separated lesion should be replaced in preference. The primary problem of patellar instability should additionally be dealt with if it coexists with the rare condition of patellar osteochondritis dissecans (Pfeiffer *et al.* 1991). Bradley and Dandy (1989) have questioned whether true osteochondritis dissecans ever appears at sites other than the classic site and consider that distal femoral ossification patterns (Caffey *et al.* 1958) are unrelated to the condition.

Blount's disease (tibia vara)

In rare instances the normal bow-leg 'deformity' of a toddler fails to correct and the medial tibial growth plate collapses rather than being stimulated under compression. The deformity is discussed in Chapter 4 as one of the paediatric angulatory conditions that require treatment and careful monitoring. Blount (1937) described the progressive varus and internal rotation deformity of the upper tibia, noting that the medial proximal metaphysis became fragmented and then beaked with a distal curvature. Undiagnosed trauma or infection may cause the unilateral adolescent form, but the classical bilateral condition is developmental and poorly understood (Greene 1993).

In the toddler it is customary to observe the child with serial measurements and radiographs over a period of 2–3 years. Bracing is difficult to apply for prolonged periods and is poorly tolerated by the child. Therefore by the age of 4–6 years, a proximal tibial valgus osteotomy is advised, in order to correct the internal rotation and to produce 5–10° of valgus (Langenskiöld 1981).

If a medial growth plate tether develops between the ages of 8 and 10 years, it should be excised and the site of the resected bony bar filled with fat, Silastic or dental cement. Osteotomy alone at this age is unlikely to succeed, but may be combined with excision of the bar. Tomography or computed tomography (CT) will define the size of the bar, and external fixation, with distraction using the Ilizarov frame, is tolerated by the older child.

As the child nears adolescence, the proximal tibial surface may be severely tented. Function is further impaired by the presence of ligament laxity, which allows a coronal rocking movement. The medial tibial plateau may then require elevation and support (Siffert 1982) using bone graft or an excised segment of fibula (Figure 4.14, p. 67). Lateral proximal tibial epiphysiodesis is combined with this reconstruction if the child has 2 or more years (over 1 cm) of longitudinal growth at that site. In unilateral cases, a contralateral proximal tibial epiphysiodesis will control the leg-length discrepancy which complicates the unilateral condition.

Tumours

▪ Soft tissue swellings

The knee joint may be the site of a neoplastic growth, either in the soft tissues or in bone. Any anatomical structure forming part of the knee can enlarge abnormally. Thus fat may produce a lipoma, and fibrous tissue a sarcomatous tumour, including fibrosarcoma or a neurofibroma if there is a neural element in the tissues. Tumours of muscle (leiomyoma, leiomyosarcoma and rhabdomyosarcoma), vascular tumours, such as angiomas and various forms of angiosarcoma (haemangioendotheliomas and haemangiopericytomas) and several fibromatous conditions within bone as well as in the surrounding tissue will produce lumps around the knee, although they are rare. These have to be distinguished from the more common proliferative, inflammatory lesions such as pigmented villonodular synovitis and bursitis. Synovioma is a relatively rare but malignant tumour of the synovial lining; aggressive treatment is required in the form of radical excision (Novelli and Redner 2010).

Cystic lumps around the knee (Figure 9.11; see also Figure 2.1, p. 13) generally develop insidiously. In contrast, trauma produces more rapid swellings, such as a haematoma, arteriovenous fistula or abnormalities in the contour of the muscle as a result of rupture or avulsion from a bony attachment. Infective conditions may result in abscesses and enlargement of soft tissues. Chronic inflammatory conditions such as gout and rheumatoid arthritis produce tophi and rheumatoid nodules respectively, usually over the extensor surface of the knee.

▓ Bone tumours

Bone tumours involving the distal femur and proximal tibia are relatively common, and account for between 20 per cent and 25 per cent of all skeletal primary neoplasias. Gerhardt *et al.* (1990) reviewed 199 cases of neoplasia affecting the knee in childhood, noting that the lesions were referred more commonly in the older child. Benign tumours accounted for half the cases, and in decreasing order of frequency were osteochondroma, non-ossifying fibroma, chondroblastoma, osteoid osteoma, aneurysmal bone cyst, giant cell tumour, chondromyxoid fibroma, simple bone cyst and fibrous dysplasia. Benign lesions tend to be small and well marginated, with minimal or no cortical alteration and no soft tissue mass adjoining them. Benign 'latent' tumours such as fibrous cortical defect or dysplasia should be differentiated from active lesions, for example aneurysmal bone cyst or chondroblastoma (Lodwick *et al.* 1980).

Radiographically, these lesions produce slightly different appearances, as shown in Figure 9.12, but quite often the diagnosis cannot be made with certainty and a histological examination is essential (Vajnar 2010). Non-ossifying fibroma, or fibrous cortical defect, is very common in the end of a long bone during growth, and these are rarely of any concern. Other benign tumours encountered in the younger patient (chondromyxoid fibroma, fibrous dysplasia, benign chondroblastoma (see Figure 9.13) and diaphyseal aclasis) may give cause for concern and therefore merit follow-up.

Investigation of a malignant tumour should include:

* CT (including 3–1)
* MR imaging
* Angiography
* Soft tissue and bone biopsy.

As with soft tissue tumours, the cell of origin of bone tumours can usually be defined and hence the following classification is of some histological value:

Osteogenic:
* Osteoid osteoma
* Osteochondroma

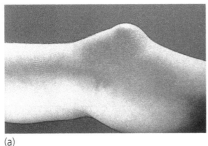
(a)
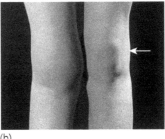
(b)

Figure 9.11 (a) The discrete swelling of prepatellar bursitis ('housemaid's knee'); (b) a left quadriceps ganglion.

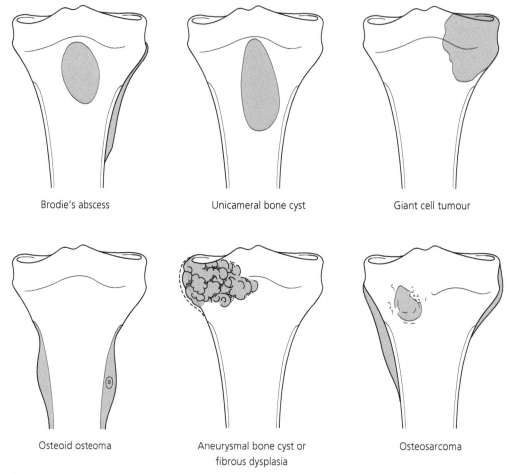

Brodie's abscess   Unicameral bone cyst   Giant cell tumour

Osteoid osteoma   Aneurysmal bone cyst or   Osteosarcoma
fibrous dysplasia

Figure 9.12 Radiographic features of the more common lesions affecting the proximal tibia.

     – Single: sessile or pedunculated
     – Multiple
- Osteosarcoma
- Parosteal sarcoma

Chondrogenic:
- Chondroma (or enchondroma)
- Benign chondroblastoma
- Chondromyxoid fibroma

Fibrogenic:
- Non-osteogenic fibroma
- Fibrous dysplasia
- Fibrosarcoma
- Malignant fibrous histiocytoma

Bone 'cyst':
- Unicameral
- Aneurysmal
- Giant cell tumour

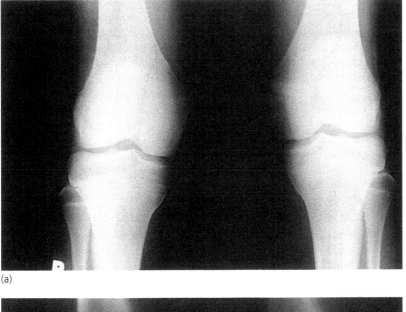

(a)

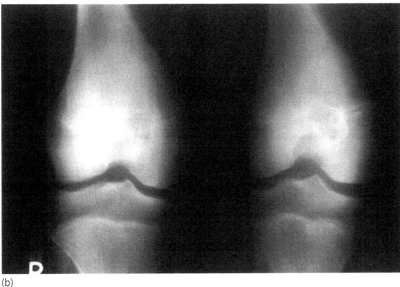

(b)

Figure 9.13 Chondroblastoma of the right distal femur (a), only apparent on tomography (b).

- Ewing's sarcoma
- Brown tumour of hyperparathyroidism
- Metastasis from other site.

The treatment of these bone tumours is beyond the scope of this book, but they should be recognized in the differential diagnosis of the painful knee, and always suspected in cases where the history is non-specific or where there is progressive swelling and tenderness of the femur or tibia.

Many benign tumours will heal or remain asymptomatic. Treatment is only directed to those that become symptomatic, usually because of an incipient stress fracture, enlargement (Figures 9.14, 9.15) or developing malignancy. The sarcomas of bone can sometimes be treated 203

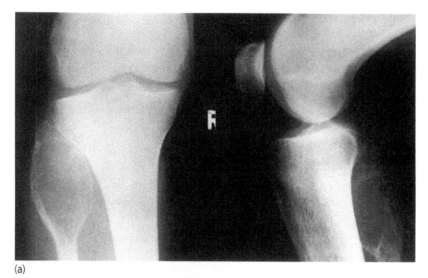

(a)

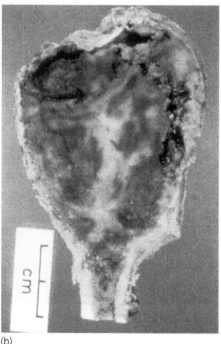

(b)

Figure 9.14a,b A giant cell tumour of the proximal fibula.

by radical resection and chemotherapy, thus saving the leg. All too often, however, the only surgical recourse is segmental resection, an upper thigh amputation or hip disarticulation.

Compartment syndrome

Exercise-induced compartment syndrome

The muscle compartments of the calf are shown in Figure 9.16. Those that commonly affect the athlete are the anterior compartment and the deep posterior compartment. After 10–20 minutes of strenuous exertion, pressure can be shown to rise within the anterolateral compartment, from a normal resting level of approximately 4 mmHg to more than 10 times this value. These changes are less well documented in the deep posterior compartment, and here the pathological cause of the pain is not understood. The compartment syndrome affects the function of the knee indirectly because of its influence upon the use of the leg generally and the local pain experienced within the calf.

Although rest, alteration in training patterns and attention to shoe wear may prevent the symptoms of both 'shin splints' (or medial tibial syndrome) and compartment syndrome, certain cases will only respond to surgical decompression by means of a fasciotomy. This is very effective in the anterior compartment syndrome, but the results of surgery for 'shin splints' are less predictable.

Radionuclide or MR scanning is usually negative, ruling out the presence of a tibial stress fracture. However, the deep compartment syndrome may be caused by a periostitis or chronic inflammatory condition along the medial tibial border where the tibialis posterior muscle attaches to bone. In these cases the bone scan may be positive. Surgical release of the deep fascia can be effective in relieving some or all of the pain, but may have no effect on muscle compartment pressure. On the other hand, the reduction in tissue pressure after fasciotomy of the anterior tibial compartment has been well documented.

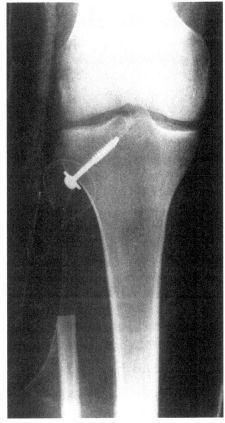

Figure 9.15 Radiographic appearances after excision of the tumour. The lateral (fibular) collateral ligament and biceps tendon have been reattached to the proximal tibia.

◼ Acute, post-traumatic compartment syndrome

Following fractures of the tibia, an acute compartment syndrome may affect the muscles of the calf, particularly if the fascia remains intact and there is no compounding wound at the fracture site. Soft tissue pressure can be measured after tibial fractures and may increase to approximately 100 mmHg. If this is present for more than a few hours the function of muscle and nerve within the affected compartment will be seriously and permanently impaired.

The pathophysiology of the acute compartment syndrome involves a combination of:

- Arterial occlusion secondary to an increase in extravascular pressure brought about by haemorrhage
- Subsequent venous occlusion and stasis
- A superimposed soft tissue oedema.

The last process is produced in part by the release of vasoactive amines, and these will compound the problems of the circulatory stasis by producing dilatation and increased capillary permeability. Muscle wet weight increases by over 50 per cent and pressure receptors within the muscle fibres may in turn cause further arterial spasm.

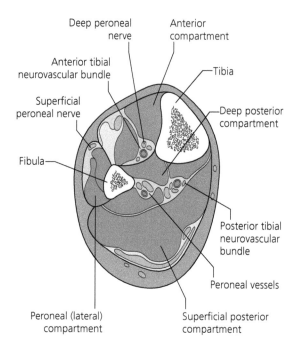

Figure 9.16 Cross-section of the calf to show the fascial boundaries of the muscle compartments.

Deep peroneal nerve

Anterior compartment

Anterior tibial neurovascular bundle

Tibia

Superficial peroneal nerve

Deep posterior compartment

Fibula

Posterior tibial neurovascular bundle

Peroneal vessels

Peroneal (lateral) compartment

Superficial posterior compartment

The compartment syndrome is aggravated by systemic hypotension, increased metabolic rate and elevation of the affected limb. If relief of the acute syndrome is not ensured within 6 hours, unremitting deep pain being the most significant presenting symptom, then the patient will be left with partial or complete paralysis of the affected muscles, patchy sensory loss and subsequent contractures affecting the foot. The presence or absence of a pulse cannot be used as a diagnostic feature, but pain on passive movement of the toes, distal pallor and cooling of the limb are significant additional features.

Deep venous thrombosis

Clotting (thrombosis) within the deep and superficial veins of the calf is caused by a combination of stasis of blood flow and injury to the vessel wall. Lower limb fractures and other forms of significant trauma increase the likelihood of deep venous thrombosis. In addition, at least 50 per cent of patients after lower limb surgery may also develop venous thrombosis. Calf tenderness and swelling, with later chronic pain, are the presenting features, and the girths of the legs should be carefully compared. Oedema of the ankle and foot may develop and function of the knee and ankle is impaired.

If the thrombosis spreads proximally to involve the iliofemoral segment, there is an increased risk of a propagated clot, with subsequent pulmonary embolism. Lower limb injuries of any sort can produce thrombosis as far proximally as the pelvic veins, and the very real danger of a pulmonary embolism must be anticipated. Clinical detection of venous thrombosis is made possible by the use of venography, radioactive fibrinogen counting or Doppler ultrasound. However, many cases of deep vein thrombosis either go unnoticed or are missed, despite clinical examination.

If there is significant symptomatology and swelling of the leg, then anticoagulation is advisable with intravenous or subcutaneous low molecular weight heparin initially for at least 48 hours until the concurrent use of oral warfarin affects the prothrombin time. In the older patient some degree of anticoagulation can be obtained with aspirin or dextran, although their prophylactic action is not marked. The details of deep vein thrombosis prophylaxis are well covered in the surgical guidelines of hospitals.

Pressure sores

These may be produced by tight plasters around the knee and lower leg. Local ischaemia produces microscopic changes within the skin and underlying tissues within 30 minutes, and shearing stress will extend the necrosis. At first the skin becomes erythematous. After 2 hours the changes become irreversible and the skin will then blister and become increasingly indurated.

The pressure sore extends deeply down to the underlying bone, such that a tetrahedron of necrotic fat underlies the affected skin. The necrosis may progress no further than to form a sterile abscess, but if infection occurs an osteitis of bone may also develop. The skin ulcerates and its edges gradually become undermined. Major, excisional surgery may be necessary.

The simplest remedy for bed sores is to prevent their development. Tight plasters must be avoided and the regular turning of comatose or immobilized patients is an essential part of nursing and medical care of the injured.

References

Ahlbäck S, Bauer GCH and Bohne WH (1968) Spontaneous osteonecrosis of the knee. *Arthritis Rheum* **11**, 705–33.

Aichroth PM (1971) Osteochondritis dissecans of the knee. *J Bone Joint Surg Br* **53**, 440–7.

Baker ADL and Macnicol MF (2007) Haematogenous osteomyelitis in children: epidemiology, classification, aetiology and treatment. *Paediatr Child Health* **18**, 75– 84.

Blount WP (1937) Tibia vara: osteochondrosis deformans tibiae. *J Bone Joint Surg Am* **19**, 1–29.

Bradley J and Dandy DJ (1989) Osteochondritis dissecans and other lesions of the femoral condyles. *J Bone joint Surg Br* **71**, 518–22.

Caffey J, Madel SH, Roger C, *et al.* (1958) Ossification of the distal femoral epiphysis. *J Bone Joint Surg Am* **40**, 467–74.

Carey RPL (1983) Synovial chondromatosis of the knee in childhood. *J Bone Joint Surg Br* **65**, 444–7.

Coolican MR and Dandy DJ (1989) Arthroscopic management of synovial chondromatosis of the knee. Findings and results in 18 cases. *J Bone Joint Surg Br* **71**, 498–500.

Daniel D, Akeson W, Amiel D, *et al.* (1976) Lavage of septic joints in rabbits: effects of chondrolysis. *J Bone Joint Surg Am* **58**, 393–5.

Edwards DH and Bentley G (1977) Osteochondritis dissecans patellae. *J Bone Joint Surg Br* **59**, 58–63.

Flower C (2007) Severe hemophilic arthropathy of the elbow and knee. *J Rheumatol* **34**, 1356–61.

Garrett JC (1991) Osteochondritis dissecans. *Clin Sports Med* **10**, 569–93.

Gerhardt MC, Ready JE and Mankin HJ (1990) Tumours about the knee in children. *Clin Orthop* **225**, 86–110.

Giron V, Ganel A and Heim M (1991) Pigmented villonodular synovitis. *Arch Dis Chtldh* **66**, 1449–50.

Goldenberg DL, Brandt KD, Cohen AS and Cathcart ES (1975) Treatment of septic arthritis: comparison of needle aspiration and surgery as initial modes of joint drainage. *Arthritis Rheum* **18**, 83–90.

Greene WB (1993) Infantile tibia vara. *J Bone Joint Surg Am* **73**, 130–43.

Hughston JC, Hergenroeder PT and Courtenay BG (1984) Osteochondritis dissecans of the femoral condyles. *J Bone Joint Surg Am* **6**, 1340–8.

Ivey M and Clark R (1985) Arthroscopic debridement of the knee for septic arthritis. *Clin Orthop* **199**, 201–6

Jacobs MA, Loeb PE and Hungerford DS (1989) Core decompression of the distal femur for avascular necrosis of the knee. *J Bone Joint Surg Br* **71**, 583–7.

Jarrett MP, Grossman L, Sadler AH and Gravzel Al (1981) The role of arthroscopy in the treatment of septic arthritis. *Arthritis Rheum* **24**, 737–9.

Joyce MJ and Mankin HJ (1983) Caveat arthroscopos: extra-articular lesions of bone simulating intra-articular pathology of the knee. *J Bone joint Surg Am* **65**, 289–92.

Juhl M and Krebs B (1989) Arthroscopy and synovial haemangioma or giant cell tumour of the knee. *Arch Orthop Trauma Surg* **108**, 250–2.

Kistler W (1991) Synovial chondromatosis of the knee joint: a rarity during childhood. *Eur J Pediatr Surg* **1**, 237–9.

Klein KS, Aland CM, Kim HC, *et al.* (1987) Long-term follow-up of arthroscopic synovectomy for chronic hemophilic synovitis. *Arthroscopy* **3**, 231–6.

Koshino T (1982) The treatment of spontaneous osteonecrosis of the knee by high tibial osteotomy with and without bone-grafting or drilling of the lesion. *J Bone Joint Surg Am* **64**, 47–58.

Koshino T and Okamoto R (1985) Resection of painful shelf (plica synovialis mediopatellaris) under arthroscopy. *Arthroscopy* **1**, 136–41.

Kraenzlin ME, Graf C, Meier C, *et al.* (2010) Possible beneficial effect of bisphosphonates in osteonecrosis of the knee. *Knee Surg Sports Traumatol Arthrosc* **18**, 1638–44.

Langenskiöld A (1981) Tibia vara: osteochondrosis deformans tibiae. *Clin Orthop* **158**, 77–82.

Limbird TJ and Dennis SC (1987) Synovectomy and continuous passive motion (CPM) in hemophiliac patients. *Arthroscopy* **3**, 74–9.

Lindholm S and Pylkkänen P (1974) Internal fixation of the fragment of osteochondritis dissecans in the knee by means of bone pins: a preliminary report on several cases. *Acta Chir Scand* **140**, 626–9.

Lodwick S, Wilson AJ, Farrell C, *et al.* (1980) Determining growth rates of focal bone lesions from radiographs. *Radiology* **134**, 577–83.

Macnicol MF (1986) Osseous infection and immunodeficiency. In: Hughes SPF and Fitzgerald RH (eds) *Musculoskeletal Infections*. Chicago: Year Book, pp. 68–79.

Macnicol M F (2001) Patterns of musculoskeletal infection in childhood (editorial). *J Bone Joint Surg Br* **82**, 1–2.

Motohashi M, Morii T and Koshino T (1991) Clinical course and roentgenographic changes of osteonecrosis in the femoral condyle under conservative treatment. *Clin Orthop* **266**, 156–61.

Novelli EM and Redner RL (2010) Knee pain: ACL, MCL, or CML (Chronic Myeloid Leukaemia)? *Blood* **115**, 5287–91.

Ohl MD, Kean JR and Steensen RN (1991) Arthroscopic treatment of septic arthritic knees in children and adolescents. *Orthop Rev* **20**, 894–6.

Paget J (1870) On the production of some of the loose bodies in joints. *St Bartholomew's Hosp Rep* **6**, 1–4.

Paley D and Jackson RW (1986) Synovial haemangioma of the knee joint: diagnosis by arthroscopy. *Arthroscopy* **2**, 174–7.

Patel D (1986) Plica as a cause of anterior knee pain. *Orthop Clin North Am* **17**, 273–8.

Petterson H, Ahlberg A and Nilsson IM (1980) A radiological classification of haemophilic arthropathy. *Clin Orthop* **149**, 153–9.

Pfeiffer WH, Gross ML and Seeger LL (1991) Osteochondritis dissecans of the patella. *Clin Orthop* **271**, 207–11.

Schoen RT, Aversa JM, Rahn DW and Steere AC (1991) Treatment of refractory chronic Lyme arthritis with arthroscopic synovectomy. *Arthritis Rheum* **34**, 1056–60.

Siffert RS (1982) Intraepiphvsial osteotomy for progressive tibia vara: case report and rationale of management. *J Pediatr Orthop* **2**, 81–5.

Skeith L, Jackson SC and Brooks J (2010) Assessing baseline joint hypermobility as a risk factor for arthropathy development in moderate and severe haemophilia. *Haemophilia* **16**, 698–700.

Skyhar MJ and Mubarak SJ (1987) Arthroscopic treatment of septic knees in children. *J Pediatr Orthop* **7**, 647–51.

Smillie IS (1957) Treatment of osteochondritis dissecans. *J Bone Joint Surg Br* **39**, 248–60.

Smith JB (1990) Osteochondritis dissecans of the trochlea of the femur. *Arthroscopy* **6**, 11–17.

Stanitski CL, Harvell JC and Fu FH (1989) Arthroscopy in acute septic knees. Management in pediatric patients. *Clin Orthop* **241,** 209–12.

Stewart JW, Matthew JB, Morganti V (2008) Large osteochondral fracutres of the lateral femoral condyle in the adolescent: outcome of bioabsorbable pin fixation. *J Bone Joint Surg Am* **90**, 1473–8.

Thomson NL (1987) Osteochondritis dissecans and osteochondral fragments managed by Herbert compression screw fixation. *Clin Orthop* **224**, 71–8.

Twyman RS, Desai K and Aichroth PM (1991) Osteochondritis dissecans of the knee: a long-term study. *J Bone Joint Surg Br* **73**, 461–4.

Vajnar J (2010) Imaging and biopsy hold the key to knee pain diagnosis. *JAAPA* **23**, 54–5.

Verma N, Valentino LA, Chawla A (2007) Arthroscopic synovectomy in haemophilia: indications, technique and results. *Haemophilia* **13**(Suppl 3), 38–44.

Weidel JD (1990) Arthroscopy of the knee in hemophilia. *Prog Clin Biol Res* **324**, 231–9.

Wilson JN (1967) A diagnostic sign in osteochondritis of the knee. *J Bone Joint Surg Am* **49**, 477–80.

Zywiel MG, McGrath MS, Seyler TM, *et al.* (2009) Osteonecrosis of the knee: a review of three disorders. *Orthop Clin North Am* **40**, 193–211.

Treatment of soft tissue injuries

Acute injury

Acute soft tissue injuries occur from direct (extrinsic) or indirect (intrinsic) trauma. Collision with another player, the ground or a fixed object will produce typical patterns of damage, although the precise extent of the injury may be difficult to ascertain initially. Indirect injuries from forced rotation and rapid stretch or deceleration may be hard to diagnose, although the site of discomfort is usually localized. A third category of injury is the 'overuse syndrome', where repetitive submaximal stresses exceed the resilience of structures comprising the joint.

Whenever ligament, tendon, muscle or bone are injured acutely, blood vessels are disrupted at the site of the tear or fracture. The resultant haemorrhage within the confined space produces a haematoma, from which spring the cells of regeneration or repair. Whether the deficiency is made good by scar or by a restitution of the normal tissue, the cellular response still progresses through the stages of inflammation, proliferation, remodelling and maturation. Excessive early movement and inappropriate loading may retard this process, as will the presence of gapping, inadequate nutrition and oxygenation, and infection.

■ Inflammation

The central and peripheral mediators of inflammation interact in a complex fashion, their concentrations being controlled by the activation of precursors, often through cascade reactions, and the subsequent recruitment of inhibitors and inactivating enzymes. The vasodilatory response is mediated by histamine, bradykinin, prostaglandin and other evanescent substances such as 5-hydroxytryptamine. Blood clot acts as an early scaffold, filling the gap in a ligament tear with coagulum which gradually builds up collagen type III, and later collagen type I as the long-term matrix (Woo and Buckwalter 1987). Chronic inflammatory tissue subsequently aggregates glycosaminoglycan, fibronectin and DNA, and these in turn delineate the early formation of the host tissue.

Proliferation

Differentiation of the cellular morphology progresses in parallel with the establishment of a definitive blood supply. Although water content remains elevated compared with normal tissue, there is a progressive change in the constituents of the tissue, including increased concentrations of type I collagen and extracellular matrix. The architecture of the healing tissue remains immature, as in callus formation at a fracture site, but a gradual reorientation of the constituent fibres occurs, particularly if subjected to controlled loading.

Remodelling and maturation

Over several months the collagen turnover rate returns to normal and the macroscopic shape of the healing tissue becomes better defined. The extracellular matrix is restored, although it may never return entirely to normal (Figure 10.1). A mature and efficient blood supply is established, allowing the return of gliding movement to ligament and tendon if scarring is broken down progressively. However, the regrowth of a competent nerve supply of afferent neurones is rarely achieved in full (Johansson *et al.* 1991), so that the repaired tissue may remain chronically susceptible to reinjury. This should be remembered when the patient is advised about a return to sport after ligament reconstruction, and emphasizes the importance of training other components of normal lower limb function.

Wasting of the type I muscle fibres, the so-called 'slow' fibres which are responsible for muscle tone, results from disuse and characterizes injuries to the knee where there is loss of joint movement or a lack of exercise owing to pain. Rupture of ligaments such as the anterior cruciate will also reduce the proprioceptive input (Barrett 1991; Corrigan *et al.* 1992) and the stimulus for muscle development. Occasionally, a primary abnormality of muscle is present, such as a myopathy or myositis ossificans, and wasting is also associated with conditions such as rheumatoid arthritis, haemophilic arthropathy and certain neurological disorders.

Type I muscle fibre

The type I or slow-twitch fibre is low in adenosine triphosphatase (ATPase) and glycolytic enzymes, and is dependent on aerobic metabolism. This reliance on oxidative metabolism is demonstrated histologically by an increase in mitochondrial enzymes, and the large number of capillaries that supply this muscle type. Although type I fibres are more resistant to fatigue, they atrophy rapidly if the knee is immobilized and are not well preserved by isometric contractions. The population of type I fibres within a muscle seems to be genetically determined and is probably little influenced by physical training.

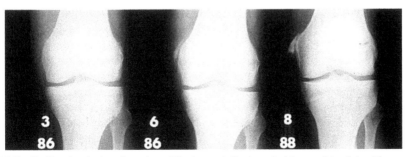

Figure 10.1 Ossification developing after a tear of the femoral attachment of the medial collateral ligament.

■ Type II muscle fibre

The type II or fast-twitch fibre is characterized by a high ATPase content and a greater degree of glycolytic enzymic activity than is seen in the type I fibre. Type II fibres have been subdivided into groups A, B, C and M (Gauthier 1986). The fast-twitch type IIA (fast/red myosin) fibres possess some oxidative capacity owing to the presence of mitochondria and myoglobin and are therefore more resistant to fatigue than the type IIB (fast/white myosin) fibres which are completely glycolytic (anaerobic). Type IIC are intermediate fibres comprising a mixture of types A and B, while a recently identified type IIM ('superfast') fibre contains a specific myosin.

Training by means of specific muscle exercises will produce variable improvement in strength and endurance. High-tension, low-frequency contractions stimulate hypertrophy, particularly of the type II fibres (Faulkner 1986), and the stimulus of stretch is also beneficial. Eccentric contraction (activation of the muscle while it is being lengthened by an opposing force greater than the force in the muscle) replicates the demand placed on muscle very effectively and is recognized to be a vital component of rehabilitation or training. The tension developed in eccentrically loaded muscle is greater than during isometric loading, and considerably greater than in concentric contraction. Hence muscle is frequently injured during peaks of eccentric contraction (Figure 10.2), usually failing in the region of the myotendinous junction. Conversely, metabolic efficiency is greatest with concentric and least with eccentric contraction.

Low-tension, repetitive exercise improves endurance, but when training is discontinued, the number of oxidative fibres regresses to the control value within weeks. Although isometric exercises may prevent the atrophy of type II fibres, particularly the type II B group, endurance training has no effect on cross-sectional size of muscle. Instead, it increases the number of capillaries per muscle fibre, and possibly the levels of oxidative enzymes. Conversely, resistive training using weights increases the size of muscle fibres and thereby their strength, but there is no increase in their oxidative capacity.

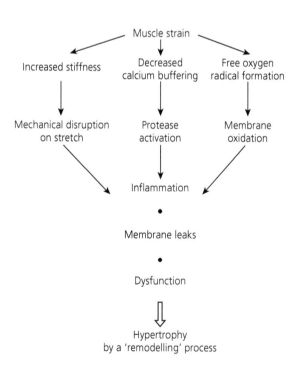

Figure 10.2 The pathophysiology of a muscle strain. Muscle stretching and microtears usually result from the rapid lengthening of activated muscles (eccentric contraction). Injury is proportional to the maximum tension generated and the extent of muscle fatigue.

Principles of therapy

■ The rule of 12s

- In the first *12 seconds* after injury the decision is made to stop a player from participating further. The assessment must be hurried but informed, and may involve the team coach, physiotherapist or doctor. Pain, laxity, swelling and deformity are judged as accurately as possible. Inability to weightbear and loss of movement are absolute contraindications to continuing with the sport.
- During the next *12 minutes* the player is reassessed off the field. Generally the decision to stop playing is consolidated and severe injuries should be protected with a temporary splint. Haemorrhage, whether revealed or concealed, is controlled with compression and cooling.
- Over the ensuing *12 hours* rest, ice, compression and elevation ('RICE') are time-honoured remedies. Fractures should be ruled out by radiographs, the injured knee or other part magnetic resonance (MR) scanned and the player referred to a surgeon if skeletal or soft tissue injuries merit this.

Cooling by indirect ice packs or a packet of frozen peas, a silicone gel bag, or cold water compresses limits the inflammatory response, principally by constricting the capillaries supplying the injured tissue. Use of Cryo Cuff will also ensure gentle compression. Alternatively, pressure may be applied evenly over the knee by Tubigrip or bandaging. Rest and elevation are ensured by instructing the athlete to keep the leg with 'toes above your nose', since this makes up for the lack of muscle pump in the resting limb. Splintage with a backshell canvas support or light brace will relieve pain when abnormal laxity is present, and anti-inflammatory analgesics are prescribed. Crutches may be required to allow mobility and to reduce symptoms.

The first *12 days* after the injury are spent controlling the inflammation further and preserving the range of movement without incurring additional damage. With haematoma and swelling limited, the joint should be reassessed. Many injuries occur on a Saturday and therefore this examination is carried out on a Sunday or a Monday. Pain is inhibitory and Hilton's law of rest and pain (Hilton 1863) is still valid, requiring the patient to remain at rest at least over the weekend. The therapist gains further insight into the severity of the injury over these 12 days, and referral for a surgical opinion is best achieved during this time.

The *12-week* phase concentrates on regaining mobility, power and normal function. The speed of recovery will vary according to the injury (Durand *et al.* 1993) and the rapport established between the patient and physiotherapist. Important characteristics of the patient are motivation, expectations, general fitness and physique. Hypermobility or lack of flexibility should be noted, together with alignment of the leg and foot posture. Training and return to sport is usually achieved even if surgical intervention has been necessary.

Following severe injuries, particularly cruciate ligament disruption and displaced fractures, a *12-month* rehabilitation period is usual before sport can be continued. Loss of agility, coordination and confidence takes time to recover, even if the range of movement and muscle bulk have been restored more rapidly. The complex interplay between psyche and motor skills will be understood by the experienced coach and therapist. Communication, reassurance and altered training patterns help towards full rehabilitation.

In summary, the aims of therapy are to:

- Preserve strength without undue stress to the injured part
- Maintain or restore the normal range of motion
- Preserve patellar mobility
- Regain proprioception and agility

- Recover endurance and confidence
- Return to full functional activity.

Specific elements in physiotherapy have become better defined in the last few years, particularly the postoperative regimen following anterior cruciate ligament reconstruction (Box 10.1). Based on the premise that a relatively rapid return to full movement and normal gait is beneficial, this 'accelerated rehabilitation' (Shelbourne and Nitz 1990) was conceived

---

Box 10.1 Monitoring progress after anterior cruciate ligament reconstruction

As swelling decreases, movement should increase; the Cryo Cuff hastens this phase

Weightbearing and 'closed kinetic chain' exercises return the limb to normal use:

- 0–4 weeks – partial weightbearing with 10–90° flexion arc
- 4–16 weeks – increase to full weightbearing and 0–135° of flexion

Normal gait should be achieved by 4–6 weeks

The appearance of the scar offers a monitor of the degree of graft maturation

The KT-1000 arthrometer (Figure 10.3) allows the assessment of residual laxity at 6–18 months postoperatively (ideally 5 mm or less compared to the normal knee)

A graduated return to sport is permitted over 6–18 months postoperatively in the expectation that 90 per cent of patients will achieve this

---

Figure 10.3a,b The KT-1000 arthrometer.

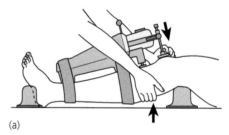

(a)

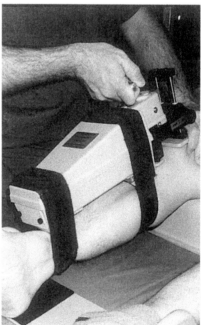

(b)

in response to the observation that 'non-compliant' patients made a more rapid and complete recovery than those who followed the suggested protocol of a guarded and delayed return of movement and power. It was also noted that complications such as stiffness and anterior knee pain were uncommon in those who recovered rapidly. However, it is equally possible that those who progressed quickly were a self-selected group where motivation, problem-free surgery and muscle recovery combined to produce a good result. Unless prospective trials reveal the long-term results to be convincingly better, accelerated physiotherapy cannot be supported unconditionally. Therefore, the following represents a basic rehabilitation programme:

A varying amount of 'open kinetic chain' activity is now permitted with the judicious use of weights. Emphasis is placed upon rebalancing other muscle groups acting across the spine, hip and hindfoot. The use of a fixed bicycle will increase strength and endurance safely. Exercises to improve balance, coordination and proprioception are vital in the later stages of recovery, before sports-specific drills, full training and competitive sport are permitted.

▨ Pain

The relief of pain in the immediate post-injury or postoperative period can be achieved by oral non-steroidal anti-inflammatory medication, epidural or regional anaesthesia, opiate analgesia and by continuous passive motion (CPM) (Noyes *et al.* 1987; Paulos *et al.* 1991). If a CPM machine is used when there is potential anterolateral laxity, anterior translation of the proximal tibia should be minimized by avoiding the use of a support behind the upper calf (Drez *et al.* 1991). Transcutaneous electrical nerve stimulation (TENS) and cooling the joint with a Cryo Cuff (Aircast) will also give temporary pain relief. Since the majority of ligament, chondral and meniscal procedures are carried out as daycase surgery, the patient has to be capable of walking with crutches and under no risk on returning home. This means that careful preoperative preparation should be ensured, the patient being fully briefed about the possible obstacles to rapid recovery.

▨ Strength

Muscle strength is maintained by active-assisted, range of movement exercises initially, which may be all that a painful lesion will permit. Co-contraction of the extensor and flexor muscle groups is encouraged as a means of stabilizing the joint where pathological laxity is present, or as a means of protecting a graft reconstruction of a ligament. Each therapist will develop an individualistic approach to the stages of rehabilitation, but it is now widely recognized that supervised movement should be allowed immediately. Strength is later developed by bringing in eccentric as well as concentric muscle contraction.

Quadriceps 'setting' can be achieved with both isometric and isotonic exercises, agonists and antagonists being encouraged to work together. In the early stages, taping or strapping (Figure 10.4) will lessen pain by improving patellar tracking (McConnell 1986) or knee stability. 'Inner range' quadriceps drill, emphasizing vastus medialis power, is achieved by combining knee extension with adduction of the externally rotated leg. Retropatellar pain is controlled by confining the early stages of therapy to isometric contraction of vastus medialis with the knee flexed at varying angles and the thigh rotated externally. A graduated approach to regaining power is particularly important in patellar pain syndromes where confidence must be restored if lasting relief of pain is to be achieved.

Eccentric contraction stimulates muscle hypertrophy, essential in sports requiring sudden deceleration such as jumping, downhill 'fell' running and cycling. Plyometrics encourages

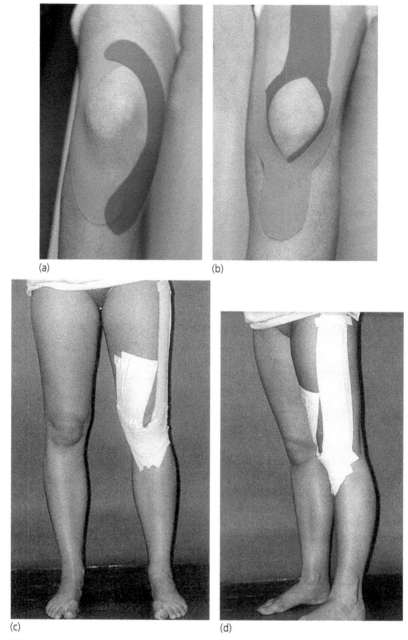

(a)   (b)

(c)   (d)

Figure 10.4 Supportive taping (a,b) or strapping (c,d).

eccentric power and control, but may not be appropriate for bulky athletes engaged in power sports. This decision lies with the physiotherapist and emphasizes the importance of tailoring exercises to the physique and sporting demands of the patient.

Electrically induced co-contraction of the thigh muscles (Wigerstad-Lossing *et al.* 1988; Snyder-Meckler *et al.* 1991) has yet to find a significant role in rehabilitation, and as a general principle conscious effort by the patient is preferable. Nevertheless, if an impasse is reached in the early stages of an exercise programme, both electrical stimulation and CPM may have a limited role to play. Manipulation under anaesthesia may also regain motion in the later stages of recovery if stiffness and a block to extension or flexion become established. The changing concepts in rehabilitation after anterior cruciate reconstruction have been described by Reid (1993). There has been a move away from unloaded, knee extension work. These 'open kinetic chain' exercises were conducted with the foot in a free (non-stationary) position and placed considerable anterior tibial translational and patellofemoral forces through the knee (Grood *et al.* 1984). Closed kinetic chain exercises, with the foot fixed, are therefore preferred as they promote maximal joint stability and co-contraction of the quadriceps and hamstring groups (Palmitier *et al.* 1991). It is also preferable to increase the time spent on these exercises rather than emphasizing progressive loading. Leg presses are preferred to standard knee extension drill against resistance (Grood *et al.* 1984) and the dangers of single episodes of excessive loading or cyclical shearing stress guarded against (Reid 1993).

Closed chain exercises are a more natural means of training and markedly improve endurance. Stair climbing, stationary bicycling, the rowing machine and jogging offer individual patients a welcome relief from repeated single exercises and encourage a sense of improvement. Step-ups, both forwards and sideways, with eyes open and then closed, provide a simple means of monitoring the return of precision activity (Macnicol 1992) and agility can be improved with the use of a wobble board or small trampoline. Initially the patient concentrates on simple balance, but later in the programme a second activity, such as catching and throwing a ball, is introduced, while the patient stands on the injured leg.

Compression bandaging is permissible if this gives confidence and a greater sense of knee control. When discomfort and insecurity are marked, exercises in a warm swimming pool are confidence-boosting and reduce loading and torque stress through the knee. General fitness should be developed, especially power in the opposite leg, upper body strength and cardiorespiratory reserve.

Flexibility

Alongside muscle strengthening should be a programme of stretching tight structures such as the iliotibial band, the hamstrings and the calf. The tensor fasciae latae muscle (Figure 10.5) is often adaptively shortened, and distal contracture of the iliotibial band is reversed by medial patellar translocation with the patient in a side-lying position. Stretching exercises should also be taught routinely as part of a 'warm-up' and a 'warm-down'. Once again, closed and monitored open chain exercises and a progressive return to weightbearing are recognized as important components of restoring flexibility, taken in conjunction with the minimal use of external splint or brace support.

Warm-up is known to reduce muscle viscosity, manifest by both improved contraction and greater elasticity. Stretching should be conducted after a warm-up, slowly and regularly over time. This will gradually ease muscle tightness and will enhance conditioning. Musculotendinous tears are more common in the two joint units (hamstrings, rectus femoris and gastrocnemius), so particular attention should be paid to their stretching, both after warm-up and during cool-down. In this way soft tissue injuries should be minimized (Ekstrand and Gillquist 1982; Garrett *et al.* 1984).

Gait

Re-education will involve a change in gait pattern which has developed in response to a chronic instability. Adaptation following ligament injury was investigated by Perry *et al.* (1980) when they reviewed the intended effects of pes anserinus transfer, using gait analysis and electromyography. Stride length, single limb support time and walking speed were uniformly reduced, and the effects of pesplasty were not considered to be significantly therapeutic.

A 'quadriceps-avoidance' gait was observed by Berchuck *et al.* (1991) in patients with an absent anterior cruciate ligament. The magnitude of flexion was appreciably reduced during walking or jogging, thus preventing anterior translation of the proximal tibia by the relatively unopposed effect of quadriceps contraction. Climbing stairs was unaffected by this alteration and 25 per cent of their patients did not adopt a quadriceps-avoidance gait. The combination of anterior cruciate deficiency and varus alignment leads to an abnormally high moment of adduction with medial shift of loading through the joint (Noyes *et al.* 1992), Quadriceps inhibition was also noted, with a reduction of extensor muscle force and enhanced hamstring muscle activity in approximately half of the group under study. Degenerative changes are more likely, therefore, when laxity is combined with varus deformity.

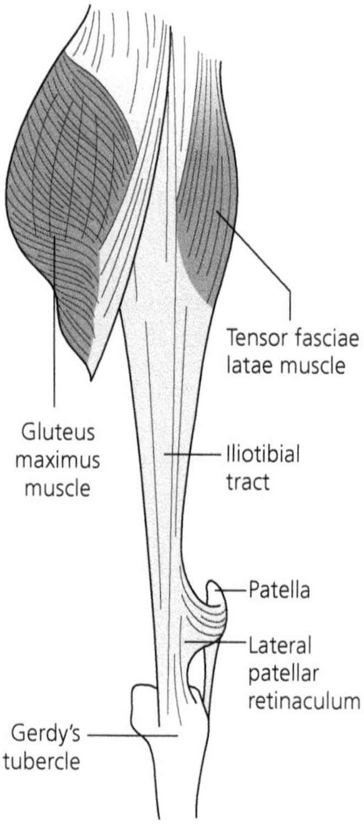

◼ Isokinetics

Over the past 40 years isokinetic devices have been developed into complex machines such as the Biodex, Cybex and KinCom. The principle behind isokinetic exercise is that an accommodating resistance should be applied to a limb moving at a fixed speed or angular velocity. Maximal or submaximal load can therefore be ensured at all angles in the range of movement.

Muscle function can be quantified by providing data on peak torque, average torque, work expended and power developed.

Figure 10.5 The tensor fasciae latae (and gluteus maximus) inserts into the tibia and also into the patella and the lateral femoral condyle.

Labels on figure: Tensor fasciae latae muscle; Iliotibial tract; Gluteus maximus muscle; Patella; Lateral patellar retinaculum; Gerdy's tubercle

Muscle contraction can be divided into the concentric and eccentric phases (Figure 10.6) with a high degree of retest reliability. The objective measurements allow comparison between the normal and abnormal limb after injury, and offer the physiotherapist both the means of monitoring recovery and of providing a structured and progressive programme of resisted exercises. Hence the patient can be closely supervised after injury or reconstruction of the anterior cruciate ligament, as a common example, and an optimum ratio between quadriceps and hamstring power is established. Hamstring strength of some 70 per cent of quadriceps strength may be increased by hamstring drill if residual anterolateral knee laxity requires

Figure 10.6 A KinCom read-out, comparing the quadriceps power of the normal left leg and the injured right leg.

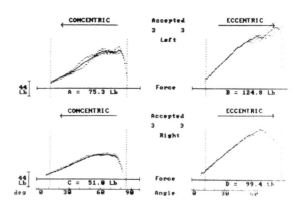

greater dynamic control. Accessories for each machine also allow closed kinetic chain exercises as a means of enhancing rehabilitation. The aim is to restore power in the injured leg to within 10 per cent of the normal side.

Knee bracing

The value of knee braces is unproven, and their use prophylactically, as has been suggested for children in certain sports, is unwarranted (Grace *et al.* 1988). Much depends on the compliance of the patient and the brace may offer little more than an improvement in proprioception (Cook *et al.* 1989). Stark (1850) is reported to have made the first knee brace, describing, in an Edinburgh journal, the use of a steel spring for two patients. The success of this treatment was unclear. The problems inherent in bracing include:

- Restrictive of flexion and rapid movement
- Friction over points of contact
- Compression and the production of localized oedema
- Translation down the leg.

Migration of the orthosis remains a significant problem and can only be minimized by custom-made braces. Beck *et al.* (1986) studied seven brands of functional knee braces and found that anterior tibial translation could not be prevented when peak forces were applied to a level typical of strenuous sport. Control of rotational forces is enhanced, but this effect is greater at 60° than at 30° of flexion (Wojtys *et al.* 1987), and therefore the derotational effect on the extended, weightbearing joint is probably minimal.

Modern braces (Figure 10.7) impede activity less, in contrast to earlier concerns about their constraints on normal knee motion (Wright and Fetzer 2007; Thijs *et al.* 2010). Approximately

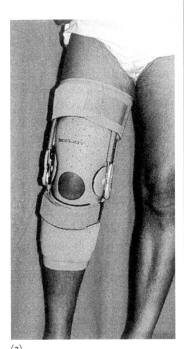 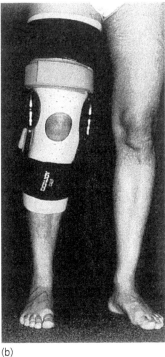

(a)   (b)

Figure 10.7 A Don Joy brace designed to support the knee after anterior cruciate ligament reconstruction (a) and to control posterior cruciate chronic laxity (b).

one-half of anterior cruciate-deficient knees are improved by bracing, judged by the protection against episodes of giving way, swelling and pain. Combined ligament injuries may also be supported effectively in the early stages of recuperation. Cawley *et al.* (1991) reviewed a large number of papers dealing with the previous use of braces, noting that at least 25 commercial braces were available at that time. Objective assessment and scientifically convincing data were rare, but the overall impression gained then, and currently, is that properly applied bracing is of value both as a means of improving proprioception and by a stabilizing effect (Figure 10.8).

Figure 10.8 Therapeutic effects of bracing.

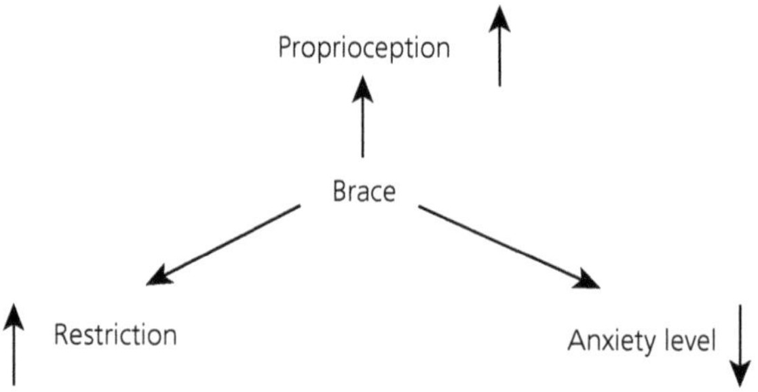

Ultrasound

Ultrasound produces a local increase in tissue temperature and may alter the biochemical structure of collagen. This improves flexibility and the treatment is therefore valuable in the later stages of management of soft tissue trauma, such as sprains and strains, tendonitis, bursitis and joint stiffness. A combination of ultrasound and electrical muscle stimulation may speed recovery after a limb has been immobilized, but muscle re-education still depends largely on voluntary effort. There are also legitimate concerns about the possibly injurious effect of ultrasound on the skeletal growth plate.

Interferential therapy

Deeper, and more directed, electrical therapy can be provided by the 'crossfire' effect of two currents directed at right angles to each other. This is thought to inhibit the parasympathetic system if high frequencies (over 4000 Hz) are used. At lower frequencies the muscle may be stimulated to contract, and this is not necessarily of value. Both interferential therapy and ultrasound have a part to play, but must not be used by unskilled attendants.

Massage and manipulation

The use of massage is controversial and it may often be abused. Frictional massage, where the fingertips apply firm pressure across the line of a muscle or tendon, may break down adhesions and can be combined with stretching exercises. Vibratory massage may also be beneficial, if only to relieve symptoms; but deep and firm massage can be injurious to inflamed or recovering muscles. In the early stages of the rehabilitation after injury, therefore, massage must be used with care.

Manipulation of a stiffened knee joint is sometimes justified and may restore a better range of movement if adhesions are broken down. However, other causes of restricted movement should be ruled out since forced manipulation may damage a meniscus, chondral surface or other structure within the knee. Fracture and displacement of the growth plate have also been reported. Complete relaxation of the patient is necessary and therefore general anaesthesia is usually indicated. The technique is not recommended in the athlete and great care must be taken to avoid further injury.

Heat

Heat in the form of short-wave diathermy, which allows a deeper permeation of the rays, is occasionally recommended when a muscle is recovering from injury. However, radiant heat (hot water bottles, heat lamps or liniments) and short-wave diathermy are not appropriate in the early stages after an injury as they may increase the hyperaemic response. It is far better to rely on rest and cooling of the tissues initially.

When scar tissue has formed, there may be a place for increasing tissue temperature, improving blood flow and the possibility of scar breakdown. Heat also has a sedative and analgesic effect, which may allow greater muscle stretching to reduce spasm.

Analgesic therapy

Apart from the use of anti-inflammatory analgesics with their known effect on the inflammatory process (Figure 10.9), transcutaneous electrical stimulation can also reduce the perception of pain. The small nerve fibres conducting pain impulses are thought to be blocked at the level of the spinal cord and there may be an increased release of pain-inhibiting substances, such as endorphins and encephalins.

The lessening in pain experienced by the patient after injury will permit an earlier return to exercise and joint movement, but there is always the risk that further damage may be incurred. The same criticism can be levelled at the use of ice or various other forms of cryotherapy,

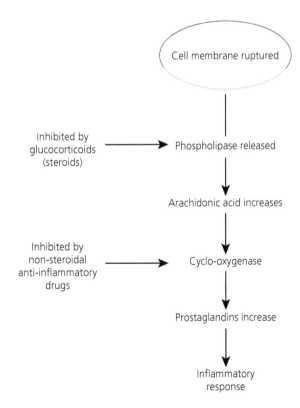

Figure 10.9 Mode of action of anti-inflammatory drugs.

including ethyl chloride 'cold' spray, which may deaden the sensitivity of nerves but at the same time make the knee more vulnerable to further injury.

Platelet-rich plasma

Platelet-rich plasma (PRP) therapy is claimed to improve the process of tissue repair through the local delivery of autologous bioactive agents. Injections of this natural derivative are considered to influence critical reactions such as inflammation, angiogenesis and extracellular matrix synthesis. However, there is no convincing level 1 evidence in favour of PRP (Redler *et al.* 2011). The early studies were impressive (Sánchez *et al.* 2007), but well-performed randomized controlled trials in the Netherlands (de Vos *et al.* 2010) and Sweden (Schepull *et al.* 2011) show that it is at best of no use, and possibly harmful.

Pathological conditions affecting muscle

◼ Partial tear or complete rupture of muscle

Partial tear or complete rupture of the belly or musculotendinous region of a muscle is not uncommon and may affect the quadriceps, hamstring, adductor or calf muscle groups. Magnetic resonance scanning offers a clear image of the extent of the injury. The formation of an interstitial haematoma, or a more extensive intramuscular bleed, will obviously restrict the function of that muscle and produce pain. Indirectly, the knee is thus involved. Rarely, muscle may also be avulsed from its point of attachment in bone, and occasionally it should therefore be reattached, particularly significant apophyseal avulsions at the anterior inferior iliac spine and the ischial tuberosity in skeletally immature patients. Suturing a muscle rupture is ineffective and will not benefit the patient.

Treatment should be directed at reducing the formation of scar by rest and local cooling. Later, when the scar has become mature, it can be gently stretched and muscle function returned to a near-normal level.

◼ Contracture of muscle

Contracture occurs when the muscle is allowed to shorten, and hence works from a reduced resting length. Contracture is common after disuse or inflammatory conditions involving joints, and will also occur if there is a muscle imbalance, as is seen in certain neuromuscular abnormalities. With the passage of time, the contracture tends to worsen and although physiotherapy may partially correct the shortened length, a residual deficit is usually present.

◼ Compartment syndrome

This may be either acute or chronic. In the former, trauma produces an increased pressure within the fascial compartment surrounding muscle, part of the haemorrhage commonly occurring as a result of a fracture. Tissue pressure increases as a result of arterial haemorrhage, venostasis and the resultant oedema. Intravascular pressure is rapidly exceeded and muscle and related segments of nerve become ischaemic (Crist *et al.* 2010).

In the chronic form, repetitive activity produces pressure, inflammation and possibly a metabolic acidosis in muscle. This in turn results in swelling. If the muscle is not free to expand, pressure rises and will impair the blood supply to the muscle with increasing pain as metabolites build up within the muscle. Although symptoms are quickly relieved by rest, they may prove very limiting. An adhesive tendonitis may be difficult to differentiate from chronic muscle compartment syndrome (Frink *et al.* 2010).

Myositis ossificans

Myositis ossificans describes a pathological process whereby calcification takes place, leading eventually to mature bone formation within the damaged area of a ruptured or partially torn muscle. Calcium deposits within the haematoma progress to bone, a pathological alteration that may be increased by a rapid resumption of activity. In particular, the stretching of muscle may stimulate the ossification process and lead to increasing disability (Aronen *et al.* 2006).

The phenomenon is one of the presentations of heterotopic ossification and has been divided into localized, circumscripta and progressiva forms. Two aetiological processes have been advanced. The first suggests that haemorrhage triggers the formation of heterotopic bone in proximity to damaged muscle and its associated periosteum and bone. Muscle fibre necrosis induces an invasion of macrophages which in turn stimulates the release of osteogenic growth factors such as platelet-derived growth factor, tumour necrosis factor and interleukin 1. The second hypothesis implicates muscle spasticity which leads to the generation of free oxygen radicals. These trigger the differentiation of mesenchymal stem cells into osteoblasts, at the expense of fibroblasts.

Excision of 'mature' ossified deposits is occasionally advocated, but there is a tendency for the myositis ossificans to recur. Although the process may be affected by certain drugs, the principal treatment of the condition is the restriction of its occurrence by using a graduated and careful programme of convalescence (Chidel *et al.* 2001).

Occasionally muscle may be infected by ill-advised injections, or cysts and fibrocytic nodules may form within the thigh. The principal method of treatment is prevention, but if these do occur, medical attention is essential and a surgical drainage or excisional procedure may be required.

Muscular dystrophy

Muscular dystrophy may be a cause for muscle wasting, and various neurological and muscular conditions should always by considered in a patient whose recovery appears abnormal, or if wasting of groups of muscles become progressive.

Reflex sympathetic dystrophy (complex regional pain syndrome)

Reflex sympathetic dystrophy is now termed complex regional pain syndrome (CRPS), type I being reflex sympathetic dystrophy, and type II replacing 'causalgia', where additional peripheral nerve injury is present (see also Chapter 4). The condition has also been known as algodystrophy or Sudeck's atrophy. Injury or surgery are precipitants and it is characterized by a burning pain, often widespread around the knee, which persists at night. Numbness, stiffness, mechanical symptoms and swelling may occur in varying degrees to confuse the clinical picture (Tietjens 1986). Skin changes include discolouration, sweating, change in temperature and sensory alteration. The vasomotor changes involve deeper tissues so that stiffness and radiographic rarefaction of bone occur (Seale 1989).

Knee stiffness and weakness initially result from the pain produced during muscle action and joint movement, but eventually oedema and fibrosis lead to a more morbid process. The nociceptive nerve fibres contain substance P, which can be mapped by immunohistochemistry (Wotjys *et al.* 1990), while an inflammatory process is confirmed by increased uptake on radioisotope bone scanning, especially during the first six months of the condition. The anterior knee pain syndromes may also be associated with a positive scan and these sympathetically-mediated symptoms are best dealt with non-surgically. Thermography (Figure 9.5, p. 194) in the vasodilatory, acute stage of the condition confirms an increase in temperature of 2–3 °C and may be used to monitor the response to treatment (Rothschild 1990).

Complex regional pain syndrome (reflex sympathetic dystrophy) is conventionally divided into an acute, early phase characterized by pain, then by a dystrophic phase where stiffness and sympathetic over-activity are obvious, and a final, often intractable stage. Stiffness may become established and is complicated by the secondary changes of muscle wasting and arthrofibrosis. In some patients a gradual improvement occurs with time, with a slow return to normal activity. In others, the joint becomes permanently restricted and painful, compounded by anxiety or depression.

Treatment of the dystrophy will be more successful if it is recognized early. Inpatient physiotherapy, non-steroidal anti-inflammatory analgesia and sometimes counselling are important components in preventing the progression of the stages towards irreversible stiffness. Intervention and forcible manipulation are contraindicated but arthroscopic irrigation and sympathetic blockade by pharmacological agents should be considered if an extensive exercise programme fails. Continuous epidural anaesthesia using an indwelling catheter for 4 days was described by Cooper *et al.* (1989), who were then able to establish CPM. This form of management relieves the symptoms in approximately two-thirds of patients although its timing may be critical. Regional intravenous guanethidine blocks are also effective (Bonelli *et al.* 1983).

Conclusion

Throughout this book emphasis has been placed upon the importance of a practical approach to pathological conditions and injuries of the knee, basing this on anatomical knowledge and an appreciation of the interrelationship between muscle, ligament and joint function. When a soft tissue injury or fracture occurs there is a concomitant loss of movement and of muscle power during the stages of healing. Treatment should be directed towards a return of normal movement and muscle strength, but should not hasten events to the extent that an effusion recurs or ligament laxity is promoted. Obstructive lesions within the knee should be recognized early, by careful clinical examination and appropriate investigations, and removed before the articulating surfaces of the knee are damaged. Abnormal laxity and angulatory deformity similarly imperil the knee and may require surgical intervention to preserve function.

The experienced coach, physiotherapist or doctor will have learnt that recovery from injury also depends on the general fitness and motivation of the athlete or patient. Success attends the two-way process when the patient respects the skills and recommendations of the therapist, and where the therapist in turn trusts to the efforts of his or her charge.

References

Aronen JG, Garrick JG, Chronister RD, *et al.* (2006) Quadriceps contusions: clinical results of immediate immobilization in 120 degrees of knee flexion. *Clin J Sport Med* **16**, 383–7.

Barrett DS (1991) Proprioception and function after anterior cruciate reconstruction. *J Bone Joint Surg Br* **73**, 833–7.

Beck C, Drez D, Young J, *et al.* (1986) Instrumental testing of functional knee braces. *Am J Sports Med* **14**, 253–5.

Berchuck M, Andriacchi TP and Bach BR (1991) Gait adaptations by patients who have a deficient anterior cruciate ligament. *J Bone Joint Surg Am* **73**, 871–7.

Bonelli S, Conoscente F, Morilia A, *et al.* (1983) Regional intravenous guanethidine vs stellate ganglion block in reflex sympathetic dystrophies: a randomised trial. *Pain* **16**, 297–307.

Cawley PW, France P and Paulos LE (1991) The current state of functional knee bracing research. *Am J Sports Med* **19**, 226–33.

Chidel MA, Suh JH and Matejczyk MB (2001) Radiation prophylaxis for heterotopic ossification of the knee. *J Arthroplasty* **16,** 1–6.

Cook FF, Tibone JE and Redfern FC (1989) A dynamic analysis of a functional brace for anterior cruciate insufficiency. *Am J Sports Med* **17**, 519–24.

Cooper DE, De Lee JC and Ramamurthy S (1989) Reflex sympathetic dystrophy of the knee. Treatment using continuous epidural anaesthesia. *J Bone Joint Surg Br* **71**, 365–9.

Corrigan JP, Cashman WF and Brady MP (1992) Proprioception in the cruciate deficient knee. *J Bone Joint Surg Br* **74**, 247–50.

Crist BD, Della Rocca GJ and Stannard JP (2010) Compartment syndrome: surgical management techniques associated with tibial plateau fractures. *J Knee Surg* **23**, 3–7.

de Vos RJ, Weir A, van Schie HT, *et al.* (2010) Platelet-rich plasma injection for chronic Achilles tendinopathy: a randomized controlled trial. JAMA **303**, 144–9.

Drez D, Paine RM, Neuschwander DC and Young JC (1991) *In vivo* measurement of anterior tibial translation using continuous passive motion devices. *Am J Sport Med* **19**, 381–3.

Durand A, Richards CL, Malouin F and Bravo G (1993) Motor recovery after arthroscopic partial meniscectomy. *J Bone Joint Surg Am* **75**, 202–14.

Ekstrand J and Gillquist J (1982) The frequency of muscle tightness and injuries in soccer players. *Am J Sports Med* **10**, 75–8.

Faulkner JA (1986) New perspectives in training for maximum performance. *J Am Med Assoc* **205**, 741–6.

Frink M, Hildebrand F, Krettek C, *et al.* (2010) Compartment syndrome of the lower leg and foot. *Clin Orthop Relat Res* **468**, 940–50.

Garrett WE Jr, Califf JC and Bassett FH (1984) Histochemical correlates of hamstring injuries. *Am J Sports Med* **12**, 98–103.

Gauthier GF (1986) Skeletal muscle fiber types. In: Engel AG and Banker BQ (eds) *Myology*, vol. 1. New York, NY: McGraw-Hill, pp. 255–84.

Grace TG, Skipper BJ, Newberry JC, *et al.* (1988) Prophylactic knee braces and injury to the lower extremity. *J Bone Joint Surg Am* **70**, 422–7.

Grood ES, Suntag J, Noyes FR and Butler Dl. (1984) Biomechanics of the knee extension exercise. Effect of cutting the anterior cruciate ligament. *J Bone Joint Surg Am* **66**, 725–34.

Hilton J (1863) *The Influence of Mechanical and Physiological Rest.* London: Bell and Daldy.

Johansson H, Sjolander P and Sojka P (1991) A sensory role for the cruciate ligaments. *Clin Orthop* **268**, 161–78.

McConnell J (1986) The management of chondromalacia patellae: a long-term solution. *Aust J Physiother* **32**, 215–24.

Macnicol MF (1992) The conservative management of the anterior cruciate ligament-deficient knee. In: Aichroth PM and Dilworth Cannon W (eds) *Knee Surgery: Current Practice.* London: Martin Dunitz, pp. 217–21.

Noyes FR, Mangine RE and Barber S (1987) Early knee motion after open and arthroscopic anterior cruciate ligament reconstruction. *Am J Sports Med* **15**, 149–60.

Noyes FR, Schipplein OD, Andriacchi TP, *et al.* (1992) The anterior cruciate ligament-deficient knee with varus alignment. An analysis of gait adaptations and dynamic joint loadings. *Am J Sports Med* **20**(6), 707–16.

Palmitier RA, Kai-Nan A, Scott SG and Chao EYS (1991) Kinetic chain exercise in knee rehabilitation. *Sports Med* **II**, 404–13.

Paulos LE, Wnorowski DC and Beck CL (1991) Rehabilitation following knee surgery. *Sports Med* **II**, 257–75.

Perry J, Fox JM and Boitano MA (1980) Functional evaluation of the pes anserinus transfer by electromyography and gait analysis. *J Bone Joint Surg Am* **62**, 973–80.

Redler LH, Thompson SA, Hsu SH, *et al.* (2011) Platelet-rich plasma therapy: a systematic literature review and evidence for clinical use. *Phys Sportsmed* **39**, 42–51.

Reid DC (1993) Current concepts in rehabilitation of the anterior cruciate deficient knee. *Curr Orthop* **7**, 101–5.

Rothschild B (1990) Reflex sympathetic dystrophy. *Arthritis Care Res* **3**, 144–53.

Sánchez M, Anitua E, Azofra J, *et al.* (2007) Comparison of surgically repaired Achilles tendon tears using platelet-rich fibrin matrices. *Am J Sports Med* **35**, 245–51.

Schepull T, Kvist J, Norrman H, *et al.* (2011) Autologous platelets have no effect on the healing of human achilles tendon ruptures: a randomized single-blind study. *Am J Sports Med* **39**, 38–47.

Seale K (1989) Reflex sympathetic dystrophy of the lower extremity. *Clin Orthop* **243**, 80–5.

Shelbourne KD and Nitz P (1990) Accelerated rehabilitation after anterior cruciate ligament reconstruction. *Am J Sports Med* **80**, 292–9.

Snyder-Meckler L, Ladin Z, Shepsis AA and Young JC (1991) Electrical stimulation of the thigh muscles after reconstruction of the anterior cruciate ligament. *J Bone Joint Surg Am* **73**, 1025–36.

Stark J (1850) Two cases of rupture of the crucial ligaments of the knee joint. *Edinb Med Surg* **74**, 267–71.

Thijs Y, Vingerhoets G, Pattyn E, *et al.* (2010) Does bracing influence brain activity during knee movement: an MRI study. *Knee Surg Sports Traumatol Arthrosc* **18**, 1145–9.

Tietjens B (1986) Reflex sympathetic dystrophy of the knee. *Clin Orthop* **209**, 234–43.

Wigerstad-Lossing I, Grimby G, Johsson T, *et al.* (1988) Effects of electrical muscle stimulation combined with voluntary contractions after knee ligament surgery. *Med Sci Sports Exerc* **20**, 93–8.

Wojtys EM, Goldstein SA, Redfern M, *et al.* (1987) A biomechanical evaluation of the Lenox Hill knee brace. *Clin Orthop* **220**, 179–84.

Woo SLY and Buckwalter JA (eds) (1987) *Injury and Repair of the Musculoskeletal Soft Tissues.* Rosemont, IL: American Academy of Orthopaedic Surgeons, pp. 114–17.

Wotjys EM, Beaman DR, Glover RA, *et al.* (1990) Innervation of the human knee joint by substance-P fibres. *Arthroscopy* **6**, 254–63.

Wright RW and Fetzer GB (2007). Bracing after ACL reconstruction: a systematic review. *Clin Orthop Relat Res* **455**, 162–8.

Appendix I   Stages in recovery after injury

1	Reduce inflammation	Compression
		Cooling
		Anti-inflammatory agent
2	Maintain movement	Active assisted exercise
		Joint and muscle massage
		Stretching
3	Increase power*	Isometric exercise through a pain-free range
		Co-contraction of quadriceps and hamstrings
		Resisted exercise (antigravity, Theraband, springs, weights)
		Closed chain activity
4	Regain fitness	Graded strengthening (closed and open chain)
		Cardiovascular work (hydrotherapy, jogging, arm ergometer)
		Progression of sport-specific skills

*Monitor the knee by avoiding the production of effusion and pain.

Appendix II
Assessment rating scales

TEGNER ACTIVITY SCALE

10 Competitive sports
   Soccer – national or international level
 9 Competitive sports
   Soccer – lower divisions
   Ice hockey
   Wrestling
   Gymnastics
 8 Competitive sports
   Bandy
   Squash or badminton
   Athletics (jumping, etc)
   Downhill skiing
 7 Competitive sports
   Tennis
   Athletics (running)
   Motocross or speedway
   Handball or basketball
   Recreational sports
   Soccer
   Bandy or ice hockey
   Squash
   Athletics (jumping)
   Cross-country track finding (orienteering)
       both recreational and competitive
 6 Recreational sports
   Tennis or badminton
   Handball or basketball
   Downhill skiing
   Jogging, at least 5 times weekly
 5 Work
   Heavy labour (e.g. construction, forestry)
   Competitive sports
   Cycling
   Cross-country skiing
   Recreational sports
   Jogging on uneven ground at least twice weekly
 4 Work
   Moderately heavy work (e.g. truck driving, scrubbing floors)
   Recreational sports
   Cycling
   Cross-country skiing
   Jogging on even ground at least twice weekly

3 Work
    Light work (e.g. nursing)
    Competitive and recreational sports
    Swimming
    Walking in rough forest terrain
2 Work
    Light work
    Walking on uneven ground
1 Work
    Sedentary work
    Walking on even ground
0 Sick leave or disability pension because of knee problems

LYSHOLM KNEE SCORES

Limp	
None	5
Slight or periodic	3
Severe and constant	0

Support	
None	5
Stick or crutch needed	2
Weight bearing impossible	0

Locking	
None	15
Catching sensation, but no locking	10
Locking occasionally	6
Locking frequently	2
Locked joint at examination	0

Instability	
Never	25
Rarely during athletic activities	20
Frequently during athletic activities	15
Occasionally during daily activities	10
Often during daily activities	5
Every step	0

Pain	
None	25
Inconstant and slight during strenuous activities	20
Marked during or after walking more than 2 km	10
Marked during or after walking less than 2 km	5
Constant	0

Swelling	
None	10
After strenuous activities	6
After ordinary activities	3
Constant	0

Stairs

No problem	10
Slight problem	6
One step at a time	3
Impossible	0

Squatting

No problem	5
Slight problem	4
Not beyond 90° of flexion of the knee	2
Impossible	0

CINCINNATI KNEE RATING SYSTEM

Symptom rating scale
Normal knee

Strenuous work/sports

Jumping	
Hard pivoting	10

Moderate work/sports

Running, turning, twisting	
Symptoms with strenuous work/sports	8

Light work/sports

No running, twisting jumping	
Symptoms with moderate work/sports	6

Daily living activities

Symptoms with light work/sports	4
Moderate symptoms (frequent, limiting)	2
Severe symptoms (constant, not relieved)	0

Sports activities

Level 1	(participates 4–7 days per week)	
	Jumping	
	Hard pivoting	
	Cutting (basketball, volleyball, football gymnastics, soccer)	100
	Running	
	Twisting	
	Turning (tennis, racquetball, handball baseball, ice hockey, field hockey, skiing wrestling)	95
	No running, twisting, jumping (cycling, swimming)	90
Level II	(participates 1–3 days per week)	
	Jumping	
	Hard pivoting	
	Cutting (basketball, volleyball, football, gymnastics, soccer)	85
	Running	
	Twisting	
	Turning (tennis, racquetball, handball, baseball, ice hockey, field hockey, skiing, wrestling)	80
	No running, twisting, jumping (cycling, swimming)	75

Level III   (participates 1–3 times per month)
    Jumping
    Hard pivoting
    Cutting (basketball, volleyball, football, gymnastics, soccer)   65
    Running
    Twisting
    Turning (tennis, racquetball, handball, baseball, ice hockey, field   60
      hockey, skiing, wrestling)
    No running, twisting, jumping (cycling, swimming)   55
Level IV   Daily living activities (No sports)
    Without problems   40
    Moderate problems   20
    Severe problems – on crutches, full disability   0

ASSESSMENT OF FUNCTION

Walking
    Normal, unlimited   40
    Some limitations   30
    Only 3–4 blocks possible   20
    Less than one block, cane, crutch   0

Stair climbing
    Normal, unlimited   40
    Some limitations   30
    Only 11–30 steps possible   20
    Only 1–10 steps possible   0

Squatting, kneeling
    Normal, unlimited   40
    Some limitations   30
    Only 6–10 possible   20
    Only 0–5 possible   0

Sports
    Straight running
      Fully competitive   100
      Some limitations, guarding   80
      Run half-speed, definite limitations   60
      Not able to do   40

    Jumping/landing on affected leg
      Fully competitive   100
      Some limitations   80
      Definite limitations, half-speed   60
      Not able to do   40

    Hard twisting/cutting/pivoting
      Fully competitive   100
      Some limitations, guarding   80
      Definite limitations, half-speed   60
      Not able to do   40

Glossary

Abrasion A deep grazing of the skin caused by friction; further injury of the underlying soft tissue should always be suspected.

Actin–myosin coupling The energy-dependent process by which the components of muscle contract.

Aponeurosis A sheet of thin connective tissue overlying muscle or bone.

Apophysis A growth centre in juvenile bone at which a musculotendinous unit attaches, and thus a site for traction injuries and 'growing pains'.

Arthralgia A painful inflammatory condition of one or more joints, generally secondary to a systemic condition.

Arthrodesis A deliberate, surgical procedure that fuses the bones on contiguous sides of a joint, leaving the joint pain-free but functionally impaired.

Arthroscopy A relatively non-invasive procedure, which is carried out under local, regional or general anaesthesia, with insertion of a sterile telescope through different portals, thus affording a good view of the joint

Articular Pertaining to a joint, and in particular to the cartilage surfaces.

Atrophy Wasting or loss of bulk (and strength).

Axial Along the line of a limb (the adjective is also used to describe structures composing and linked to the spine).

Axonotmesis A disruption of the axon, causing Wallerian degeneration, but the nerve sheath is preserved.

Backshell splintage A posterior splint or plaster of Paris 'shell' that affords support to a joint or limb when bandaged into place for temporary control

Blister A collection of clear fluid (serum) below the superficial layer of the skin caused by repeated friction and the resultant inflammation of the tissues.

Blumensaat's lines On the lateral radiograph of a knee in 30° of flexion the patella normally lies below a line defined by the extension of the epiphysial 'scar' proximally and a distal line extended from the intercondylar fossa

Cancellous (metaphyseal) bone The 'spongy' network of bone which forms the ends of long bones in adults, and which lies between the diaphysis (shaft) and epiphysis of a juvenile long bone; cancellous bone also forms the bulk of discrete bones such as the patella, calcaneum and the vertebra.

Chondral abrasion Articular (hyaline) cartilage lesions can be smoothed over with the rotating, cutting end of a motorized shaver under arthroscopic control, but this abrasion may produce results that are relatively short-lived.

Compartment syndrome An increase in tissue pressure within a relatively inelastic fascial space, leading to serious neurovascular compromise (see pp. 204–6, 222).

Concentric contraction Contraction of a muscle (such as the quadriceps group) against load, allowing the muscle to shorten progressively

Continuous passive motion (CPM) Avoidance of splintage of a joint, such as the knee post-operatively, by means of an external motor that passively moves the knee from extension to approximately 90° of flexion, and back again, over many cycles

Contraction The active process of actin-myosin coupling, causing muscle shortening and hence movement of the related limb.

Contracture Adaptive shortening of muscle and connective tissue that occurs when a joint ceases to move through its full range; this shrinkage can prove difficult to reverse and must therefore be prevented.

Coronal The side-to-side plane of the body (right/left).

Cortical bone Compact, lamellar bone making up the surface and diaphyses (shafts) of the skeleton.

Crepitus A grating feeling or sound produced either by the fractured ends of bone rubbing against each other or by friction of soft tissue (such as occurs in tenosynovitis or osteoarthritis).

Dislocation Complete separation of one articular surface from its comrade surface.

Eccentric contraction Although the muscle (group) contracts. it does so only to allow controlled lengthening of the muscle under load, rather than shortening (such as in descending stairs).

Ecchymosis A deep and widespread discolouration of skin and tissue produced by haemorrhage from a torn ligament, articular injury or fracture.

Embolization Blockage of arteries or arterioles, used therapeutically to reduce the vascular supply to a neoplasm by introducing small, sterile particles into the regional circulation.

Epiphyseal plate (the physis) The cartilaginous, highly cellular growing end of a young bone, between the metaphysis and the epiphysis.

Equinus foot The toe-down, relatively fixed position of the foot and ankle produced by calf or ankle contracture, or by neurological conditions where the powerful posterior calf muscles (plantar flexors) dominate the weaker dorsiflexors.

Esmarch compression Exsanguination (removal of blood by compression) is achieved by wrapping an elastic bandage or rolling on a rubber sleeve from the foot proximally to the upper thigh, prior to inflating a proximal tourniquet.

Fascia A sheet or band of strong connective tissue, often linking muscle to bone.

Feedback loop The sensory and motor reflex arc which maintains balance, muscle tone and joint integrity (see p. 2).

Fibrosis The production of scar tissue as an end stage of chronic or repeated inflammation; contracture of a joint or loss of muscle function may result.

Fixed flexion deformity A loss of joint extension, usually permanent, which has been produced by soft tissue contracture or deformity of bone.

Gait The walking pattern of an individual, comprising alternating strides at a particular cadence; gait may be antalgic (painful), short-leg or Trendelenburg (due to abnormal hip mechanics), or altered as a result of a stiff knee.

Genu recurvatum Hyperextension deformity of the knee, sometimes a manifestation of generalized ligament laxity but also seen in pathological conditions.

233

Genu valgum Knock-knee deformity where the knee joint is characterized by lateral deviation of the lower tibia and inward (medial) angulation.

Glide Forward-back or side-to-side movement of one joint on another without any pivoting around the fulcrum of the joint; some glide is normal and necessary, but an excess of this movement results from pathological laxity and makes a joint feel unstable.

Growth plate (or physis) The region of rapidly dividing cells, in different zones of metabolic activity, lying between the metaphysis and the epiphysis.

Hamstring drill A combination of hamstring stretching and active contraction, with the aim of improving both flexibility and power.

Haematoma A deep but localized bruise, generally involving muscle.

Haemophilia A genetically determined coagulation disorder, mainly affecting males.

Hyperpathia Increased and unpleasant perception of sensation, usually pain, in an area where the sensory nerves have been injured and are now recovering.

Hyperpression A syndrome characterized by excessive pressure exerted by the patella laterally against the lateral femoral condyle.

Hypertrophy Increased size of muscle fibre or other soft tissue as a result of regular use.

Hypopression Loss of the normal articulating pressure between joint surfaces (such as the medial patellar facet), which may affect the nutrition of the articular cartilage.

Instability The feeling of weakness or giving way that results from abnormal joint or muscle function.

Isokinetic A type of contraction or exercise where the resistance applied varies but the speed of movement is constant.

Isometric A type of contraction or exercise where the speed of movement is held constant but the resistance varies.

Isotonic A type of contraction or exercise where no movement is made by the limb against a fixed resistance.

Joint lubrication A process of reducing friction in joints, which is dependent on the fluid–film characteristics of synovial fluid and the biological characteristics of articular cartilage.

Juvenile chronic arthritis An autoimmune inflammation of one or many joints related to rheumatoid arthritis; previously known as Still's disease.

Kinesiology The study of motion of the human body and its limbs.

Laxity Inherited or post-traumatic looseness of a joint owing to ligament incompetence.

Ligamentum mucosum A thin, connective tissue structure that suspends the fat pad in the knee.

Locking A loss of the extremes of joint movement (see p. 6) as a result of an obstruction between the articular surfaces.

Magnetic resonance (MR) scanning Non-invasive imaging of the deeper structures, both soft tissue and osseous, relying upon their different densities.

Medial tibial syndrome (junior leg) An adhesive or occasionally a compressive syndrome affecting the lower tibialis posterior muscle and its tendon, principally in young athletes. It should be differentiated from tibial stress fracture and compartment syndrome.

Myositis (ossificans) A traumatic, inflammatory condition of muscle, which may result in the deposition of calcified and then ossified tissue in the site of a muscle bleed.

Neuroma A thickening of the nerve resulting from the sprouting of axons at the site of injury, and the fibrotic nature of the healing process.

Neurapraxia A temporary interruption of nerve conduction caused by oedema of the axon, but without any break in the continuity of the axon or its sheath.

Neurotmesis Disruption of both the axon and its sheath, resulting in a variable gap between the nerve ends and the formation of a neuroma.

Osteoarthritis The destruction and ineffectual inflammatory repair of articular surfaces of a joint produced by abnormal wear, and resulting in stiffness and deformity of the joint.

Osteochondritis dissecans A pathological process affecting subchondral bone, classically in the medial femoral condyle, which may cause an osteochondral fragment to separate (see pp. 72–8).

Pannus Synovial tissue invasion and subsequent damage of the articular surfaces of a joint that is chronically inflamed as a result of conditions such as rheumatoid arthritis and haemophilia.

Paratenon The filmy connective tissue that surrounds a tendon.

Paraesthesia Abnormal perception of sensation, usually with a painful component.

Patella alta (high patella) A description of the position of the patella in relation to the femoral condylar groove. (see Blumensaat's lines)

Patella baja (low patella) A rare, inferiorly positioned patella.

Pes anserinus ('goose's foot') A group of muscles (sartorius, gracilis and semitendinosus) which helps to stabilize the medial side of the knee in dynamic fashion and also internally rotates the tibia.

Proprioception The sense of feeling in a joint or muscle that depends on a feedback loop.

Pseudo-locking A feeling of restricted joint movement, particularly flexion, which is not caused by an intra-articular obstruction (often the result of patellar instability).

Q-angle The angle between the axis of the pull of the quadriceps muscle (defined as a line from the anterior superior iliac spine to the centre of the patella) and the patellar tendon (approximately 10–15° normally).

Quadriceps inhibition A reflex prevention of quadriceps muscle contraction produced by serious pathology in the knee, mainly as a result of pain and capsular distention.

Recurvatum Hyperextension or a bending backwards of the knee joint, often seen in those with ligament laxity or following trauma.

Reflex arc Similar to a feedback loop, comprising afferent and efferent nerves (see p. 2).

Rheumatoid arthritis An autoimmune systemic disease of connective tissue involving the synovial joints, characterized by remissions and exacerbations.

Rotatory instability A complex instability resulting from abnormal rotation of the femur upon the weightbearing tibia, and perceived by the patient as a knee that is not 'true'.

Sagittal The anteroposterior (forward-back) plane of the body; knee flexion and the drawer tests occur in this plane.

Shin splints An exercise-induced (and therefore reversible) compartment syndrome involving the anterior compartment of the calf; also used loosely to describe the medial tibial syndrome and tibial stress fracture.

Soft tissue reefing The suturing of soft tissues such as fascia and muscle aponeurosis, in an attempt to tighten lax structures and realign patellar or tibiofemoral positioning.

Sprain A partial tear of a ligament.

Strain A tear involving the muscle fibres.

Subluxation A partial dislocation in which some contact between the articular surfaces is still maintained.

Synovium The highly cellular inner lining of the joint which contributes to nutrition and lubrication but may also become chronically inflamed.

T_1/T_2-weighted Variations in the magnetic resonance scanning frequency allowing different structures and pathological processes to be identified (see pp. 40–5).

Tenosynovitis An inflammatory condition of a tendon within its synovial sheath, causing pain, crepitus and loss of function.

Tilt An abnormal angulation of a joint at right angles to its normal plane of movement, and therefore usually in the coronal plane.

Tinel sign A tingling feeling (paraesthesias) transmitted down a nerve when the site of an axonotmesis is tapped lightly.

Tophi Hard, subcutaneous urate deposits encountered over the extensor surfaces of a limb affected by gout.

Torsion An axial deformation of a long bone (generally the femur or tibia) or a rotating movement at a joint (better termed rotation or twisting).

Tracking The normal movement of a structure within a groove or reciprocal surface, such as tracking of the patella between the femoral condyles.

Valgus A lateral deviation of the peripheral segment of the joint (the knock-knee deformity).

Varus A medial deviation of the peripheral segment of a joint (the bow-leg deformity).

Vascular Pertaining to blood vessels and the supply of blood to a part of the body.

Wasting A colloquial term for the atrophy of a muscle secondary to disuse or disease.

Index

Illustrations are comprehensively referred to from the text. Therefore, significant material in illustrations (figures and tables) have only been given a page reference in the absence of their concomitant mention in the text referring to that illustration. Appendix references are followed by (A) and glossary reference by (G).

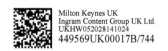